# Ayurvedic Perspectives
# on Selected Pathologies

# Other Books by Vasant D. Lad

Ayurveda: The Science of Self-Healing. 1985

The Complete Book of Ayurvedic Home Remedies. 1998

The Textbook of Ayurveda: Fundamental Principles,
Volume One. 2002

Strands of Eternity: A Compilation of
Mystical Poetry and Discourses. 2004

The Textbook of Ayurveda: A Complete Guide
to Clinical Assessment, Volume Two. 2006

Secrets of the Pulse: The Ancient Art
of Ayurvedic Pulse Diagnosis. 2nd ed., 2006

Pranayama for Self-Healing. DVD, 2010.

The Textbook of Ayurveda: General Principles
of Management and Treatment, Volume Three. 2012

Applied Marma Therapy Cards. 2013


The Yoga of Herbs: An Ayurvedic Guide to Herbal Medicine. 1986
by Vasant Lad and David Frawley


Ayurvedic Cooking for Self-Healing. 2nd ed., 1997
by Usha and Vasant Lad

Ayurvedic Cooking for Self-Healing. Hardcover, 2016
by Usha and Vasant Lad


Marma Points of Ayurveda: The Energy Pathways
for Healing Body, Mind and Consciousness with a
Comparison to Traditional Chinese Medicine. 2008, 2015
by Vasant Lad and Anisha Durve


Ayuryoga: VPK Basics. 2014
by Vasant Lad and Maria Garre

# Ayurvedic Perspectives on Selected Pathologies

*An Anthology of Essential Reading*
*from* Ayurveda Today
*Third Edition*

by
Vasant D. Lad, BAM&S, MASc

Anthology Compiled by Vasant D. Lad
First Edition Compiled by Glen Crowther

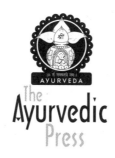

The
Ayurvedic
Press

Albuquerque, New Mexico

Although the information contained in this book is based on Ayurvedic principles practiced for thousands of years, it should not be taken or construed as standard medical diagnosis or treatment. For any medical condition, always consult with a qualified physician.

Traditional Ayurvedic medicine may contain botanicals (herbs), minerals, animal substances or any combination of them. The remedies in this book follow the traditional Ayurvedic pharmacopoeia and may contain substances that modern science and conventional medicine do not consider to be safe or effective. Consult with a qualified physician before using any of the formulations listed in this book.

This book is printed on acid-free paper.

Cover design by Michael Quanci.
Project management and layout by Laura Humphreys.

First Edition 2005
Second Edition 2012, revised and expanded
Third Edition 2018, revised and expanded
ISBN 978-1-883725-24-2
Printed in the United States of America

**Library of Congress Cataloging-in-Publication Data**

Names: Lad, Vasant, 1943- author.
Title: Ayurvedic perspectives on selected pathologies : an anthology of
  essential reading from ayurveda today / by Vasant D. Lad, B.A.M.&S.,
  M.A.Sc. ; anthology compiled by Vasant D. Lad ; first edition compiled by
  Glen Crowther.
Description: Third edition. | Albuquerque, New Mexico : The Ayurvedic Press,
  2018. | Includes bibliographical references and index.
Identifiers: LCCN 2018051704 | ISBN 9781883725242 (pbk. : alk. paper)
Subjects:  LCSH: Medicine, Ayurvedic.
Classification: LCC R605 .L25 2018 | DDC 615.5/38--dc23
LC record available at https://lccn.loc.gov/2018051704

Published by **The Ayurvedic Press** • P.O. Box 23445 • Albuquerque, NM 87192-1445
*For more information on Ayurveda, contact:*
The Ayurvedic Institute • 11311 Menaul Blvd. NE • Albuquerque, NM 87112
(505) 291-9698 • Fax 505.294.7572 • www.ayurveda.com

# Table of Contents

## Rasa/Rakta Vaha Srotas

## Mamsa Vaha Srotas

## Meda Vaha Srotas

## Asthi/Majjā Vaha Srotas

## Majjā Vaha Srotas

## Shukra Vaha Srotas

## Ārtava Vaha Srotas

## Purisha Vaha Srotas

## Mano Vaha Srotas

# Editor's Preface

IN THIS EDITION, Dr. Lad selected the additional titles for the book from the numerous articles that he has written in the ensuing six years' publication of *Ayurveda Today*. Dr. Lad has grouped the articles according to srotāmsi, the bodily channels, and this is noted in the Table of Contents. Oriented to the practitioner and student of Ayurveda, these articles give in-depth descriptions of pathologies from an Ayurvedic understanding along with detailed recommendations to correct these imbalances.

There are hundreds of substances used for healing mentioned in this text. The appendix has a comprehensive list of the herbs and their Latin names. Additionally, there are illustrations in the appendix for the marma therapy protocols recommended within the text as well as photos of the yoga poses mentioned. Instructions for some of the simple remedies that can be done by the practitioner or at home are included as well.

Meditation is an important part of health for body, mind, and spirit. Dr. Lad suggests several meditation techniques in the text. Instructions for Empty Bowl and So'hum Meditation are available on our website at https://www.ayurveda.com/resources/general-information. He also mentions prāṇāyāma (breathing exercises) as a form of self-healing. These can be learned from qualified yoga instructors. Also available is a DVD, *Pranayama for Self-Healing,* with full instructions by Dr. Lad, available on our website. He talks about beneficial yoga postures many times in the text, most often with their English names. They are shown in the Appendix.

***Sanskrit.*** Knowledge of Ayurveda originates in the Sanskrit language. Sanskrit is a precise phonetic language that uses a set of written symbols not familiar to most Westerners. The phonetic representation of Sanskrit words using the English alphabet is called transliteration. We can transliterate Sanskrit to English characters, but not every sound translates directly. There are quite a few sounds that do not exist in the English language, requiring special characters to represent them accurately.

One example is वात ,which translates to vāta. The first 'a' in vāta is a 'long a,' as in "father"; it is held for two beats. The second 'a' is a 'short a,' as in "what." Another example is a sound somewhere between an 'i,' a 'u' and an 'r' that occurs in the word प्रकृति.

i

This word is transliterated as prakṛti. The 'ṛ' is pronounced as the 'ri' in the English spelling of the word Krishna. To make things even more complicated, among those who use Sanskrit the 'ṛ' is pronounced in northern India as the 'i' in "it" and in southern India as the 'u' sound in "root." Because of the regional variations in pronunciation, in this book both ru and ri are found in place of the technically correct 'ṛ'.

Another consideration is that the trailing 'a' in Sanskrit words is sometimes omitted because of the influence of the Hindi language. It is included in many of the words in this book. The trailing 'a' is also subject to grammatical changes depending on the letters that follow it and, for simplicity's sake, we generally ignore these rules. For example, the word *meda* (fat) can be transliterated as *medo, medas,* and meda depending on the word following it. Ordinarily, we use the most common form, meda, so that you, the reader, will have to learn only the one word. Of course, it would be wonderful if all our readers began the study of Sanskrit, inspired by the knowledge available in these ancient texts, but it is not our purpose here to teach that language.

In *Ayurvedic Perspectives*, we have chosen to use transliteration characters only for long vowels, denoted by an overscore or macron character, and for the 'nya' sound denoted by 'ñ'. The pronunciations of the vowels are:

a as in about; ā as in father

i as in ink; ī as in fee

u as in put; ū as in food

e as in pay; ai as in I

o as in corn; au as in loud

In all of our texts, we have elected to italicize only the first occurrence of the Ayurvedic terms used in the text,[1] since they are used repeatedly throughout the text.

## Acknowledgements

The idea for the first edition of this book originated with Glen Crowther, Dr. Lad's long time editor and student. He selected the articles and helped edit them to fit within the publication. He brings creativity, precision, and a deep knowledge of Ayurveda to his work. We are grateful to him for his long association with The Ayurvedic Press and Dr. Lad.

Photos listed here are © 123rf.com: page 70, designua, page 189, obencem, page 194, psoriasishriana, page 196, anamariategzes, page 200, benedamiroslav, rehtse, page 202, koolsabuy, page 208, roxanabalint, page 209, designua, joshyabb, alila, joshyabb, page 213, jarun011, jarun011, ratmaner, page 265, rob3000, page 266, rob3000, page 320, koldunov, page 321 sifotography, page 324, designua, page 327, rob3000Page 329 nattapanpis, page 333, idealnabrajpage 337, rob3000, tahi, page 339, alila, page 340, alila, page 341, rob3000, page 342, designua, page 344, rob3000, page 349, paha_l, page 359, dolgachov, page 361, rob3000, page 362, designua, rob3000, page 389, joshyabb, page 454, byheaven, fizkes, and page 455, szefei. Copyright format for illustration creators is "*name*/123rf"; for brevity the "/123rf" is not included.

All other illustrations are by Vasant D. Lad, BAM&S, MASc, © copyright 2012. Photos on pages 181, 266, 267, 300, 440 and 450-454 are © copyright The Ayurvedic Institute.

1. *The Chicago Manual of Style,* 16th ed. (Chicago: University of Chicago Press, 2010), 364.

# Chapter 1

# Causative Factors of Āma

Fall 1999, Volume 12, Number 2

ऊष्मणोऽल्प बलत्वेन धातुमाद्यमपाचितम् ।
दुष्टमामशयगतं रसमामं प्रचक्षते
वाग सु १३.२५

Ushmano 'lpa balatvena dhātum ādyama pāchitam
Dushṭam āmashaya gatam rasam āmam prachakshate

*The first dhātu (rasa) which by the weakness of the (digestive) fire remaining uncooked and becoming vitiated accumulates in the stomach and small intestine is known as āma.*

Vāg. Su. 13.25

THESE SUTRAS DESCRIBE the formation of āma in the body and mind. You should learn this first *sūtra* by heart. The first line of the sūtra means: because of the low, inner fire, *āhāra rasa*—the food precursors of all subsequent *dhātus*—remains *apachita,* remains undigested, unprocessed and raw.

In the second line of the sūtra, the raw, unprocessed āhāra rasa, which is disturbed by āma, goes into the *āmāshaya,* the stomach. The drawing on the next page illustrates the lesser curvature of the stomach and its blood vessels as well as the greater curvature and its many blood vessels. Also shown are *jāthara agni* and the thoracic duct or chyle duct

*ushmano:* ushma means heat referring to inner heat, fire, agni
*'lpa:* 'lpa means low, little, scanty
*balatvena:* by the strength
*dhātum:* the tissue
*ādyāma:* the first; first dhātu, the rasa
*pachitam:* undigested, unprocessed, unassimilated
*gata:* to go
*rasam:* it goes to the rasa dhātu
*āmāshaya:* stomach
*chaksa:* to look
*prachaksa:* means not only looking but knowing

which contains *ādyām apachitam rasam,* the undigested food precursors. Ādyām apachita rasa refluxes back into the stomach through the blood vessels because of low agni. This means that āma formation takes place when the end product of previously eaten food contains materials that have not been fully digested. This end product, whether fully digested or not, is the food precursor for the dhātus. This food precursor is the *ādyā*hāra

1

rasa which is not digested completely or processed properly because of low jāthara agni. Because it is undigested, it is called āma which is *dushtam*—disturbed—by quality. Translating the entire sūtra: *Because of the low inner fire, the first food precursors of the dhātus remain unprocessed. Those disturbed, unprocessed, raw food precursors then enter the stomach instead of going to feed the dhātus, at which point they are called āma.*

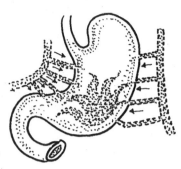

Āma formation due to low agni causes unprocessed micro-chyle to regurgitate back into the stomach.

This first sūtra is one of the beautiful definitions of āma. It puts emphasis on jāthara agni, the gastric fire. Because of the low strength of inner fire, agni, the first āhāra rasa remains undigested and disturbed. That undigested and disturbed āhāra rasa enters back into the stomach for further digestion because the tissue does not accept and cannot process anything raw. This is the intelligence of the body. This is the reason a person's tongue looks coated. Before eating look at your tongue in the mirror. If the tongue is coated because of āma, that means undigested, unprocessed rasa is regurgitating back into the stomach. You should not eat if your tongue is coated. That is going against the intelligence of the body. Modern medicine does not give any importance to a white coating; they say do not worry, it is there. However, Ayurveda says this is the root cause of all disease; that disease is born out of āma. That is why disease is called *āmaya*. It means that which is born out of āma.

A white coating on the tongue indicates āma in the gastrointestinal tract.

आमं अन्नरसं केचित् केदित्तु मल संचयं ।
प्रथम दोष दुष्टिं च केचित् आमं प्रचक्षते ॥

अनाम

Āmam annarasam kechit kedittu mala sanchayam
Prathama doṣa dushṭim cha kechit āmam pracakshate

*According to some, accumulated wastes are āma but, according to others, undigested* āhāra rasa *is āma and according to others the previously disturbed dosha is called āma.*

Anon.

The second definition is more complete. This sūtra is not in the classical texts; it is from an enlightened master, *kechit*. Kechit can even be translated as "someone" or "some authority." *Amam* is āma and *anna rasam* means undigested food juice. Therefore, according to an authority, āma is undigested food juice. That is the whole meaning of this first phrase, *amam annarasam kechit.* The second phrase, *kedittu mala sanchayam*, means that when a person does not sweat properly, then this unexpressed sweat will make the body impure. If a person does not urinate for three days then non-eliminated urine will make the body impure. It is the same if a person does not defecate for four or five days, those constipated feces make the body impure. When the *malas* stay in the body for too long they make the body impure. Mala means the impurities of the body, which are urine, sweat, and feces. These are the three malas.

According to this sage, āma is simply accumulated impurities, malas. Meaning that when a person has constipation, scanty urination or no perspiration, then those impurities become āma. This is a very beautiful definition. This sūtra also says āma is undigested food juice and that āma is due to previously disturbed *dosha*. This is a very complete definition.

In the first sūtra, āma is defined as undigested āhāra rasa because of low agni. According to the next sūtra, āma is accumulated, stagnated impurities or malas because of improper elimination of urine, feces or sweat. This sūtra also says that āma is nothing but previously disturbed dosha. These sūtras are good explanations of the sources of āma. They give us a complete, three-dimensional picture of the formation of āma in the body.

*amam:* Ām
*annarasam:* the food juice, the end product of digested food juic
*kechit:* according to someone, according to some authority; the repeated reference, *kedit*, means according to another authority
*tu:* but
*mala:* the three *mala* — urine, feces and sweat; that which makes the body impure if it is accumulated
*samchayam:* accumulation, stagnation
*pratamama:* previous, the first, the one before
*dosha:* vāta, pitta, kapha
*dushtim:* disturbed
*cha:* and
*prachakshate:* is called

स्रोतोरोध बल भ्रंश गौरवानिल मूढताः ।
आलस्यापक्ति निष्ठिव मलसङ्गारुचि क्लमाः ॥

अष्ट हृ सु १३ २३

Sroto rodha bala bhramsha gauravānila mūḍatāḥ
Ālasyāpakti nishthiva malasaṅgāruchi klamāḥ

*The signs and symptoms of āma are clogging of channels, sense of heaviness, low energy, restlessness, lethargy, indigestion, kapha type congestion (expectoration), accumulation of the three malas (wastes), loss of taste and sexual debility.*

Aṣṭ Hṛd. Su. 30.23

This third sūtra is important and supplements the previous two. The first word is *sroto rodha*. Sroto rodha is blocking the channels. In this sūtra, they are using this very beautiful, specific phrase: Whenever āma is formed in the system, it creates clogging of the channels. These blocked channels can mean many things: coronary occlusion, pulmonary embolism, stagnation, venous engorgement or lymphatic obstruction. For all these, they are using just one phrase: sroto rodha which is due to āma in the system.

*Bala bhramsha* refers to having low energy or strength. This can manifest as someone having chronic fatigue syndrome which is due to too much āma in the liver. If you feel tired and weak, drink agni tea. It will burn āma and you will get energy. This first phrase, sroto rodha bala bhramsha, refers to low energy, fatigue and tiredness. *Gaurava* is a sense of heaviness. The person feels heavy subjectively—heaviness in the body, hands, belly or head. Whenever you feel heaviness anywhere, it is due to āma.

*Anila mūdhatā* means the *vāta* channels are blocked. Vāta starts moving about seeking an open channel and, in its constant movement, gains momentum due to the pressure

*srotas:* channels
*rodha:* blocked, blockage, blocking the channels
*balā:* strength, energy
*bhramsha:* low, lack of energy, fatigue
*gaurva:* sense of heaviness
*anila:* vāyu
*mūdhatā:* restlessness and confusion of vāta dosha
*ālasya:* lethargy, malaise
*apakti:* indecision. *Pakti* means decision; *apakti* no decision
*malasanga:* accumulation of impurities
*aruchi:* lack of taste
*klamaha:* means sexual debility, or sexual weakness

created by the blockage. These efforts to find its own way around that blockage cause vāta to become restless. This restlessness of vāta creates breathlessness, tingling and numbness, burping, flatulence, and hyper-peristalsis. Mental confusion and restless or excessive thinking are signs of blocked vāta. Anila mūdhatā is as if a heavy storm has happened in the body because of āma, creating ringing in the ear, insomnia, "ungroundedness," confusion, constipation, vague intestinal pain, increased peristalsis, tremors, ticks, or spasms.

It is as if vāta becomes hyperactive because of being blocked by āma. Another meaning of the phrase anila mūdhatā refers to mental confusion, lack of clarity, and poor perception. This restlessness and confusion cause the mind to become foggy resulting in mental āma.

In the second sentence, the person has no enthusiasm to do anything because of *ālasya* and the inability to decide whether to take an action, caused by *apakti*. *Nishthiva* has a very significant meaning. A meaning of the word *nishtha* is faith, but because of āma, it becomes nishthiva, which means faithlessness. One hidden meaning of the word nishthiva is lack of mental faith. The disciple who has a lot of āma in his or her mind loses faith, because faith is trust, clarity and love. When there is mental āma the person does not trust, so nishthiva means doubt or delusion. That is one meaning of nishthiva.

Another meaning of nishthiva is to spit out or expectorate *kapha*. *Kapha nishthivanam* means pulmonary congestion. When veins are clogged with kapha that is also āma. Āma and kapha are very similar in quality. They are both heavy, oily, sticky and cloudy. Āma creates nishthiva, congestion, adhesions and fibrocystic changes in the breasts. Even when you do oil massage, if there is too much āma the person's body will ache. In a case like this, have them take trikatu and ginger tea to burn that āma and the pain will go away.

*Malasanga* is the accumulation of malas—urine, feces, sweat—but can also mean the accumulation of mental mala—conclusion, judgment, criticism. When the suppression of unresolved anger, fear or frustration accumulates in the mind, it becomes polluted and that is another form of malasanga or mental āma. *Aruchi,* which means a lack of taste or flavor, can also mean a lack of interest or enthusiasm. *Klamaha* means sexual debility or weakness. The accumulation of malas is a sroto rodha and it leads to a lack of enthusiasm and sexual debility, which is the result of āma.

A modern definition of āma could include high cholesterol, high triglycerides, high sugar and increased white blood cells—leukocytosis—or decreased white blood cells—leukocytopenia. Āma also is indicated by an accumulation of antibodies, increased blood urea, increased platelet count and increased red blood cell count—called polycythemia, which is āma resulting from aggravated *pitta*. Stagnant bile in the gallbladder is āma, which can create gallstones. Increased liver enzymes (SGOT, SGPT) are indications of āma in the liver, leading to chronic fatigue syndrome. Āma in the eye increases intraocular pressure creating glaucoma. According to the definition of āma in the second sūtra, even the accumulation of bacteria leading to bacterial infection is pittagenic āma. These examples help us to understand the role āma plays in terms of modern science and in Ayurveda.

We can see from these sūtras that āma can be classified according to the doshic disturbance, to improper digestion of the āhāra rasa and to the blockage of the *srotas* or channels of the body. There can also be mental āma. It is interesting that āma creates mūdhatā, restlessness because restlessness also creates āma. The cause becomes the effect and the effect then becomes a cause.

I would like to add one more. According to my observations, āma is also formed from unresolved emotion. If you have unexpressed anger, emotions or fears, it will create mental āma. So, I can add one more sūtra and say: According to a kechit or an authority who lives in Albuquerque, āma could be formed by unresolved, unexpressed emotions.

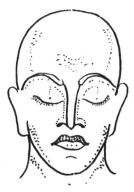

Mental āma is formed from unresolved emotions.

To be one with the present moment is clarity, but we live in the past or we live in the future. Because of its sticky, gluey qualities, āma creates attachment to the past and, because of its liquid, slimy qualities, it causes us to skate or slide into the future. It is the past and the future that gives meaning to life. The present moment is deeply connected to the past and when you stay with the present moment, you can see the past clearly.

To be in the present moment is to be with agni and agni is clarity, love, digestion. When we are stuck with the past, our emotion never gets digested or processed into love or intelligence. So, be in the present moment! In the present moment, when an unresolved emotion or thought from the past comes up and you are in the present moment, you are looking at it with clarity, with love. Then you can act from that clarity, call your friend or loved one and ask for forgiveness. By remaining in the present moment, you can heal your past. Getting stuck with the past is mūdhatā. It is apakti when you remain with the past; then there is no digestion of the past hurt and you blame yourself. Do not blame yourself. Love yourself and forgive yourself. Forgiving happens in the present moment.

In the present moment, you can see the beauty of the blue sky, the lonely shadow of a tree, marvel at the beautiful face of a child, or the innocent face of your wife or husband. When you are here, be here, at this moment. Buddha taught this meditation: eating mindfully, sitting mindfully, sleeping mindfully. If you really practice mindfulness, you live in the present moment. This awareness brings perfect digestion of our moment-to-moment experiences. By practicing this art of being one with this present moment, we can easily burn mental āma. Practicing mindfulness burns āma.

Thank God, we are given one moment at a time, not two, not three! One moment at a time, but even so we cannot live that moment completely. We are either stuck with past grief, sadness and emotions, or we are worried about the divine future. If I live fully, completely this moment, this moment will make my future. Therefore, instead of saying, "make my day" you can say, "make my moment." Meditation is the simplest thing to do, there is nothing as simple as breathing, there is nothing as simple as paying attention to this very moment. So, when you live in the present moment, a tremendous energy comes to you, you become the central focus of the entire universe. If you stay in the present moment, the Universe is blessing you, showering a benediction upon you from all directions. This moment is called *pakti*. Pakti means digestion. In the present moment there is no āma. The present moment is poetry, the present moment is art, and it is ecstasy and joy. So, my dear friend, let us learn this art of living mindfully every moment, not to judge, not to criticize, but to be one with this moment.

# Chapter 2

# Shat Kriyā Kāla: Vāta

## Management of the Six Stages of Samprāpti for Vāta

Spring 2010, Volume 22, Number 4

THE FIVE CLINICAL barometers used in Ayurvedic medicine in order to study a disease are called *nidāna pañchakam*. These are *nidāna,* etiology, *pūrva rūpa,* prodromal signs and symptoms, *rūpa,* the cardinal signs and symptoms, *upashaya,* therapeutic trial and *samprāpti,* pathogenesis.

We have discussed this topic numerous times and most students are very familiar with the six stages of samprāpti. In this article, we will see how the *shat kriyā kāla,* the six important stages of samprāpti, can be effectively managed when we pay complete, undivided attention to the signs and symptoms of the patient.

Each individual has his or her unique *prakruti,* personal genetic code, which maintains his or her unique psycho-physiological balance. This balance can be disturbed by environmental changes, seasonal changes, change within a relationship and the moment-to-moment changes of emotions. Due to the influence of these factors, the doshas undergo qualitative and quantitative changes. The *gunas* (qualities, attributes) related to each stage of samprāpti, beautifully explained in volume two of the *Textbook of Ayurveda* series, are shown in the table below.

## Table 1: Gunas (Qualities) Relating to Each Stage of Samprāpti

| Stage | Vāta | Pitta | Kapha |
|-------|------|-------|-------|
| Sanchaya (accumulation) | Cold | Liquid, Sour | Heavy, Cool |
| Prakopa (provocation) | + Dry, Light | + Hot, Pungent | + Liquid, Slow, Dull |
| Prasara (spread) | + Mobile | + Spreading, Oily | + Oily |
| Sthāna Samshraya (deposition) | + Subtle | + Sharp | +Sticky, Slimy |
| Vyakti (manifestation) | + Rough | + Light | + Cloudy, Soft |
| Bheda (complication) | + Clear | + Fleshy smell | +Hard, Dense, Static, Gross |

If we look closely at these qualitative expressions of the doshas in the stages of samprāpti then one can see that it is beneficial to use the opposite quality to oppose the aggravation by using the table of the pairs of opposites.

## Vāta Management and the Stages of Samprāpti

In this article, we will attempt to cover the management of vāta in the various stages of samprāpti.

In the *sanchaya* stage, the cold quality accumulates in the anal canal and the rectum producing constipation, lower abdominal distention and gas. In this case, we can apply our theory of using the opposite quality to oppose or balance the aggravated quality by placing a hot castor oil heavy compress on the abdomen or a hot water bottle followed by a warm sesame oil *basti*. (see Appendix for more about basti, page 449)

In the *prakopa* stage, the cold, dry and light qualities cause vāta to become aggravated in the colon. These will require more space and produce fullness in the flanks, increased peristalsis and pressure under the diaphragm accompanied by difficulty in breathing. To compensate for this, a warm dashamūla tea basti can be used. Prepare this by boiling 1 Tbs. of dashamūla powder in 1 pint of water. Then strain and allow to cool. While it is still warm, add ½ cup of sesame oil then administer the basti. This type of basti will conquer vāta in its second stage. To prevent further prakopa, use triphalā guggulu 300 mg in capsules three times a day (TID) or gandharva harītakī, 1 tsp. at bedtime with warm water as necessary.

| |
|---|
| T.I.D. = from the Latin means *ter in diem*, three times a day |
| B.I.D. = from the Latin means *bis in diem*, two times a day |

With the *prasara* stage, the mobile quality helps vāta to leave the gastrointestinal (GI) tract. Any dosha entering circulation comes into contact with the heart, the capillary layer, *rakta dhātu* and the topmost layer of the skin, *rasa dhātu*. During this stage, vāta creates dry skin, goose bumps, poor circulation, cold hands and feet, palpitations, ringing in the ears, and abnormal pulsations in the veins. This stage requires abhyanga (massage) or *snehana* (self-massage with oil) and *svedana* (sudation) to stabilize vāta. The vāta types can use sesame oil, pitta can use sunflower oil and kapha can use olive oil. This should be followed by svedana. For vāta types a few drops of nirgundī oil can added to the steam box; a couple of drops of sandalwood oil for pitta types and three to five drops of eucalyptus oil can be added for the kapha types. For the palpitations that occur during this stage, take a dashamūla tea with ½ tsp. of arjuna. For the ringing in the ears, *karna pūrana* is well indicated.

As for the abnormal pulsation in the veins, a formula consisting of equal parts of manjishthā, rakta chandana, and jatamāmsi can be taken ½ tsp. TID with warm water until the symptom subsides.

### Sthāna Samshraya and the Dhātus

In *sthāna samshraya,* the addition of the subtle quality of vāta in the process of samprāpti allows vāta to enter any weakened dhātu (tissue) or to impair the *agni* (metabolic fire) of the dhātu. If all *dhātu agnis* are healthy then vāta is not able to enter into any dhātu and will return to the colon. This is a state called *prashama avastha,* in which all dhātu agnis are healthy and there is no *khavaigunya* (defective space). However, it is very rare for this to happen. It is far more usual for vāta to enter the tissues or to skip one dhātu and move to the subsequent one, wherever the agni is impaired.

*Rasa Dhātu.* When *rasa dhātu agni* is low, vāta enters this tissue creating fever with chills, dry dark skin, malaise, fatigue, general body ache, acne, palpitations, goose bumps and dehydration. This is the textbook picture of *vāta jvara* (fever) and is best treated by using a formula with dashamūla 500 mg, tribhuvan kirti 200 mg, or sudarshan gana vati 200 mg with tulsi tea.[1] In the west, we can use dashamūla

### The 20 Paired Opposite Gunas

| Heavy | Light |
|---|---|
| Slow / Dull | Sharp |
| Cold | Hot |
| Oily | Dry |
| Slimy / Smooth | Rough |
| Dense | Liquid |
| Soft | Hard |
| Static (stable) | Mobile |
| Subtle | Gross |
| Clear | Sticky / Cloudy |

500 mg, tagara 200 mg, and mahāsudarshan 200 mg with ginger, cinnamon, and basil tea. The person should be wrapped in a warm blanket and, to correct dehydration, given a homemade dextro-saline solution made by adding 5 tsp. of sugar, ½ tsp. of salt, and the juice of ½ lime to a pint of water.

*Rakta Dhātu.* If the mobile and subtle qualities of vāta encounter a strong rasa dhātu agni and are warded off, then vāta attempts to enter rakta dhātu. If rakta dhātu is low, then *rakta gata vāta* occurs.[2] In this case, there will be poor circulation and cold hands and feet. This vāta condition will create very small red blood cells (microcytic anemia), blood clots, varicose veins, craving for meat, and aneurism.

For the poor circulation, massage briskly, creating friction, with mahānārāyana oil to improve circulation. Afterwards, soak in a bath containing cup each of ginger powder and baking soda for at least 5-10 minutes. This can be done daily until the condition subsides.

In the case of microcytic anemia, one should use 1 tsp. of mahatikta ghrita before each meal, take 4 Tbs. of kumārī āsava with equal amounts of water after lunch and dinner, or take loha āsava in the same way. Additionally, add supplements such as vitamin $B_{12}$, 500 mg per day, and folic acid, 60 mg per day.

In the case of blood clots, Ayurveda recommends the use of kaishore guggulu, 200 mg TID, or trikatu in the same dosage. This regimen would be very similar to the use of 85 mg of aspirin to prevent clotting.

The craving for protein can be met by having chicken broth, liver soup, fried rabbit blood, or blood sausage sautéed with ghee. Alternatively, a vegetarian could consume beet juice, carrot juice, barley greens, blue green algae, spinach, or red cabbage, which are also sources of the iron that the body is craving.

Varicose veins can be aided by taking ½ tsp. TID of a formula containing kaishore guggulu 200 mg, trikatu 200 mg, and pushkaramūla 200 mg. Foods like garlic, onions, turmeric, and ginger will help the blood fluidity. Apply mahānārāyana oil to the varicose

---

1. Vati are tablets, usually flattened.
2. Gata means 'gone;' in this context, entering into.

veins, then keep the legs elevated or in the *viparīta karanī* (legs up the wall) yogic posture at least once daily. (see yoga poses in Appendix page 450)

**Māmsa Dhātu.** In the case that both the rasa and the rakta dhātu agnis are functioning properly and not allowing vāta to enter the dosha, then *māmsa dhātu* will be the next to be affected, if its agni is not strong. When vāta enters this tissue, it creates *māmsa gata vāta,* which will manifest as muscle spasm, muscle pain, tics and tremors, muscle wasting, and low muscle power, tone and coordination, which can lead to paralysis, foot drop, restless leg syndrome, or even dancing chorea (involuntary dancing).

For the muscle pain, simply do abhyanga or snehana with mahānārāyana oil, followed by a svedana with nirgundī oil. Furthermore, it would be beneficial to take internally ½ tsp. TID a formula containing equal proportions of yogarāja guggulu, mustā, and tagara with warm water.

In case of emaciation, a formula containing ashvagandhā 500 mg, balā 400 mg and vidārī 300 mg can be given with milk in the dosage of ½ tsp. TID. Additionally, increasing the consumption of cashews, almonds or almond milk, protein intake, and/or eating meat will generally reverse muscle wasting.

To enhance power and coordination, use a formula containing sarasvatī 500 mg, brahmī 300 mg, and jatamāmsi 300 mg. Take ½ tsp. of this TID with either dashamūla arishta, ashvagandhā arishta, or balā arishta. These are Ayurvedic herbal wine preparations that kindle *māmsa dhātu agni*. If not available, use warm water as the *anupāna*.

For cases of paralysis, paraplegia or foot drop in India, highly potentized compounds are given such as mahāyogaraja guggulu 200 mg TID or mahā vāta vidvamsa 200 mg tablets TID. Another option is to administer a *madhu tailam basti* (honey and oil basti). For this, mix ½ cup of honey and ½ cup of warm sesame oil and retain the mixture to strengthen the muscles. Nutritive foods such as quinoa, amaranth, milk, tofu, almond milk, goat cheese, and medicated ghee such as balā ghrita (ghee) or shatāvarī ghrita should be favored.

The mobile quality of vāta creates abnormal muscular movements resembling dance (dancing chorea). Use a formula of dashamūla 500 mg, ashvagandhā 400 mg, balā 300 mg, vidārī 200 mg, yogarāja guggulu 200 mg, and sarasvatī 200 mg. Take ½ tsp. TID with almond milk. Additionally, the person should do self-massage, applying balā tailam or ashvagandhā oil as the massage oil, and use vacha-medicated *nasya* oil.

**Meda Dhātu.** If all the dhātu agnis prior to *meda dhātu agni* are strong and meda dhātu agni is impaired, vāta will enter this tissue instead, creating *meda gata vāta*. Lack of lubrication, lack of sweat, dry skin, lumbago, displacement of organs such as descending kidneys or spleen, osteopenia, and dislocation of the joints are some of the signs and symptoms of vāta entering *meda dhātu*. When this occurs, the first line of treatment is plenty of deep oil massages using oils like ashvagandhā tailam, dashamūla oil, dhanvantari tailam (an oil preparation with balā in it), or balā tailam. Internally to support meda dhātu, medicated ghees are given such as shatāvarī ghee, balā ghrita, vidārī ghee, or yashthi madhu ghrita in a dosage of 1 tsp. TID before food.

Additionally take ½ tsp. TID after meals of a formula containing dashamūla 500 mg, ashvagandhā 400 mg, balā 300 mg, and vidārī 300 mg with shatāvarī ghee. A special soup, called *mahasneha* soup, is recommended as well. It contains ghee, animal fat and bone marrow. Use an oil enema or make a tea of dashamūla and ashvagandhā vidārī and combine with oil for a tea and oil enema.

In the case of organ displacement, the classic formulas use ½ tsp. of a mixture of ashvagandhā, vidārī, balā, kākolī, and kshirakākolī in milk TID. It is also recommended to bandage the organ site to support the ligaments. A similar protocol is used in the case of dislocation of the joints.

As for osteopenia, Ayurveda uses a mixture of herbs and bhāsmas, so the typical formula would contain dashamūla 500 mg, pravāl pañchāmrit 200 mg, moti bhāsma 200 mg, and kaishore guggulu 200 mg; ½ tsp. of this mixture TID with goat's milk.

***Asthi Dhātu.*** Cracking and popping of the joints, osteoporosis, spinal misalignment, scoliosis, lower back ache, neck ache, splitting hair ends, receding gums, hair loss, thyroid dysfunction, and ringing in the ear are all signs that vāta has entered *asthi dhātu.*

Mahānārāyana oil is widely used topically for local lubrication in this case. Internally, for osteoporosis, a formula containing dashamūla 500 mg, yogarāja guggulu 300 mg, and pravāl pañchāmrit 200 mg is used in the dosage of ½ tsp. TID with milk. For spinal misalignment, the internal formula is dashamūla 500 mg, ashvagandhā 400 mg, and balā 300 mg. In India, this formula would be supplemented with a bone supporting tablet called asthi poshaka vati, which contains egg shell ash, coral ash, and calcium from antlers, among other ingredients.

For lower backache, application of mahānārāyana oil in a *kati basti* (pooling of oil on the lower back) is indicated as well as massage with mahānārāyana oil. Dashamūla tea basti is also commonly advised. Internally, take a formula containing ashvagandhā 400 mg, yogarāja guggulu 200 mg, tagara 200 mg, and pravāl pañchāmrit 200 mg, ½ tsp. TID with warm water.

In the case of receding gums, chew sesame seeds in the early morning and massage the gums. *Gandūsha,* filling the mouth with oil, swishing it, and retaining it before spitting it out, is also very useful.

With irregular thyroid function, there is a deficient calcium metabolism, so the person looks chubby but the bones are weak. To support the system, classic Ayurveda recommends the use of kaishore guggulu and pravāl pañchāmrit and, in modern Ayurveda, kelp is also recommended. Bhrāmarī prānāyāma and ujjāyi prānāyāma are very good tools as well and can be added to the protocols used in the vāta sanchaya and prokopa stage.

***Majjā Dhātu.*** When vāta enters *majjā dhātu,* there is tingling and numbness in the extremities. *Majjā gata vāta* creates habitual ticks, spasms, muscle tremors, and gradual muscle wasting. As majjā dhātu includes the brain, spinal cord, eyeball, and articular surface of the joint, majjā gata vāta can create cluster headaches, spinal pain (pain along vertebra), nystagmus (involuntary eye movement), and stiffness in the joints. As vāta runs along the tract of the nerve, it can then cause classic conditions such as neuralgia, trigeminal neuralgia, and sciatica. According to the Ayurvedic system of medicine, majjā dhātu is the substratum of consciousness, thoughts, feelings, and emotions. Due to high vāta in majjā, there can be rushing of thoughts, mood swings, poor memory, forgetfulness, anxiety, fear, and insomnia.

In general, for *majjā gata vāta samprāpti* the herbal protocol is dashamūla 500 mg, sarasvatī 300 mg, brahmī 200 mg, shankha pushpī 200 mg, and tagara 200 mg, ½ tsp. TID with warm water. For *virechana* (purgation), 1 tsp. of plain harītakī at night in hot water is recommended. For nasya in the morning, use 5 drops per nostril of brahmī ghee, vacha tailam, or anu tailam. *Shirodhāra* three times a week is beneficial and rub brahmī or bhringarāja oil on the skull at night before bed. Karna pūrana (filling of the ear with warm oil) with a medicated vacha oil can also calm vāta in majjā. Dashamūla basti should be administered daily in the vāta time of day until symptomatic relief has been achieved.

In the case of trigeminal neuralgia, mahā yogarāja guggulu should be added to the above general herbal protocol and a local application of mahānārāyana oil with massage to the area would be ideal.

With majjā gata vāta in the eye, *netra basti* with plain ghee is advised in addition to the recommendations above.

For muscle tremors and wasting, the formula changes to dashamūla 500 mg, ashvagandhā 400 mg, vidārī 300 mg, and balā 200 mg. Take ½ tsp. TID with warm milk. For abhyanga or snehana, use ashvagandhā or balā tailam.

For neuro-psychiatric disorders such as anxiety, fear, memory loss, etc., the formula is dashamūla 500 mg, brahmī 200 mg, jatamāmsi 200 mg, and sarasvatī 200 mg, ½ tsp. taken TID with brahmī ghee.

Unfortunately, long lingering majjā gata vāta can lead to Parkinson's and Alzheimer's. In these cases, add 200 mg of ātma guptā to the general majjā gata vāta neuro-psychiatric herbal protocol.

***Shukra Dhātu.*** Vāta in *shukra dhātu* can produce oligospermia (scanty formation of semen), temporary or permanent deficiency of spermatozoa in seminal fluid, erectile dysfunction, premature ejaculation, dyspareunia (painful coitus), sexual impotency, lower back ache, fear associated with sex, or even deformed sperm leading to cleft palate, spina bifida, talipes equinovarus (club feet), depleted *ojas,* difficulty in conception, multiple miscarriages that affect the offspring and partner.

For general management, the herbal protocol requires dashamūla 500 mg, ashvagandhā 400 mg, vidārī 300 mg, ātma guptā 200 mg, and tagara 200 mg; take ½ tsp. TID with milk. Additionally, a dashamūla, ashvagandhā, balā, or madhu tailam basti can be done every day to protect ojas. Take ashvagandhā ghee, ashvagandhā arishta, or dashamūla arishta TID. Topical application to the glans penis of ashvagandhā or balā oil or a vidārī and nutmeg ointment are encouraged. Foods to favor include goat testicle soup, bone marrow soup, or chicken soup, accompanied by red wine.

***Ārtava Dhātu.*** Vāta in *ārtava dhātu* gives rise to infertility, sterility, amenorrhea, irregular menses, pain during ovulation, constriction of the cervix, cervical dysplasia, dryness in the vagina, dyspareunia, irregular menstruation, vaginal and uterine prolapse, retroverted uterus, and/or premature orgasm. These conditions can be alleviated by a general herbal protocol of dashamūla 300 mg, shatāvarī or ashvagandhā 300 mg, tagara 300 mg, and ashoka 300 mg. Take ½ tsp. internally TID with warm water. Traditionally a *pichu* (vaginal tampon) using shatāvarī ghee or dashamūla ghee is inserted at least twice a week. Also, take ashokarishta or kumārī āsava twice a day before each meal, 4 Tbs. with an equal amount of water. To lessen vāta in ārtava, perform a kati basti with sesame oil, a warm massage to the lower back, or apply a warm oil compress to the abdomen.

### Vyakti Stage

In the *vyakti* stage the rough qualities of vāta will create the full manifestation of the disease, *vyādhi darshana,* and basically the treatment protocols are the same as those provided in the sthāna samshraya stage.

### Bheda Stage

In the *bheda* stage of samprāpti where the clear quality of vāta manifests, there are more complications. Bheda stage in rasa dhātu creates severe dehydration; in rakta dhātu, it generates severe anemia; in māmsa, muscle wasting, emaciation, and atrophy occur; in meda, the depletion of normal, healthy fatty tissue leads to degenerative changes; in asthi, osteoporosis, spontaneous fractures, deposition of calcium in soft tissue, and reduction of height manifest. Vāta in bheda stage penetrating the majjā dhātu creates a loss of function of cerebral activity, epileptic convulsions, severe Parkinson's, Alzheimer's with total memory loss, loss of consciousness, and coma. If instead the vāta in bheda stage moves to the shukra or ārtava dhātu, there is total loss of libido, total reproductive dysfunction, and loss of secondary sexual characteristics.

## Management in Bheda Stage

Critical care is needed at this stage and, in most incidences, hospitalization is required. The following guidelines are given for each tissue so that you can prevent additional aggravation of the dosha and dhātu.

For rasa dhātu, maintain water electrolyte balance and avoid dehydrating herbs like punarnavā, gokshura, or triphalā. Cleansing therapies and even mild virechana should not be administered. For rakta dhātu, blood-building foods can be eaten such as beets, red cabbage, black raisins, currants, and blueberries. In India, loha āsava is recommended. For māmsa dhātu, give a gentle yet deep massage with ashvagandhā and balā medicated oils, followed by svedana, daily for three to four weeks. In terms of food guidelines, meat soup, chicken broth, almond milk, and milk with ashvagandhā are favored.

For meda dhātu, this is the time when Ayurveda recommends fatty fried food and internal consumption of shatāvarī ghee, balā ghee, or licorice ghee, all preceded by a pinch of rock salt or trikatu to aid the digestion. For asthi dhātu, calcium, magnesium, and zinc supplementation may be needed. In India, a typical medicine is asthi poshaka vati, which in essence is very similar to coral calcium. Gentle weight-bearing exercises and yoga are also advised.

For majjā dhātu, shirodhāra and *shiro basti* are the therapies that bring the most benefit. Nasya with vacha tailam and *prānāyāma* are helpful as well.

For shukra, in India, strong *rasāyanas* are used such as mākaradvāja 200 mg twice a day, kapikacchū vati 300 mg TID, or ashvagandhā vati 300 mg TID. For ārtava, licorice tea *uttara basti* is recommended daily, then weekly. For both shukra and ārtava, yogic postures like *vajrāsana* (thunderbolt pose), *utthita padmāsana* (elevated lotus pose), *halāsana* (plow pose), *bhujangāsana* (cobra pose) and *balāsana* (child's pose) are very beneficial at this stage. Beneficial *mudras* are *vāyu mudrā* and *agni mudrā,* and y*oni mudrā* for women. (see yoga poses in Appendix page 450)

# Chapter 3

# Shat Kriyā Kāla: Pitta
## Management of the Six Stages of Samprāpti for Pitta

Summer 2010, Volume 23, Number 1

AS PROMISED IN the previous chapter, in this article we will cover the management of *pitta dosha* in the various stages of samprāpti.

In the sanchaya stage, the liquid and sour qualities (see Table 1 on page 7) cause umbilical pain, intense hunger, and yellow discoloration of urine and sclera. In this condition, we can use one teaspoon at night of āmalakī, to counteract the increased liquid quality, with aloe vera juice, to counteract the sour or in India,[3] they would use shanka vati, a *bhasma* of calcinated shell.

In the prakopa stage, the hot and pungent qualities mingle with the liquid and sour qualities that were already present and give rise to acid indigestion, hyperacidity, heartburn, nausea, and gastric pain. In this condition, use a mixture of shatāvarī or gudūchī 500 milligrams (mg), gulvel sattva 200 mg, shanka bhasma 200 mg, and kāma dudhā 200 mg, ½ teaspoon three times a day (TID) before meals with cup of milk.

Up to this stage, the doshas are excited, overwhelmed, and filling their organs completely. Vāta inflates the colon, pitta overwhelms the small intestines, and kapha is ready to overflow the stomach. Now is the crucial time for proper management because, if not handled with treatment, the dosha will leave its site and start traveling throughout the body. It will start by trying to enter rasa and rakta dhātu in the prasara stage. In the prasara stage, the qualities of pitta are spreading and oily, which precipitates pitta aggravation and leads it to sthāna samshraya. These two qualities actually help the entry of pitta into the dhātus. As long as the doshas are in the gastrointestinal (GI) tract, it is fairly easy to remove them from the system. However, once they enter the *bāhya mārga,* then management and removal becomes more complicated as it progresses to the sthāna samshraya stage. (see Vyādhi Mārga Illustration page 16)

---

3. There are herbs, compounds, and bhasmas that are available only in India or are no longer made. Lad includes these to give a complete picture of the recommended remedies in the ancient texts.

## Sthāna Samshraya

*Rasa Dhātu.* If sthāna samshraya occurs in the rasa dhātu—the plasma tissue (serum, white blood cells, lymphatic system)—the individual gets repeated hives, rash, urticaria, hyperpyrexia (high fever), acne on the face or on the body, dermatitis, eczema, and psoriasis. Even melanin cells under the skin become irritated, leading to red spots under the skin that can turn into multiple moles. A person with *sthāna samshraya pitta* in the rasa dhātu may become subject to skin cancer or malignant melanoma, a highly metastasizing cancer, and for that reason entry of pitta into the rasa dhātu should not be taken lightly.

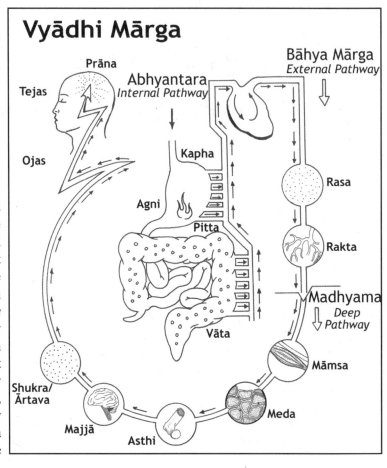

The protocols for sthāna samshraya pitta in the rasa dhātu vary according to the condition. For high fever, one can use ½ teaspoon TID of an herbal compound containing mahāsudarshan 300 mg, gulvel sattva 200 mg, kāma dudhā 200 mg, and pravāl pañchāmrit[4] 200 mg with either lemongrass tea or cinnamon, ginger, sandalwood, and mustā tea where the ingredients are combined in equal proportion. Also, one should sponge the forehead with a tepid mixture of rose and camphor water TID and away from food. Should the person in question be a child, the caregiver should grate one onion. Take half of the grated onion, wrap in a cotton cloth and apply it to the forehead; wrap the other half and apply it to the belly button. This type of *lepa,* application of paste, is also quite common in cases of febrile convulsions. Externally onion is cooling and can have an immediate effect on body temperature.

One should never undergo virechana, purgation, during high fever and the person should stay hydrated to avoid dehydration. In India, they use sutshekhar pills 200 mg TID

---

4.  A compound of coral, conch, oyster, pearls and cowrie shells processed in aloe vera and rose water.

and 4 Tbs. of mahāsudarshan qwath (an alcoholic preparation of mahāsudarshan) with equal amounts of water, two times daily (BID).

> T.I.D. = from the Latin means *ter in diem,* three times a day
>
> B.I.D. = from the Latin means *bis in diem,* two times a day

For hives and rashes, a lepa consisting of equal proportions of sandalwood, rose, and manjishthā and prepared with milk can be applied topically at night or early morning. Allow the lepa to dry then rinse off. Juice fresh cilantro and drink this TID. You can then use the pulp residue as an additional topical application. Should the rash be an allergic reaction due to contact, for example, with poison oak or ivy, then tikta ghrita can be applied on the rash. Internally take ½ tsp. TID of an herbal mixture consisting of equal proportions of gudūchī, manjishthā, and turmeric.

For urticaria, active dermatitis, take ½ tsp. TID of a bitter herbal combination comprising shatāvarī 500 mg, kutki 200 mg, manjishthā 200 mg, and neem 200 mg. The anupāna (vehicle) can be pomegranate juice or even milk.

For chronic, long-lingering pitta, sthāna samshraya of pitta in the rasa dhātu can create eczema and psoriasis. In these conditions there is burning, itching, red lesions of inflammatory changes, and there can also be bleeding in spots. In India for this type of condition, one is given ārogya vardhini capsules of 200 mg and capsules of sutshekhar 200 mg and kāma dudhā with moti 200 mg. Since these medicines are not available here in the United States, we use a mixture of shatāvarī 500 mg, gudūchī 200 mg, manjishthā 300 mg, neem 200 mg, and turmeric 200 mg. Use this combination ½ tsp. TID with aloe vera gel. Aloe vera gel has a sustained action versus the short acting juice.

Acne, a common problem in teenage boys and girls who are arriving at the pitta time of life, may be due to hormonal changes. Young boys have excess testosterone in their blood stream and girls have excess estrogen; as a result, they break out in the form of acne. In pitta-predominant prakruti and *vikruti,* stress can also trigger sthāna samshraya pitta in the rasa dhātu, which may manifest as acne.

In India, the internal treatment protocol is very similar to that prescribed for eczema and psoriasis. In the west we can differentiate and for the female use a mixture of shatāvarī 200 mg, gudūchī 300 mg, manjishthā 200 mg, neem 200 mg, and harītakī 200 mg, taken ½ tsp TID with aloe vera juice. For males, the mixture would consist of ashvagandhā 500 mg, vidārī 400 mg, gudūchī 300 mg, manjishthā 200 mg, neem 200 mg, and harītakī 200 mg, taken ½ tsp TID with milk.

For external treatment, wash the affected area with neem soap or sandalwood soap to remove all the oil and then apply a simple turmeric-sandalwood paste, an almond-nutmeg-milk paste, or a multani mitti-sandalwood-manjishthā-rose paste for skin healing. Allow to dry and then rinse to remove. In some serious cases of acne, the best recommendation is *rakta moksha,* blood letting, which can be done easily by donating blood to the blood bank. This method can clear acne within one week.

Generally, pitta prakruti/vikruti individuals tend to get multiple moles on the skin. As a rule, they should avoid long exposure to sun light. Usually when the mole has clear-cut margins, is round or oval in shape, the boundaries are cleanly distinguished, and surface is smooth, it is a benign mole. You can apply a mixture of coconut oil and castor oil, half and half, to the mole area. However, if mole looks puckered, the margins have merged into the peripheral tissue, the mole has discoloration spots or brownish areas, and/or the surface looks granular, then this type of mole can create more itching and slight bleeding. Additionally, it may be malignant. You should immediately go to the dermatologist for an expert opinion and biopsy. If they want to remove the mole, let them do so.

***Rakta Dhātu.*** If rasa dhātu agni is strong and healthy then pitta has no chance to deposit into the rasa dhātu, red blood cells. Such angry and irritated pitta will then go to the rakta and, if the *rakta dhātu agni* is weak and impaired, pitta will enter the rakta dhātu. Pitta and rakta…they have very similar qualities. Pitta is *ushna* (hot), rakta is ushna. Pitta is *tīkshna* (sharp), rakta is tīkshna. Pitta is *sūkshma* (subtle), rakta is sūkshma. Pitta is *sara* (spreading), rakta is spreading. The condition of sthāna samshraya of pitta in the rakta is called *rakta pitta.*

Pitta gives its hot, sharp, sour qualities to rakta; and rakta gives its red fleshy smell and spreading quality to pitta. This condition creates bleeding disorders. Due to the hot and sharp qualities of pitta and rakta, the platelet count diminishes. When platelet count diminishes, the prothrombin[5] and thrombin[6] clotting factors are affected and the blood becomes thinner, easily rupturing the peripheral capillaries or blood vessels and creating bleeding disorders.

If rakta pitta is pushed upward by *udāna vāyu* then the person gets bleeding from the upper pathways, i.e., the nose, gums, eyes, and ears. If rakta pitta is pushed downward by *apāna vāyu* then the individual can get bleeding from the lower pathways, i.e, the urethra, vagina, and rectum. If rakta pitta is pushed inward or outward by *samāna vāyu* or *vyāna vāyu,* the person can get petechial hemorrhage or hemophilia purpura. Charaka states a very important sūtra in the *Chikitsā Sthāna* that says, *pratimārgam cha haranam cha rakta pittam vidhiyate,* meaning that bleeding disorders are treated with herbs that encourage the opposite flow of direction of the disorder. Hence, with an upward flow of blood to the nose, gums, or teeth, we use a sweet, mild virechana like āmalakī that will give an opposite downward pull to the dosha. For the downward flow of bleeding, we have to induce a mild emetic, which creates an upward pull on the dosha, using licorice, neem, or madana phala with either pomegranate juice or milk. In both cases, virechana and *vamana* are not expected; we want only to change the vector.

When samāna pushes rakta pitta creating petechial hemorrhage, one can use gulvel sattva, kāma dudhā, manjishthā, lodhra, and sandalwood in equal proportions, ½ tsp TID with aloe vera juice. Then give a mild virechana of bhumi āmalakī. Externally apply sandalwood-rose paste or sandalwood-rose-camphor paste. Camphor is cooling. You can use mustā in place of sandalwood, in case sandalwood is too expensive.

If there is severe bleeding with sputum, then use iced water, sip by sip. This will also stop bleeding. In general, ice is not nice but here ice is nice because it helps to clot the blood. It is observed that if there is bleeding and you put ice on it, it will freeze the blood,

---

5. A coagulation (clotting) factor that is needed for the normal clotting of blood.
6. A key clot promoter, thrombin is an enzyme that presides over the conversion of a substance called fibrinogen to fibrin, creating the right conditions for a clot.

acting as a hemostatic; conversely, when you apply heat, it will increase the bleeding. So bleeding time increases by application of heat and bleeding time reduces by application of cold.

Another condition of pitta sthāna samshraya in the rakta is inflammatory arthritis such as gout, where high uric acid levels create crystals, which go into the joint and irritate the synovial membrane, creating inflammation, deformity, and pain in the interphalangeal joint. In this case, vāta is pushing pitta in the *rakta vaha srotas* and rakta dhātu, creating gout. This condition is called *vāta rakta* in Ayurvedic literature. The treatment protocol is a mixture of kaishore guggulu 200 mg, amrita guggulu 200 mg, kāma dudhā 200 mg, and pravāl pañchāmrit 200 mg. Take ½ tsp. TID with aloe vera juice. Use a topical application of an anti-inflammatory paste of red sandalwood and turmeric.

For any kind of bleeding disorder, use *pitta-rakta* soothing and pacifying herbs. They are shatāvarī, gulvel sattva, manjishthā, neem, turmeric mixed with neem, rose, red sandalwood, white sandalwood, lodhra, and mocha rasa. These herbs will separate pitta from rakta and act as a hemostatic, acting to arrest bleeding or hemorrhaging.

The next condition of sthāna samshraya pitta in the rakta is hot flashes. This condition occurs as a woman enters perimenopausal and menopausal stages. Lack of estrogen hormone may push pitta in the hematopoietic system. The treatment protocol for hot flashes is a mixture of shatāvarī 500 mg, kāma dudhā 200 mg, gulvel sattva 200 mg, and moti bhasma 200 mg. Take ½ tsp. TID with aloe vera juice, which is also a source of estrogen. To further maintain estrogen balance, use evening primrose oil 500 mg, one capsule after dinner for 15 days on, 15 days off.

Sthāna samshraya of pitta in the rakta dhātu may create weeping eczema. Use a topical paste of equal proportions of catechu, neem, manjishthā, and sandalwood, twice daily. Internally take a mixture of shatāvarī 200 mg, gudūchī 200 mg, neem 200 mg, manjishthā 200 mg, and kāma dudhā 200 mg, ½ tsp. TID with aloe vera gel.

***Māmsa Dhātu.*** If the rakta dhātu agni is strong, it will never allow pitta to enter its territory. One could say this disappoints pitta, since pitta thought that rakta was a brother and yet was sent away. Pitta then travels to māmsa dhātu and, if māmsa dhātu agni is low, enters the muscle tissue where it can create fibromyalgia or fibromyositis. In fibromyalgia, there are nine bilateral trigger points (18 points in all, see page 20) that are exceptionally sensitive to the touch; they feel like sensitive *marmāni*. Generally, 11 points must be sensitive for three months before one can diagnose fibromyalgia. The treatment protocol is a mixture of ashvagandhā 500 mg, as a vehicle to carry the medicine to the māmsa dhātu, shatāvarī 400 mg, as *pitta pratyanika,* specific to the dosha, then gudūchī 300 mg, kaishore guggulu 200 mg, both as anti-inflammatory, mustā 200 mg, a muscle relaxant and analgesic, and tagara 200 mg, analgesic. Take ½ tsp. TID with warm water. Topically one can apply mahānārāyana oil to the troubled area. For fibromyositis, the treatment protocol is the same as for fibromyalgia.

Another condition of sthāna samshraya pitta in the māmsa is bursitis, an inflammation of the bursa around the joints and ligaments. The treatment protocol for this is a mixture of ashvagandhā 500 mg, kaishore guggulu 200 mg, mustā 300 mg, and tagara 200 mg taken orally ½ tsp. TID with warm water. Topically apply mahānārāyaṇa tailam for any inflammatory muscle disorder.

## The Bilateral Trigger Points of Fibromyalgia

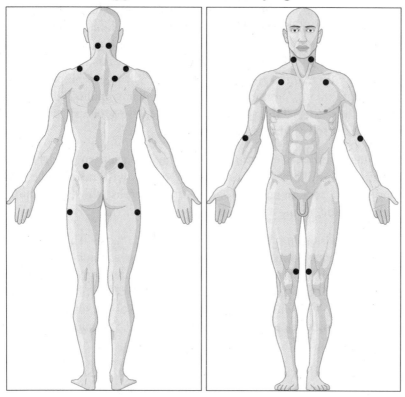

*Māmsa gata pitta,*[7] another name for sthāna samshraya pitta in the māmsa, can create bleeding and spongy gums like scurvy. For that, Ayurveda recommends a triphalā tea gargle with a pinch of alum or a neem oil *kavala gandūsha.* Kavala gandūsha is to fill the mouth with oil, swishing it for several minutes, and retain it before spitting it out. One tsp. of āmalakī at night is good source of Vitamin C.

Long lingering pitta in the sthāna samshraya stage of māmsa dhātu can cause multiple boils and abscesses. In my experience, when a patient comes with multiple boils and abscesses, we must first rule out diabetes.

The abscess and boil is an inflammatory condition called *pacāmana avasthā,* which is a stage of inflammation. The next stage is the ripe stage or *pakvāsthā,* which is suppuration with pus formation. For a boil, we can apply local heat like ginger, black pepper, or piper longum as a paste. This will help should the boil still need to ripen and it will increase the suppuration. Once ripe, the pus will come out easily. Internally one can give a natural, herbal antibiotic like sūkshma triphalā, available in India. Here in the west, we can use gulvel sattva 200 mg, neem 200 mg, turmeric 200 mg, echinacea 200 mg, osha 200 mg, and goldenseal 200 mg as an antibacterial mixture. Take this ½ tsp. TID until the infection comes under control or for a maximum two weeks.

For māmsa gata pitta creating myositis, local inflammation, one can take internally ½ tsp. TID of a mixture containing kaishore guggulu 200 mg, ashvagandhā 500 mg, and mustā 300 mg with water.

---

7. Gata means 'gone;' in this context, entering into.

*Meda Dhātu.* *Meda gata pitta* is the term given to pitta sthāna samshraya in meda dhātu, adipose tissue or fat. If māmsa dhātu agni is strong, not allowing pitta to enter the dhātu, then pitta will turn away and possibly penetrate meda's door. Meda gata pitta will create profuse sweating and excess thirst. Excess *kleda* is eliminated through human sweat as well as through the urinary tract so pitta will have access to the urinary tract and create repeated cystitis. Then high excess pitta in the meda dhātu effects fat metabolism, creating fatty degenerative changes in the liver and impairing fat metabolism in the liver, therefore the person will get fatty diarrhea and undigested fat will pass through the urine or to the stool. Furthermore, there is a connection between meda dhātu and the adrenal glands as well as meda dhātu and the thyroid gland. High pitta in the meda dhātu creates low adrenals and can produce the autoimmune thyroid disorder known as Hashimoto's thyroiditis.

For profuse perspiration, dusting therapy called *uddhūlanam* will help. Use a superfine powder of calamus, sandalwood, and jatamāmsi or chickpea flour or oatmeal powder and then gentle brushing to help minimize sweating. Internally give shatāvarī 500 mg, gudūchī 300 mg, kāma dudhā 200 mg, and kutki 200 mg, ½ tsp. TID with cool water.

For cystitis the herbal protocol calls for a mixture of punarnavā 500 mg, gokshura 400 mg, mustā 300 mg, kāma dudhā 200 mg, and fennel 200 mg. Take ½ tsp. TID with aloe vera juice or gel. As in cystitis, there is a tendency for the urine to become acidic. It is customary in India to have ushīrāsava, a self-generating alcoholic preparation whose main ingredient is ushīra. Alternatively, one can drink a tea made out of sandalwood, ushīra, and coriander in equal proportions.

For fatty liver, in India we use ārogya vardhini 200 mg TID. However, here we use a mixture of shatāvarī 500 mg, gulvel sattva 400 mg, katukā 300 mg, neem 200 mg, and shilājit 200 mg. Take ½ tsp. TID with aloe vera gel. In addition, prānāyāma can help this condition. Recommended practices are shītalī, shītkāri, and kapāla bhāti.

For low adrenals where there may be postural hypotension, fatigue, exhaustion, or development of dark circles around the eyes, we can use a compound of ashvagandhā 500 mg, vidārī 300 mg, yashthi madhu 200 mg, and ātma guptā 200 mg. Take ½ tsp. TID with either milk or warm water.

For the thyroid dysfunction of Hashimoto's disease, one can use a formula of kaishore guggulu 200 mg, gudūchī 300 mg, kāma dudhā 200 mg, and pravāl pañchāmrit 200 mg. Take ½ tsp. TID with pomegranate juice. If thyroid function is low then we can use a mixture of punarnavā 500 mg, kutki 200 mg, chitrak 200 mg, shilājit 200 mg, and kāma dudhā 200 mg. Have ½ tsp. TID with warm water.

*Asthi Dhātu.* If *meda dhātu agni* is strong then pitta cannot access the tissue during the prasara stage and will move to the next tissue, asthi dhātu, bone and cartilage tissue. Pitta sthāna samshraya in asthi will create inflammatory changes either in the periosteum or within the matrix of asthi dhātu. As a result, the *upadhātu* of asthi, *danta* (teeth), and the mala, *kesha* (hair) and *nakha* (nails), will be affected. Long lingering pitta in the asthi dhātu can enter into the articular surface of the joint, which will affect the synovial membrane, leading to inflammatory arthritis of the joints, with heat, swelling, and generalized inflammation. During the journey from superficial to deep in the asthi dhātu, pitta dosha by its ushna (hot) and tīkshna (sharp) qualities can create periostitis.[8] Pitta dosha can also cause alopecia by affecting the root of hair and creating gingivitis, tooth abscess, bleeding gums and yellowing of teeth by affecting the root of teeth.

*Asthi dhara kalā*—the periosteum, the membranous structure covering the bone, is intimately connected with calcium metabolism and indirectly governed by the thyroid gland. The glandular system is a bridge between asthi dhātu and majjā dhātu. Therefore, pitta in the asthi dhātu has access to disturbed thyroid function and hyperthyroidism, leading to generalized heat in the body, increased perspiration, and impairment of calcium metabolism.

To deal with pitta in asthi dhātu, the treatment protocol is to use shatāvarī 500 mg as *dosha pratyanika,* kaishore guggulu, or amrita guggulu 300 mg as anti-inflammatory and pravāl pañchāmrit 200 mg and kāma dudhā 200 mg also as anti-inflammatory. This mixture is to be taken ½ tsp. TID with two tablespoons of aloe vera gel. Topically one can apply bhringarāja, brahmī, or coconut oil on the joint.

The asthi dhara kala contains specialized osteo plasma,[9] which is rich in calcium, magnesium, and zinc, and produces and nourishes asthi dhātu. In my clinical practice of the last 40 years, I have found a connection between ulcerative colitis, osteo arthritis, and osteoporosis. To treat these conditions I have had success with a dashamūla and gudūchī tea *basti* and an internal herbal mixture consisting of dashamūla 500 mg, kāma dudhā 200 mg, pravāl pañchāmrit 200 mg, and swayambhu guggulu 200 mg, ½ tsp. TID with warm milk after meals.

To make the dashamūla-gudūchī basti, take 1 pint of water and add 1 tablespoon of dashamūla and one tablespoon of gudūchī. Bring to a boil and simmer for 3 minutes; allow to cool. Strain the tea before administering the basti.

For the treatment of alopecia, one must first rule out other serious illnesses such as severe depression, stress, dermatitis, exposure to radiation, an iatrogenic condition, or the process of aging. In India, one can use ārogya vardhini 200 mg, kaishore guggulu 200 mg, and brahmī 200 mg. Apply topically neem, brahmī, or bhringarāja oil, any combination of these three.

For tooth abscess and dental disorders, Ayurveda recommends brushing the teeth with neem and gargling with ½ cup of aloe vera juice. If there is infection or gingivitis, internally take a mixture of mahāsudarshan 300 mg, neem 200 mg, manjishthā 200 mg, echinacea 200 mg, and goldenseal 200 mg, ½ tsp. TID with aloe vera juice.

For the treatment of pitta in asthi dhātu with hyperactive thyroid and excess heat we can use a mixture of shatāvarī 500 mg, gulvel sattva 200 mg, kāma dudhā 200 mg, and kaishore guggulu 200 mg, ½ tsp. TID with aloe vera gel.

In general, it is a good practice of a person suffering with *asthi gata pitta* to have shatāvarī milk, brahmī milk, or dashamūla milk at bedtime to help both bones and pitta.

---

8. Inflammation of the periosteum, a layer of connective tissue that surrounds bone.
9. Bone tissue has pathways through the cells for nutrients and waste, so even though bone is hard, there is plasma in it.

***Majjā Dhātu.*** When the *asthi dhātu agni* is strong and healthy, pitta will not be allowed to enter its territory, and pitta then tries to enter majjā dhātu, the marrow, nerve, and connective tissue. As pitta is hot, sharp, penetrating, and spreading, it will create first burning sensations, burning hands and feet, burning in the eyes, then insomnia, dizziness, nausea, and vomiting leading to pitta-type fever and, if long lingering, syncope, coma, and even death. On a psychological level, pitta may create a chemical form of depression, even suicidal depression. Pitta in majjā can also create demyelinating disorders, multiple sclerosis (MS), migraine headaches, meningitis, or encephalitis. Therefore, *majjā gata pitta* is a very serious condition.

Since the upadhātu of majjā is lacrimal secretions and *akshi vitta sneha,* the oily secretions of feces and eyes, majjā gata pitta will cause the person to wake up with sticky eyes and have mucousy yellow stool, with yellow discoloration of the sclera and photosensitivity, which may lead to ophthalmic migraine.

For burning sensation of the hands and the feet, rub coconut or castor oil on the soles of the feet and palms of the hands. Internally take TID a mixture of brahmī, bhringarāja, and gudūchī, 300 mg each.

For burning sensation in the eyes one can use a goat milk compress, a triphalā tea eyewash (see page 329), netra basti with plain ghee (see instructions page 313) or *netra bindu,* which are eye drops available in India that contain rose, camphor, and alum.

For dizziness, nausea, and vomiting, one can take internally shatāvarī 500 mg, brahmī 200 mg, and sarasvatī 200 mg, ½ tsp. TID with aloe vera juice.

For fever and migraines, one can take gudūchī 300 mg, mahāsudarshan 300 mg, and brahmī 200 mg, TID with water.

When pitta enters majjā and leads to suicidal thoughts, violence, aggression, and possible chemical depression, the situation should not be taken lightly and one should seek proper counseling. It may be necessary at some point to call for emergency care (911).

For demyelinating disorders leading to MS, *panchakarma,* abhyanga, svedana, basti, and nasya can be quite helpful. The herbal protocol for this uses a mixture of shatāvarī 500 mg, dashamūla 400 mg, kaishore guggulu 200 mg, brahmī 200 mg, and ātma guptā 200 mg, ½ tsp. TID with tikta ghrita or brahmī prash (an alcoholic preparation of brahmī).

Meningitis and encephalitis are very serious conditions that require hospitalization.

***Shukra /Ārtava Dhātus.*** When *majjā dhātu agni* is strong and pitta could not penetrate the tissue the next tissue in the pathway is shukra or ārtava dhātu, male or female reproductive tissue. Shukra and ārtava dhātu occupy the whole body. Though the top most layer of the skin represents rasa, the seventh layer is shukra/ārtava and it comes to the surface of the body at the mucocutaneous[10] junction of the lips, then at the nipple and areola, and on the skin of the penis and clitoris. These areas are very sensitive as are the throat, heart, belly button, and *linea alba.*[11] The *kama kala nādī* (an energetic pathway) passes through

---

10. A mucocutaneous zone is a region of the body in which mucosa transitions to skin.
11. "White line;" a fibrous band that runs vertically along the center of the anterior abdominal wall and receives the attachments of the oblique and transverse abdominal muscles.

these areas and kissing or touching these areas yields an intense desire to make love, as mentioned in the *Kama Sūtra,* the book on the secret science of erotic pleasure.

When pitta enters shukra/ārtava dhātu, the person will become oversensitive to touch and have irritability, anger, and even repulsion towards their sexual partner. The lips become too sensitive to kiss, the areola and nipples are tender and painful and even intercourse is painful (*sakashtha maithuna*).

Depending on how deep the pitta has gone into the shukra/ārtava dhātu, the signs and symptoms vary accordingly. In men, it will manifest as urethritis, orchitis, epididymitis, excess pitta in sperm and semen, leading to burning in the spermatic cord, urethra, and prostate. There can also be premature ejaculation. During these conditions all sexual acts are painful, irritating, and may create, as complications, outbreaks of herpes, gonorrhea, or syphilis. In women, the ovaries become sore and painful; there is pain along the fallopian tubes and repeated endometritis. There will be pitta-type pre-menstrual syndrome. The woman will suffer from tenderness in the breasts, irritability, and anger pre-menstrually and have profuse menstrual bleeding.

The pure essence of shukra/ārtava is ojas and *pitta ojo vyāpat*[12] may develop or may manifest in both individuals, where *tejas* is burning ojas and may lead to autoimmune disorder.

For generalized treatment of men suffering from *shukra gata pitta* the herbal protocol is a mixture ashvagandhā 500 mg, vidārī 400 mg, gulvel sattva 300 mg, and moti bhasma 200 mg to be taken ½ tsp. TID with milk. For women with ārtava gata pitta, the herbal protocol is a mixture of shatāvarī 500 mg, gulvel sattva 400 mg, kāma dudhā 200 mg, and ashoka 300 mg taken ½ tsp. TID with kumārī. Use a topical application of tikta ghrita on the lips, nipples, belly button, and clitoris.

For tejas burning ojas as a complication of pitta ojo vyāpat, women can take 1 tsp. BID of shatāvarī ghee, mahā tikta ghrita,[13] or shatāvarī *avaleha*[14] (syrup) orally. Men suffering from this condition can take 1 tsp. BID of ashvagandhā avaleha, 1 cup of almond milk, or have at least one ghee-soaked date per day.

## Vyakti Stage

Due to the light quality of pitta, in the vyakti stage, we will have the full-blown manifestation of pathologies and the treatment of those pathologies should follow the protocols of the sthāna samshraya stage.

## Bheda Stage

In the bheda stage, pitta will create a fleshy smell quality as at this stage there has already been inflammation, irritation, ulceration, and hemorrhage leading to abscess and gangrene. Therefore, in this stage it is crucial to have hospitalization as this stage is not to be treated at home.

---

12. Also known as ojo dushti, this is the qualitative disturbance of ojas by one or more doshas. It usually involves more than one dhatu. Ojo-vyāpat affects the entire immune system of the body.
13. A classical formula described in *Sushruta Samhitā, Chikitsā Sthāna,* chapter 9.
14. A method of medicine preparation in which herbs and/or herbal extracts are mixed into a syrup.

# Chapter 4

# Shat Kriyā Kāla: Kapha
## Management of the Six Stages of Samprāpti for Kapha

Summer 2010, Volume 23, Number 3

THE THREE DOSHAS are the three organizations of the unique human physiology. Dhātus are the constructing, cementing material of the body and malas are the impurities. The doshas govern one's unique individual psychophysiology, which is called prakruti. At the time of fertilization, the prakruti of the father and mother create a unique genetic code that determines the individual's prakruti, or nature, their unique psychophysiology.

*Dosha dhātu mala mūlam hi sharīram*

*Sushruta Samhitā,* Sharīrasthānam

These three doshas are a qualified and quantified unit. The doshas have their own unique qualities, which all Ayurvedic students are familiar with. They also have a particular ratio, such as $vāta_1$, $pitta_2$, and $kapha_3$. This is quantification, but 10 individuals with a vāta-pitta constitution are 10 unique individuals because in these 10 people there will be a unique permutation and combination of the different gunas, or qualities. Therefore, whenever we discuss shat kriyā kāla, students should pay attention to both the qualities and quantities of the doshas that undergo change.

We have discussed in detail the shat kriyā kāla of vāta and pitta doshas in previous articles. In this chapter, we will switch our attention to shat kriyā kāla of *kapha dosha.*

We know that the main site of kapha is the stomach, but there are also other subordinate sites of kapha dosha. Kapha is present in the bronchial secretions in the chest, the lymphatic secretions of the lymph system, the saliva of the oral cavity and sinus secretions of the sinuses. Kapha is also present in the lubricating material of the joint, the synovia.

## Early Stages of Samprāpti

In shat kriyā kāla of kapha, we should pay attention to the main site of kapha dosha, which is the stomach. sanchaya, or accumulation, is the first and most important stage of samprāpti. In *kapha samprāpti,* it occurs in the stomach. As we studied previously, sanchaya of vāta happens because of cold quality. sanchaya of pitta is due to liquid and sour qualities, and sanchaya of kapha takes place due to the heavy and cold qualities. Students should pay attention to these two qualities: heavy, or *guru,* and cold, or *shīta.*

Due to the heavy quality, the person will have a subjective sense of heaviness. It may be generalized heaviness or localized heaviness. Whenever there is heaviness, there is kapha. In the sanchaya stage, excess *kledaka kapha* is secreted in the stomach. The heavy quality suppresses the agni and the cold quality cools down the agni. Because agni is suppressed by these two qualities that are the opposites of the light and hot qualities of agni, then naturally the person will feel no appetite. Due to low appetite and fullness of the stomach, there is also a lethargic feeling.

These expressions of kapha: no appetite, fullness of the stomach and lethargy are symptoms of the sanchaya stage of kapha samprāpti in the stomach.

For simple management, Ayurveda talks in terms of balancing the dosha. Kapha dosha accumulates in the stomach due to certain causes. The moment kapha accumulates in the stomach and agni is suppressed, then the person will get an aversion or repulsion toward the cause. Suppose every day a person eats foods with heavy, greasy, oily, and dull qualities. This will suppress agni and on the third day even a picture of these kinds of foods will make the person nauseated. Why?

Because the body has intelligence; it has wisdom. It happens in any condition—if someone who is not accustomed to smoking smokes a cigarette, he gets an aversion towards smoking. If someone drinks too much then the next day he doesn't even like to see the bottle of whisky or wine. Aversion towards the cause is the language of the body. That means listen to the body; don't continue with the same cause.

In the sanchaya stage of kapha, the treatment is simple: to strictly avoid the cause. If there is heaviness, fullness, low appetite, lethargy, and aversion toward the cause, then don't repeat that cause. That is also a treatment, called *nidānam parivarjanam,* avoiding the cause of the increased dosha.

*Vruddhih samānyaih sarveshām, viparītair viparyayah*

Vagbhata's *Ashtānga Hridayam Sūtrasthānam*

This sūtra says vruddhih samānyaih sarveshām—like increases like. On the other hand, opposite qualities heal the body and control the dosha. We use this same principle when dealing with the first stage of samprāpti. So, pay attention to the heavy, cool qualities. The first *kriyā kāla* of sanchaya is to use the opposite quality. The opposite of heavy is light, and light quality is present in fasting, so observing a fast is one treatment. Drink only warm water or drink nothing, and don't eat anything until normal appetite comes back.

Fasting can also be done by drinking warm or room temperature juice, like apple juice for kapha prakruti, pomegranate juice for kapha and pitta, and for vāta, orange juice or sweet lime juice. A juice fast is recommended so that a person doesn't get dehydrated. It will induce the light quality in the body. In that way the heavy quality can be controlled.

Not eating means not taking something inside. Our body also encounters these universal twenty qualities in the environment, in the atmosphere, in our relationships, and in our families and homes as well as in the diet. These qualities are constantly bombarding us.

Then there is cool quality. Cool quality can calm down the agni, so to kindle agni, one can take ginger tea. Take about 1 inch of fresh ginger root, chop it into pieces, and boil it in a cup of water for a few minutes. This is a simple home remedy. Sipping ginger tea will kindle agni and calm down the cool quality of kapha. Then the lethargy, heaviness, and low appetite will go.

For lethargy due to low agni, one can kindle agni by doing *dīpana* and *pāchana*. An example of dīpana is giving ginger tea. For pāchana, you can take a pinch of chitrak with a teaspoon of honey or trikatu, which is ginger, black pepper and piper longum (pippalī) in equal proportions. One-quarter teaspoon of this mixture can be taken orally with a teaspoon of honey, and it will definitely take care of agni and burn āma. It is the āma that creates lethargy.

Due to the accumulation of kapha dosha and suppression of agni, āma is produced. This āma clogs the channels. Lethargy happens because of lack of nutrition to rasa dhātu due to āma, which is clogging the *rasa vaha srotas*. To take care of that lethargy, trikatu chūrna is used. Take ¼ teaspoon with a tsp. of honey TID. In between one can drink hot water. This management will take care of the sanchaya stage of kapha, which is induced by the heavy and cool qualities.

During the sanchaya stage, you can conquer a dosha quickly. Sushruta says *'chayo jaye dosha,'* which means you should conquer the dosha in the first stage, sanchaya. However, most people are not aware of their own dosha. They eat emotionally and because of habit, without paying attention to their bodies, doshas, *nādi* (the pulse), breath, and tongue. That is how we create our own disease process. Sushruta is a great enlightened master. His explanation of shat kriyā kāla is a very practical guide for future generations.

T.I.D. = from the Latin means *ter in diem,* three times a day

B.I.D. = from the Latin means *bis in diem,* two times a day

Next is the prakopa stage. *Kapha prakopa,* or provocation, happens because of the liquid, slow, and dull qualities. Heavy and cool qualities create accumulation, sanchaya, but if the cause still continues because the person doesn't pay attention to the aversion, then it may induce other qualities of kapha such as liquid, slow, and dull.

Liquid, slow, and dull qualities will provoke kapha dosha. The liquid quality will create excess salivation, runny nose, cold, congestion, and mucus secretion. Excess salivation can suppress agni and create nausea. The person can also get mucoid vomiting. Prakopa also creates nausea, aversion towards food, anorexia, and loss of appetite.

These symptoms are obvious but, generally, when a person has a cold, he or she takes antibiotics or a decongestant and suppresses the symptoms. Antibiotics are okay if there is an infection, but in the prakopa stage of kapha there is non-specific cold congestion; and no bacteria are involved.

In the prakopa stage, the level of the dosha rises. In the sanchaya stage, kapha accumulates in the pyloric area. In the prakopa stage, kapha comes to the fundus of the stomach. Therefore, there is more fullness. Liquid quality creates excess salivation, cold, runny nose, congestion, and nausea. Slow quality creates stagnation, and dull quality dulls agni and the mind as well as the activity of the srotas, especially anna vaha srotas.

The herbal protocol for dealing with the prakopa stage of kapha is using certain drying herbs like sītopalādi, which is an expectorant, and tālīsādi, which is a decongestant. Use 500 mg of each, TID.

To deal with the slow, dull quality we can use herbs with a sharp quality—200 mg of either pippalī or trikatu. Take either of these with honey TID to take care of the liquid, slow and dull qualities and relieve the prakopa stage of kapha dosha.

If there is a runny nose during the second stage of kapha samprapti, another treatment protocol is to inhale steam. Inhaling steam removes the liquid quality. The latent heat of the steam is much higher than boiling water, so when a person inhales steam, the liquid kapha will run out and that will help with decongestion.

In chronic runny nose or congestion, take hot water in a bowl, put a couple of drops of eucalyptus oil, cover the head with a towel, and inhale the steam. That eucalyptus steam inhalation is the opposite of liquid and dull quality, and it will relieve congestion.

When *sāma doshas*[15] are flowing out of the body, as in runny nose, let them go; don't stop them. If you use an antihistamine, decongestant, or anti-allergy medicine for a cold's congestion, it will suppress the movement of kapha and kapha will create more āma and more thick mucous. Prolonged usage of decongestants or antihistamine can create deviation of the nasal septum, nasal polyps, and thick mucus formation.

That is why Ayurveda says that to drain the nose in an acute cold, the best thing is to drink licorice tea. Boil one teaspoon of licorice in a cup of water for 3 minutes, and then add 5-10 drops of mahānārāyana oil. Take one sip of this mixture every ten minutes. It will help to drain mucous without suppressing the flow of *sāma kapha* out of the body.

If we suppress the movement of sāma dosha, then this sāma dosha accumulates in the superficial and deep connective tissue as well as the subcutaneous tissue and can create other disorders like sinus congestion or even tumor formation.

Most of the time our approach is anti, anti, anti—we try to suppress. If there is pain, we use an analgesic painkiller; if there is a spasm, we use an antispasmodic. In an emergency, I'm not against suppression of symptoms but if we suddenly jump to an antihistamine for an acute cold, it will not only suppress the symptoms. Taking an antihistamine or decongestant every time can lead to complications such as nasal polyps, nasal adenoids, or snoring. By suppressing the sāma dosha, the accumulation can move into the deep tissues, creating other complications.

For example, if a person has boils, which is sāma dosha, and it is the first formation, then don't use an anti-inflammatory, just do an incision and the pus will come out. When

---

15. Sāma means a dosha with toxins; nirāma means a dosha without toxins.

the pus comes out, the symptoms of pain and fever will go away. There is no need to do suppression therapy.

In sāma kapha, the mucus is stringy, thick, and foul smelling. If that is coming out, let it go. During the sanchaya and prakopa stages in a healthy kapha person, you can do vamana under professional direction and supervision. That involves drinking licorice tea and vomiting it out.

Even a very mild vamana will bring the kapha out. Then the symptoms of sinus congestion, nasal polyps, and deviated nasal septum will disappear. After that, we can use Super Nasya Oil® or vacha oil nasya as a decongestant. These can remove both sāma and *nirāma kapha* and protect the nasal passage from complications.

In the first two stages of kapha samprāpti, dīpana and pāchana can be done. Dīpana will kindle agni and pāchana will burn āma. If sāma doshas are leaving the body, let them go. It may be beneficial to induce vomiting.

The next stage is the prasara stage. Prasara is when the dosha's site in the gastrointestinal (GI) tract is totally full with a particular dosha—vāta in the colon, pitta in the intestine, kapha in the stomach—and that dosha becomes further aggravated, then the dosha leaves the GI tract. It then enters bāhya mārga, the external pathway, or *shākhā mārga,* the blood vessels or lymphatic system. (see Vyādhi Mārga Illustration on page 16)

The prasara stage of kapha is created by the oily quality. If you put a drop of oil on the surface of some water, the oil spreads. In the same way, kapha spreads on the surface of rasa dhātu when kapha enters the shākhā mārga. The spreading stage of kapha is due to oily quality. Because of the oily quality, kapha spreads to the deep tissues.

In prasara stage, kapha enters the rasa dhātu and can affect the top most layer of the skin so there is water retention as well as lymphatic, capillary, and venous congestion. Prasara stage will also create cold, sinus congestion, slow heartbeat, excess salivation, and generalized heaviness. A ring on the finger becomes tight, the bra becomes tight, and there is pitting of the skin upon pressure. This is the book picture of the prasara stage of kapha.

The first two stages of kapha samprāpti are in our hands, because the doshas are still in the GI tract. sanchaya is accumulation of kapha in the stomach; prakopa is aggravation of kapha in the stomach. But in prasara stage, kapha leaves the GI tract. We don't have as much control over this stage, but we can still do many things.

In prasara stage, kapha dosha travels and circulates in the body seeking a place to hide. As long as the dhātu agnis are healthy, kapha cannot enter into the dhātus and it will come back to the GI tract. However, one may be carrying a khavaigunya in some tissue, and we don't want to give kapha a chance to lodge in the khavaigunya and create a pathology.

To address this we can use 500 mg of punarnavā. Punarnavā is a dosha pratyanika as well as a diuretic. It will drain excess kapha out through the *mūtra vaha srotas.*

To kindle agni, use 200 mg of chitrak, and do pāchana using trikatu. Trikatu will kindle agni and chitrak will do *āma pāchana.* Dīpana and pāchana can be used mainly in the first three stages: sanchaya, prakopa, and prasara, because once we do dīpana and pāchana, the dosha loses its grip over the tissue and can come back to the GI tract.

One can use a formula of 500 mg punarnavā, 200 mg of chitrak, and 200 mg of trikatu, and take ½ teaspoon of this combination orally TID. It will help to liquefy kapha and take care of the prasara stage.

During the prasara stage, the oily quality is circulating in the rasa dhātu and there is not much oily quality in the GI tract, causing people to crave fatty fried food. Don't eat fatty, fried, greasy food when there is edema, swelling, lymphatic congestion, or capillary congestion. The body creates perverted desires because the bodily dosha wants to grow and enter into the dhātus.

The opposite of oily quality is dry. Dryness is created when kapha leaves the GI tract and goes into rasa dhātu. The dryness in the GI tract will attract the kapha back into the stomach. Trikatu performs dīpana and pāchana and creates more dryness in the stomach. That dryness will act like a sponge and help to pull the kapha back into the GI tract. That is why it is important during prasara stage of kapha to use punarnavā, chitrak, and trikatu. Take ½ tsp. of this combination TID with honey. The person should sip hot water in between so that āma is not produced.

These three stages—sanchaya, prakopa, prasara—belong to the first three stages of shat kriyā kāla, management of the six stages of samprāpti for kapha dosha.

## Deeper Stages of Samprāpti

Sthāna samshraya is the fourth stage. Sthāna samshraya takes place where there is a khavaigunya. If rasa dhātu agni is low, then āma and kapha have access to rasa dhātu and will get deposited there. If rasa dhātu agni is strong, then kapha cannot enter the rasa dhātu and it will attach to the next dhātu.

In sthāna samshraya stage, the dosha finds a weak spot. It may have been created by a previous trauma, a repressed emotion, a previous disease, or low *dhātu agni*. These factors, along with genetic predisposition, may be responsible for sthāna samshraya. Sthāna samshraya varies according to the site of the lesion, the site of the khavaigunya.

If sthāna samshraya happens in a vital organ, such as the heart, brain, lung, liver, or kidney then kapha will affect those areas. If sthāna samshraya happens in the bladder, the person will get polyuria, a bladder stone, or bladder atony, which is distention of the bladder. If sthāna samshraya happens in the genital organ then it will create blockage of the urethra. If sthāna samshraya happens in the testicles, it can create hydrocele. This is a bird's eye view of different types of sthāna samshraya.

Another possibility is that sthāna samshraya can happen within the GI tract itself. If sthāna samshraya of kapha happens in the stomach then it can create a tumor, or achlorhydria, which is suppression of gastric mucous secretion. If sthāna samshraya happens in the stomach itself, it will create chronic indigestion or chronic anorexia. Let us go step-by-step and look at the entry of kapha into the dhātus.

*Rasa Dhātu.* If kapha enters rasa dhātu due to low rasa dhātu agni, then in general it will create low grade fever, pallor, cough, common cold, catarrh, lymphatic congestion, edema, and hay fever. It will also create lack of nutrition and fatigue.

For low-grade fever and common cold, we can use 500 mg of sītopalādi, 300 mg mahāsudarshan, and 200 mg of abhrak bhasma. Sītopalādi is an expectorant and decongestant. Mahāsudarshan is anti-pyretic and good for low-grade fever. Abhrak bhasma is good for boosting the immune system and protecting ojas. Mahāsudarshan gana vati is good for catarrh. One can take ½ teaspoon of this herbal formula TID with a bit of honey or hot water to deal with lymphatic congestion, low grade fever, common cold, congestion, and cough.

Also in this stage, one can inhale steam and do nasya with Super Nasya Oil® or vacha oil to take care of common cold and catarrh. Punarnavā can be used if there is edema and sītopalādi is the best remedy for hay fever. This is a beneficial formula for entry of kapha into the rasa dhātu.

*Rakta Dhātu.* If rasa dhātu agni is strong and so there is no access to enter the rasa dhātu then kapha will try to enter rakta dhātu. If rakta dhātu agni is low, kapha can enter the rakta dhātu and create more swelling, plus megaloblastic anemia, high blood pressure, high cholesterol, and high triglycerides. The root of rakta vaha srotas is the liver and spleen. Excess kapha in the liver will create fatty changes in the liver and enlargement of the spleen. A person may also get hyperglycemia or any of the symptoms of diabetes.

For edema and swelling, a person can use 500 mg of punarnavā. For pallor, one can use abhrak bhasma, and for high blood pressure, one can use 200 mg each of passionflower, hawthorn berry, or rasagandha. For high cholesterol we can use 200 mg of triphalā guggulu, shuddha shilājit (purified shilājit), or trikatu.

For fatty changes in the liver, we normally use ārogya vardhini, but it may be difficult to find ārogya vardhini without mercury, so we can use 200 mg each of kutki, chitrak, and neem TID. That will take care of fatty changes of the liver as well as enlarged spleen. For diabetic patients one can use equal portions 200 mg each of turmeric and neem TID.

*Māmsa Dhātu.* These individual disorders can be treated as separate conditions created by the entry of kapha into rakta dhātu. If rakta dhātu agni is strong then kapha will leave rakta dhātu and go to the māmsa dhātu. If māmsa dhātu agni is low, kapha can enter the māmsa dhātu.

Entry of kapha into māmsa dhātu will cause māmsa dhātu agni to decrease even more. Then there will be increased *khamala* (earwax), tartar on the teeth, nasal crust, and smegma. Entry of kapha into māmsa dhātu can create myoma, or muscle tumor, muscle hypertrophy, fibroid tumor, or fibrotic changes in the breast or uterus.

We can take care of these conditions with the following herbal protocols. For earwax, clean the ear with medicated vacha oil diluted half-and-half in sesame oil and kindle māmsa dhātu agni with 300 mg of triphalā guggulu BID. For myoma, which is a muscle tumor, we should do *lekhana* (scraping) using kutki or chitrak. Vacha oil can be applied (see above) topically for myoma.

For muscle hypertrophy, one can use 200 mg each shilājit, triphalā guggulu, or chandra prabhā vati TID. For fibroid tumor, one can use 200 mg each of punarnavā, kutki, and chitrak TID. Kāñchanār guggulu, 200 mg TID, is also quite effective for fibroid tumors, uterine fibroids, and muscle hypertrophy.

If a person develops tartar on the teeth, they should get their teeth cleaned by a dentist, no doubt, but tartar on the teeth is a sign of kapha entering māmsa dhātu. People who develop excess tartar on the teeth should also check their blood sugar, as they may be pre-diabetic. Using neem or triphalā toothpaste, or gargling with triphalā tea is quite effective for treating tartar. One can also hold a mouth full of sesame oil, swish it for one minute, and spit it out.

*Meda Dhātu.* If māmsa dhātu agni is strong, then kapha will not enter māmsa dhātu. It will leave māmsa dhātu and go to meda dhātu. If meda dhātu agni is low then kapha will enter the meda dhātu and create excess weight or obesity and cause cold sweating. If apāna vāyu is pulling kapha into the lower part of the body, then the person will get distended obesity. In this condition, they have a flat chest but enlarged thighs. If samāna vāyu is pushing kapha into the peritoneum and omentum then they will get truncated obesity and have a pot-bellied abdomen. If udāna vāyu is pushing kapha upward then there will be ascending obesity. In this condition, there is an enlarged face and pendular breasts, but the thighs are not enlarged. If vyāna vāyu is distributing kapha in the periphery, a person will have peripheral obesity. They will have enlarged thighs and arms but a flatter belly and chest.

One should pay attention to the different types of obesity. They each have a different protocol. In apāna vāyu obesity, or descending obesity, one can use triphalā guggulu and do dashamūla basti. In truncated obesity, which is *samāna vāyu dushti,* one can use chitrak guggulu. This will kindle agni and pacify samāna vāyu. In ascending obesity, where obesity affects the face and breasts, one can use trikatu, because it acts on the upper part of the body. If it is peripheral obesity, then treat vyāna vāyu with arjuna and vacha, or 200 mg each of arjuna and pushkarmūla. They can also use kaishore guggulu, which has an affinity for vyāna vāyu.

When kapha goes into meda dhātu a person can get gallstones. The treatment protocol for gallstones is 500 mg of punarnavā, 200 mg of chitrak, 200 mg of trikatu and 200 mg of shilājit, taken TID orally.

*Asthi Dhātu.* If meda dhātu agni is strong, kapha will go to asthi dhātu. If asthi dhātu agni is low, kapha can enter the asthi dhātu and create osteoma, tumors of the bones, swelling of the joints, effusion, bone spur, misalignment of the spine, and lordosis. These also go together with hypothyroidism. Hypothyroidism means kapha is at the junction between asthi and majjā. The endocrine system is majjā dhātu and glandular dysfunction can happen when kapha enters the junction between these two dhātus, which is the *dhātu dhāra kalā*. When kapha passes from the *asthi dhāra kalā* to the *majjā dhāra kalā* then hypothyroidism will happen.

In hypothyroidism, the patient has calcium in the blood so there may be micro-calcification. Kapha in the asthi dhātu reduces asthi dhātu agni further and then the bone starts losing calcium. Those calcium molecules can deposit in the breast because *poshaka kapha* and lactation are by-products of rasa dhātu. Even though kapha is in asthi dhātu, it still has an affinity to *stanya,* or breast tissue. Micro-calcification in the breast can create a pre-cancerous situation.

For osteoma, or bony tumor, we can use either 200 mg of yogarāja guggulu and 200 mg of kāñchanār guggulu, or 200 mg of rāsnādi guggulu TID. For swelling of the joints, we can use punarnavā guggulu or the following lepanas topically to reduce the effusion—punarnavā lepana, gudūchī lepana, dashānga lepana. Lepanas are herbal pastes applied topically.

For bone spur, triphalā guggulu or yogarāja guggulu can be used TID. Traditionally, *agni karma* was done topically on the site of the spur. In agni karma, a red hot copper rod is used to do gentle branding. This has to be done with great skill. The counter-irritation of branding stimulates osteolytic enzyme,[16] and inhibits osteogenic enzyme.[17] This causes porosis in the spur. It also prevents spur formation by kindling asthi dhātu agni.

Misalignment of the spine may be due to kapha in asthi dhātu. Kapha is slow and sluggish, and people sitting around with bad posture develop misalignment. For that they have to correct their posture, do some yoga, and apply mahānārāyana tailam along the spine. Chiropractic manipulation or applying traction may also help.

When kapha is in the junction of asthi and majjā dhāra kalā and causes hypothyroidism, we can use 200 mg each of ārogya vardhini, chitrak, trikatu, and kaishore guggulu TID. Bhrāmarī and ujjāyi prānāyāma are also affective as well as specific *āsanas* that strengthen the spine.

***Majjā Dhātu.*** If asthi dhātu agni is strong, kapha will try to enter majjā dhātu. If majjā dhātu agni is low, kapha will enter majjā and create hypersomnia, or increased sleep, protruded eyes, hydrocephalus,[18] lethargy, and melancholy. These sound rather complicated, but they are simply kapha in the brain and nervous system.

Kapha in majjā dhātu can also create a pineal gland tumor, called pinealoma, or a pituitary gland tumor. It can also create petit mal epilepsy. These are serious conditions and they should be treated by experts.

For hypersomnia, increased sleep, we can use 200 mg each brahmī, jatamāmsī, vacha, shankha pushpī TID and vacha oil nasya. That will reduce kapha from the majjā dhātu. For a pineal or pituitary gland tumor, the dhātu treatment is the same because we are treating the dosha in majjā dhātu. For that, use 500 mg of punarnavā, 200 mg chitrak, 200 mg kutki, 300 mg brahmī, and 200 mg of shankha pushpī. One-half teaspoon of this formula TID will help. In both pineal and pituitary tumor, the following prānāyāmas are effective: bhrāmarī prānāyāma, bhastrikā prānāyāma, anuloma viloma, and kapāla bhāti.

For lethargy, one should do panchakarma with shiro basti, shirodhāra, and nasya. Internally we can use 200 mg each of punarnavā, brahmī, jatamāmsī, and shankha pushpī TID.

---

16. A bodily enzyme that breaks down bone cells.
17. A bodily enzyme that stimulates growth of the bone.
18. An accumulation of water in the subdural space or meninges.

*Shukra Dhātu.* If majjā dhātu agni is strong then naturally kapha will go to shukra dhātu. *Shukra gata kapha* can create a tumor in the testicle or epididymis, benign prostatic hyperplasia, hydrocephalus, and semen leak. In all these disorders, there is a simple line of treatment: 500 mg of punarnavā, 200 mg chandraprabhā, 200 mg ashvagandhā, and 200 mg of ātmaguptā; take ½ teaspoon of this formula TID.

A testicular tumor or benign prostatic hyperplasia could be cancer so in these conditions, one should consult with an expert to rule that out. Otherwise, benign prostatic hyperplasia has the same herbal protocol as above, and prostatic massage with medicated vacha oil or castor oil is also effective.

Shukra gata kapha can produce large amounts of semen, and the person may become sexually overactive. Even after prolonged sex, there is no satisfaction. These people may end up with depression. To strengthen shukra we can use 500 mg of ashvagandhā and 300 mg of vidārī TID. Shukra gata kapha can also produce raw, unhealthy semen that can get blocked in the prostate and produce prostatic calculi or prostatic stone. The herbal protocol for prostatic stone is 200 mg of punarnavā guggulu, 200 mg of gokshura guggulu, 200 mg of shilājit, and 200 mg of pāshana bheda TID. These herbs will help break down the prostatic calculi.

Kapha is dull and slow. In some individuals, kapha may produce low libido and premature ejaculation. The treatment protocol for low libido and premature ejaculation is 500 mg of ashvagandhā, 300 mg of balā, 200 mg of vidārī, and 200 mg of shilājit TID.

The pure essence of all bodily tissues is ojas. There are two types of ojas: *para* and *apara*. Para is superior ojas, which is present in the heart in a quantity of eight drops. There is half an *añjali* of apara ojas and it circulates throughout the body. If kapha enters shukra, it may slow down the process of dhātu metabolism and produce raw ojas. Increased raw ojas can create high cholesterol, high triglycerides, and hypertension with low libido. These people can also get albumin urea, protein in the urine.

The treatment protocol for ojovruddhi, increased raw ojas, is to treat kapha dosha with 500 mg of punarnavā, 200 mg shilājit, 200 mg of abhrak bhasma, and 200 mg of ātmaguptā TID. This herbal protocol will create healthy ojas. These people should also take 1 teaspoon of tikta ghrita, which is bitter ghee, because the bitter taste can reduce kapha dosha.

Finally, to protect ojas, Ayurveda recommends madhu tailam basti, which is ½ cup of sesame oil and ½ cup of honey mixed together and given rectally. The subject is asked to retain this for as long as he can.

*Ārtava Dhātu.* Lastly, if kapha dosha enters ārtava dhātu, it can slow down ārtava dhātu agni. The female egg becomes slow, sluggish, heavy, and enlarged, and can produce polycystic changes in the ovaries, known as polycystic ovarian syndrome or cystic ovary. This is accompanied by a hormonal imbalance with low estrogen and overproduction of testosterone. The patient develops male facial hair. This undue growth of the hair is due to male hormones, which are kapha in nature. The treatment protocol for polycystic ovarian syndrome is 500 mg of punarnavā, 200 mg of chitrak, 200 mg of kutki, and 300 mg of ashoka. Take ½ tsp. of this mixture TID. She should also do prāṇāyāma like kapāla bhāti, anuloma viloma, and bhrāmarī.

The entry of kapha in ārtava dhātu can also cause ectopic gestation, fibroid tumor, or cervical polyps. In all these disorders, the best remedy is 500 mg of punarnavā, 200 mg of chitrak, and 200 mg of shilājit TID. Don't use shatāvarī or balā in these disorders, because these are anabolic and will induce kapha further. Instead of shatāvarī and balā we can use ashoka with kumārī (aloe vera) as an anupāna.

Kapha dosha in *ārtava vaha srotas* may produce undue thickening of the endometrium, called endometriosis. Due to the increase of the heavy, thick, and stable qualities of kapha dosha, the endometrium grows through the fallopian tubes and ovaries. It can also spread into the pelvic cavity and create multiple adhesions. According to Ayurvedic principles, one should do *lekhana chikitsā* followed by 500 mg of punarnavā, 200 mg of kutki, and 300 mg of trikatu. Take ½ tsp. of this mixture TID. Also take 1 Tbs. of flax seed oil orally twice a day before breakfast and dinner.

The vyakti stage of kapha samprāpti is due to cloudy and soft qualities. Cloudy quality causes congestion and the soft quality causes discharge and oozing. During the vyakti stage, kapha can create various tumor formations related to the specific dhātu that has been affected in the sthāna samshraya stage.

In the bheda stage, we have a full-blown manifestation of pathogenesis, but the treatment of those pathogeneses should follow the protocol of the sthāna samshraya stage, because vyakti and bheda are related to the same site as sthāna samsraya. The vyakti stage may happen in any srotas or dhātu, so its signs and symptoms depend on the site of the lesion. For example, when sthāna samshraya happens in rasa dhātu, then the vyakti stage will create a growth such as lymphoma. If sthāna samshraya happens in rakta dhātu, then the vyakti stage will create will megaloblastic (pernicious) anemia or hemangioma, a tumor of the blood. Vyakti of meda dhātu will create lipoma. So, the manifestation of vyakti depends upon the dhātu. The protocol is the same as in the sthāna samshraya stage.

In the bheda stage, kapha creates structural changes in the tissue because of hard, dense, static, and gross qualities. Ultimately, the bheda stage of kapha will cause hardening, excess growth, and compactness of the tissue. There may be modified tumor, consolidation of the tissue, change of tissue structure and loss of tissue function. It can also create hard, calcified fibrotic nerves. That is why bheda stage is called *upadrava* stage, the stage of complications. The bheda stage should only be handled by a seasoned professional. Diet and lifestyle factors may help, but they will be limited, because the person has complications that may also require hospitalization, surgical intervention, chemotherapy, radiation, or other proper treatment from an oncologist.

The shat kriyā kāla opens a multi-factorial therapeutic approach. It moves students and practitioners to think about *vidhi samprāpti,* which involves the *dosha gati,* or movement of the doshas, and vyādhi mārga, the pathway of the disease. It also explains *vikalpa samprāpti,* the qualitative manifestation of the dosha. If a person follows shat kriyā kāla, they will hit the nail on the head. Their treatment will never go astray. Sometimes people think that Ayurveda takes a long time; I think that is not true. If a practitioner, student, or professional really puts these views of shat kriyā kāla into their practice, I am quite sure they will be great clinicians, healers, and practitioners. They will bring a positive result in their clinical practice.

This is my humble effort of expressing this shat kriyā kāla. It is briefly mentioned in Sushruta Samhitā but we have taken his wonderful idea and elaborated on it with our clinical data, making shat kriyā kāla a unique line of therapy.

# Chapter 5

# Pain
## Shūla

Winter 1997, Volume 10, Number 3 and Spring 1998, Volume 10, Number 4

In *Mādhava Nidānam,* one of the ancient Ayurvedic texts on clinical practice, *shūla* (pain) is treated as a separate *roga* (disease). However, many times we experience pain as a symptom of another disease. What is the difference between a disease and a symptom? A disease has its own samprāpti (pathological changes,) a definite etiology and specific signs and symptoms. It undergoes doshic changes, through the six stages of pathogenesis: accumulation, provocation, spread, deposition, manifestation and differentiation. Therefore, disease has a definite samprāpti.

On the other hand, a symptom isn't necessarily due to one particular disease process. A symptom may be caused when a dosha accumulates in its own site, without yet producing any disease. The dosha can then undergo changes and express different signs and symptoms in each stage of disease. When symptoms are incompletely manifested, they are called pūrva rūpa, which means warning bell symptoms. When signs and symptoms are completely manifested, they are called rūpa. When pain is constant, persistent and a major problem, it can itself be called a disease.

Vāta is the dosha primarily responsible for pain, because it is closely related to *prāna,* which governs the nervous system and all sensation. Vāta's main seat is in the colon and from there, vāta moves into different bodily *srotāmsi* (channels). Prāna also flows throughout the body, in every srotas (channel), organ, and *marma* point. If prāna becomes functionally disturbed, due to an imbalance in one or more of the qualities of *vāta dosha,* that results in pain in either the mind or body. Vāta is dry (*rūksha*), light (*laghu*), cold (*shīta*), rough (*khāra*), subtle (*sūkshma*), and mobile (*chala*). Extreme dryness or intense cold can create pain, as can excess roughness. The mobile quality of vāta can cause the pain to radiate, moving from one place to another.

Many times, vāta pain is seemingly causeless. The pain is mobile, radiating, fluctuating, and vague in nature. Vāta pain is aggravated at vāta times of day, which are dawn and dusk. It is also more intense during the vāta seasons, fall and winter, and is aggravated by exposure to cold, improper food combining and excessive movement. In addition, vāta pain is associated with flatulence, constipation, and bloating.

Next, look at the qualities of pitta—hot (ushna), sharp (tīkshna), spreading (sara), oily (*snigdha*), liquid (*drava*), and light (laghu). When these qualities are increased and pitta is blocking vāta, then these pitta attributes mix with vāta and create pitta type of pain. Increased hot quality causes burning and inflammation, sharp quality can create ulceration and perforation. Increased oily quality may increase congestion and produce nausea, and the spreading quality of pitta causes pain to flare, creating tenderness and pain on pressure. Pitta pain is associated with inflammation and increases during midday, midnight and during the summer season. It is often followed by nausea, vomiting and diarrhea. It is increased by exposure to heat and pacified by cooling treatments. Note that while heating treatments relieve vāta pain and increase pitta pain, both vāta and pitta pain are worsened by movement. Therefore fast walking or vigorous exercise can aggravate arthritic pain that is caused by vāta and/or pitta.

Kapha is heavy (guru), dull (*manda*), cool (shīta), oily (snigdha), sticky (*picchila*), static (*sthira*), and liquid (drava). When any of these qualities of kapha are disturbed and block vāta, the resultant pain will have kapha characteristics. Because of the heavy quality, kapha type of pain will be deep. Kapha is slow and dull, hence, kapha pain is a dull ache. It is also liquid and cool, so the skin in the affected areas will feel cold and clammy. Due to both the liquid and oily qualities, kapha pain is associated with congestion and swelling, and because kapha is static, the pain is localized, neither radiating like vāta, nor spreading like pitta. Pressure and deep massage can relieve kapha pain, as do movement and warming exercise. Kapha pain occurs more in early morning and early evening, which are kapha times of day, and during the winter and spring seasons.

Shūla is a complex subject, but we are presenting this information in a simplified way. Behind pitta or kapha pain there is always vāta, because a disturbance of vāta is always involved in any kind of pain. However, when vāta is blocked by pitta, the pain is colored by the qualities of pitta. The same is true for kapha. Pure vāta pain is pricking, gripping, spasmodic, colicky, and often excruciating. Psychologically, it creates nervousness, fever and insomnia. Pitta pain is hot, sharp and intense, and it creates irritability, anger and disturbed sleep. Finally, kapha pain is heavy, dull and static, and it creates attachment, depression and excessive sleep.

## The Qualities of Pain

Pain can be acute, subacute, chronic, radiating, and fluctuating. Whenever pain is present, we have to inquire into the qualitative changes that have occurred and determine whether the pain is mono, dual or triple-doshic.

*Mādhava Nidānam* speaks about sensory pain, motor pain and emotional pain. Sensory pain is related to prāna; motor pain to *apāna;* and emotional pain is psychosomatic. Pain is an interactive phenomenon that operates at the physical, mental, emotional and biochemical levels. It may be due to tissue damage, but remember that tissue damage is due to aggravation of the doshic qualities described above. A comfortable stimulus is called pleasure, whereas an uncomfortable stimulus is called pain.

Physiological, psychological, and social interactions can all create pain. For example, an argument with your spouse can precipitate pain. We have to see pain as a whole, having the qualities of vāta, pitta, and kapha. Understanding this basic concept helps us to deal with the pain directly.

Generally, there is a tendency for vāta pain to be acute, pitta pain to be acute or sub-acute, and kapha pain to be subacute or chronic. However this is not always true, as certain kapha pain is acute, such as a sinus headache. Kapha pain is always less intense; it doesn't create the agony caused by vāta and pitta pain. First, identify the doshic involvement: congestion is kapha; infection or inflammation indicates pitta; trauma, accident or neuralgia is vāta. Ask what time the pain occurs. Pain that worsens around midnight and midday indicates pitta. Morning and evening pain shows kapha, while pain that occurs at dawn and dusk is vāta. Also inquire about aggravating and relieving factors. Movement will aggravate vāta but relieve kapha. Application of heat, such as a warm castor oil pack, will soothe vāta but increase pitta. The usage of non- invasive measures, such as the application of heat, gentle manipulation, a splint or bandage, relaxation, yoga, prāṇāyāma, and meditation, will especially relieve vāta pain.

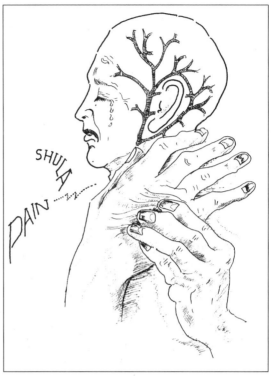

सर्वेष्वेतेषु शूलेषु प्रयेण पवन प्रभुः ।
मा. नि.

sarveṣveteṣu śūleṣu prayeṇa pavana prabhuḥ
*Mādhava Nidānam*

*Imbalanced vāta affects the other doshas, creating pain. This sensory and emotional experience is associated with the psychosomatic response to actual or potential tissue damage. In all pains, vāta is the main causative factor.*

Translation, Vasant Lad

## Associated Phenomena

Pain associated with symptoms such as fever, diarrhea, and vomiting is a sign of disturbed pitta dosha. Constipation and flatulence along with pain indicates a vāta disorder. Pain with heaviness and sleepiness is a sign of increased kapha. If there is extreme chronic anorexia (low agni) with epigastric pain, the cause may be cancer. Chronic low hydrochloric acid can also be indicative of cancer.

Vomiting is a common symptom that is associated with pain. Vomiting related to stomach or intestinal problems, such as gastritis enteritis, or peritonitis, is due to aggravated pitta. If there is also gas under the diaphragm, consider the possibility of a perforated ulcer. Vomiting may also be a sign of early appendicitis or cholecystitis, and meningitis can also cause vomiting. About ninety-five percent of vomiting is due to aggravated pitta, whereas only mucoid vomiting is a purely kapha disorder. In children, vomiting is often due to infection and projectile vomiting indicates pancreatitis. Sudden vomiting suggests an intracranial disease and if there is vomiting in the morning, during kapha time, think about pregnancy or alcoholic gastritis. Vomiting of large quantities of food in the later part of the day or night might be due to obstruction caused by a tumor, while involvement of the upper gut could be due to a pyloric obstruction.

Vomiting with heartburn could be caused by inflammation of the esophagus, another pitta disorder, and if there is regurgitation of food with pain, that might indicate an esophageal obstruction. Take the age of the person into consideration. If a man of 82 comes with a sense of obstruction while swallowing, think about cancer of the esophagus. However, if the person is in his or her twenties, the cause might be stress.

## Ayurvedic Pain Killers

*Shulāhara* or *shūlaghna* is the Sanskrit word for analgesic. Ayurveda speaks about many substances that can be used to alleviate pain.

*Opium (Papaver somniferum).* Ahiphenam or opium was used in ancient times as the most effective analgesic. Today it is a controlled substance and can only be prescribed by qualified physicians. It works as a painkiller and anti-spasmodic and it is effective for pain due to all three doshas. Even a small dose can relieve pain and insomnia, but there are many side effects. It is extremely addictive and causes severe constipation. Hence, it is vāta-aggravating. Perhaps the most serious side effect is that any form of opium is a respiratory depressant and an excessive dose can result in death.

*Dhattūra (Dhātura alba).* Although dhattūra is quite toxic to the liver and kidneys and may create extreme muscle spasm, in small doses it is a wonderful painkiller. The flower, which looks like a loudspeaker, is made into a tea. Dhattūra works best for vāta and kapha pain. Because it can create nausea and vomiting, it is not used for pitta.

*Yavānī (Trachyspermum ammi).* Yavānī is a special ajvain from Afghanistan. It is effective for vāta and kapha pain and also relieves stomach pain. Yavānī is not used for pitta, because it can create nausea and vomiting.

*Mustā (Nagar motha—Cyperus rotundus).* Mustā is effective for *tridoshic* pain. It is a muscle relaxant with an affinity for māmsa dhātu, so it is used for muscular-skeletal pain, but not for pain in the smooth muscles. Due to its diuretic action, it also relieves renal pain.

*Ashvagandhā (Withania somnifera).* Ashvagandhā pacifies vāta and kapha and it can stimulate pitta. This herb is effectively used for congestive and spasmodic pain, as well as neurologia and muscular pain. It soothes menstrual cramps caused by spasmodic dysmenorrhea, but if the cause is congestion, punarnavā is a better choice.

*Jatamāmsi (Nardostachys jatamāmsi).* This herb has an affinity for majjā dhātu and *mano vaha srotas*. Jatamāmsi is used for vāta and pitta disorders. Its actions are anti-inflammatory, analgesic and tranquilizing. It is particularly effective for pain caused by emotional or neurological or factors.

*Ajvain (Carum copticum—Wild Caraway).* Ajvain works on smooth muscles, including the muscles of the small intestine. It is heating and pungent and can be used for vāta and kapha, but it is too heating for pitta and may create bleeding. Ajvain is antispasmodic to the colon and stomach muscles and also relieves pain caused by congestion.

*Nutmeg (Myristica fragrans—jātīphalā).* Nutmeg is analgesic and a tranquilizer, similar to a mild version of opium. It may increase kapha. Therefore, excessive use can create depression. Nutmeg is used in diarrhea and it is effective for any generalized body ache, as it works on the nervous system. A pinch of nutmeg in milk, with a teaspoon of ghee added, acts on emotional pain. Nutmeg oil on the forehead will relieve a headache and it can be used in *marma chikitsā* for vāta and pitta.

*Ginger (Zingiber off.; adraka—fresh ginger; shunthi—dry ginger).* Ginger is tridoshic, but in excess may increase pitta. It has an affinity for māmsa, asthi and majjā dhātus. Note that dry ginger is more heating than fresh. Ginger paste is effective for sinus headaches and has many other uses as pain reliever. Ginger can be used if āma is lingering in rasa dhātu, as it has āma pāchana action. A ginger/baking soda bath will also help to remove this āma.

*Cinnamon (Cinnamomum zeylancium; tvak).* Cinnamon or tvak is used as a medicine for vāta and kapha, but not for pitta, because of its heating quality. It can be used internally and topically, and is good for relieving sinus headaches, stomachache and tooth pain.

*Guggulu (Commiphora mukal).* The various forms of guggulu are used for specific doshic pain. For vāta pain use yogarāja guggulu; for pitta, kaishore guggulu; for kapha, triphalā guggulu. Guggulu has a special affinity for the bones, so it is particularly good for arthritic pain.

*Jyotishmatī (Celastrus paniculatus).* This herb is used for vāta and kapha, but not for pitta dosha. Its actions are narcotic, tranquilizing and sedative. Jyotishmatī oil is used externally for arthritic pain.

*Clove (Syzigium aromaticum; lavanga).* Clove is used for vāta and kapha, but it can aggravate pitta. One drop of clove oil on an aching tooth will act as an analgesic and will also kill any bacteria. Clove is used for most types of dental pain and trigeminal neuralgia.

*Camphor (Cinnamonum camphora; karpura).* Camphor is the resin of a tree. It has an affinity to the nerve tissue and is a bronchodilator and analgesic. A pinch of edible camphor on an aching tooth will calm the pain. It is mainly used for vāta and kapha types of pain.

*Dashamūla.* This combination of ten herbal roots is widely used for vāta type of pain. Dashamūla has an affinity for asthi and majjā dhātus. Dashamūla oil can be used for massage and is effective for lower backache. Dashamūla tea basti is used to alleviate vāta pain in the abdominal area.

*Ajagandha (Cleome viscosa—Wild Mustard).* Ajagandha means male goat. This herb has a strong smell and is an aphrodisiac. It is used for vāta and kapha pain and for testicular pain in particular. Other uses include pain due to worms, parasites and indigestion.

*Kāma Dudhā.* Kāma dudhā is a compound of anti-inflammatory and analgesic bhasmas and is effectively used for pitta pain.

*Vijayā (Cannabis sativa—Marijuana).* Vijayā is marijuana. It is tridoshic when used in a small dose, but in excess it provokes all three doshas and overuse may particularly disturb vāta. Vijayā is a highly spiritual plant that is used by yogis and *tantric* people in India. It calms anxiety and gives a sense of well-being, as well as expansion of consciousness. However, it is addictive and toxic to the liver and lungs. Excessive consumption can lead to anxiety tachycardia, neurosis and schizophrenic changes. Because it slows metabolism, excessive use of this substance can also lead to weight gain. Vijayā guggulu is an effective treatment for rheumatoid arthritis and contains one-eighth vijayā.

*Bhangā.* Bhang means 'to destroy worldly nature.' A mild preparation of marijuana made from young leaves and stems of the Indian hemp plant and drunk with milk or water as a fermented brew or smoked for its hallucinogenic effects. It is similar to marijuana and gives a beautiful perception of color vision. It pacifies vāta and kapha, but in excess it can increase all doshas. Although bhangā is a strong pain killer, it is highly addictive.

*Drākshā.* Drākshā is an herbal wine and its alcohol base will increase pitta if used in excess. It acts as a diuretic and analgesic and it brings tranquility. It especially helps pain due to āma. Although drākshā can be used as a painkiller, alcohol is addictive and should be used with caution.

*Tobacco (Nicotiana tubacum; tamakhu).* Tobacco is tridoshic when used in moderation as a painkiller, but it disturbs all three doshas in excess. Tobacco goes directly into the nervous system, and it is addictive and carcinogenic. A small dose brings a mild tranquil-izing effect, causing stress-induced pain to subside. Those who smoke in moderation will hardly ever get Alzheimer's, because nicotine in a small dose is a vasodilator. However, if taken in excess, nicotine causes hardening of the blood vessels. Anything in its proper dose is medicine; anything in excess is poison.

*Arjuna (Terminalia arjuna).* This herb is used for pain due to imbalanced vāta or kapha doshas. It relieves cardiac pain by increasing cardiac circulation.

*Pushkaramūla (Inula racemosis; Elecampane).* Pushkaramūla is tridoshic. It is used for pleuritis and cardiac pain and combined with arjuna for cardio-pulmonary pain.

*Punarnavā (Boerhaavia diffusa).* This herb is used for vāta and kapha disorders, and it is slightly heating, hence, not so good for pitta. Punarnavā is particularly effective for renal colic.

*Castor Oil (Ricinus communis; eranda).* Castor oil is tridoshic when used appropriately and it is a strong laxative. A cup of ginger tea with one teaspoon of castor oil can help to relieve rheumatic pain.

Many of these substances are addictive. How and when should we use them? It depends on the skill of the physician as to the correct use of these addictive substances. The healer-patient relationship must be absolutely clear. With this clarity, the physician can use these strong herbs in small doses. The doctor-patient relationship is sacred and, unfortunately, in this modern age that relationship is rare.

For instance, ulcerative colitis responds well to a small dose of ahiphenam, but once the bleeding stops, one should gradually withdraw the drug before an addiction develops. In case of a psychic or stress headache, or even in anxiety, tobacco can be used along with nutmeg and rose. The patient can smoke three cigarettes a day with these special ingredients. Tobacco has an affinity to majjā dhātu, so in situations of stress, emotional crisis or phobias, appropriate use of tobacco induces a sense of well-being. These strong substances should be used with great caution but can be extremely helpful.

In this next section, we will discuss specific doshic treatments for various classifications of pain, as presented in *Mādhava Nidānam*.

## Part Two: Doshic Management

In the previous section, we explored the Ayurvedic concept of pain. We will now consider the management of pain according to the *doshic* involvement. The entire picture has to be considered before we can come to any conclusion about the appropriate form of treatment. The main question to ask is, "What is the nature of the pain—vāta, pitta, or kapha?"

Pain caused by vāta strikes intermittently, creating a period of time with pain followed by a period without. The symptoms may include breathlessness, tachycardia, and gas. The nature of the pain is excruciating, agonizing, colicky and intense. Vāta pain is relieved by the application of heat (svedana), oil massage (snehana), and dashamūla tea basti (medicated enema) as well as by pressure at the site of the pain.

Pitta pain is sharp, burning, and stabbing and it is increased by pressure. It is associated with nausea, vomiting, diarrhea, dizziness, and irritability. Cooling treatments, such as a cold compress or ice bag, relieves pitta type of pain. It is also relieved by virechana (purgation).

Kapha pain is dull, aching, and static. The pain is increased by bending over and lessened by standing up or otherwise moving against gravity. Movement of any kind generally relieves this type of pain, which is associated with stiffness and swelling. Kapha pain is relieved by dry and scraping treatments, such as dry brush massage or the application of dry heat, as well as vamana (therapeutic vomiting).

All types of pain can be relieved by snehana, using oils specific to the dosha involved. For vāta, use sesame oil or *ghee*. Pitta responds well to coconut, sunflower oil or ghee, all of which are cooling. For kapha, use a light and drying oil, such as corn or mustard oil. Vacha oil or dry vacha powder are also effective for kapha. In India, we use vacha oil as a nasya (nasal oil) for vāta or kapha types of sinus headache, and a vacha powder nasya is effective for kapha sinus congestion.

Essential oils can be used in svedana therapy. For pitta, use sandalwood or jatamāmsi oil added to a steam treatment. Kapha pain is helped by eucalyptus or cinnamon and vāta pain responds well to ginger, nirgundī, hina or amber in the steam.

Be sure to relieve or stop any severe pain before using the above treatments. Pain is an indication that something is wrong. One should always take it seriously and consider going to a doctor or even the hospital, especially if the pain is intense or prolonged.

# Classifications of Pain

*Mādhava Nidānam* speaks about various classifications of pain:

- *Udara shūla* – abdominal pain
- *Pārshva shūla* – pleuritic pain
- *Parināma shūla* – peptic pain during the process of digestion
- *Anna drava shūla* – pain during the process of liquefaction of food while it is still in the stomach
- *Hrid shūla or hricchūla* – pseudo-cardiac pain
- *Shira shūla* – headache[19]

## Udara Shūla

Udara shūla is abdominal pain. If it is present in the lower abdomen, the pain is usually due to vāta. Pain in the middle abdomen is generally from aggravated pitta and upper abdominal pain is often due to pitta and kapha. Whenever a patient reports abdominal pain, first determine the exact location of the pain. Pain in the right half of the epigastrium may be due to a duodenal ulcer, while pain in the left half possibly indicates a gastric ulcer. Generalized abdominal pain is commonly from āma; hence, it can be called āma shūla. In this case, there may be a history of indigestion or food poisoning and all associated symptoms need to be examined. If there is also abdominal distension and constipation, the cause may be an obstruction, which needs to be treated.

### Management

*Vāta udara shūla* occurs in the lower abdomen. First, apply a warm castor oil pack to that area. If this treatment relieves the pain, it is due to vāta dosha. Before proceeding with further treatment, one should be cautious and rule out the possibility of appendicitis. If the cause of pain is appendicitis, giving a basti could be dangerous. However, once appendicitis is ruled out, give a basti of dashamūla tea the moment the pain subsides.

If the person has had constipation for three or four days, give a basti or a glycerin suppository. If there is abdominal distension, find out if the cause is gas, constipation or an obstruction. A doctor can insert a flatus tube into the rectum and if the person passes countless bubbles, then there is no obstruction. If only a few bubbles or no bubbles pass through, send the person to hospital to determine the cause of the obstruction. Even worms in the colon can produce an obstruction, thereby creating an emergency. To treat shūla successfully may require a great deal of clinical experience.

Small stones may cause renal colic pain while passing them from the kidney into the urethra. If a stone becomes stuck somewhere, either in the beginning of the urethra near the kidney or at the end near the bladder, the entire urethra may spasm and create severe pain, causing attack after attack. It looks like vāta pain, but the pain moves from loin to groin, or vice versa. If you percuss the kidney area with your fist, it will increase the

T.I.D. = from the Latin means *ter in diem*, three times a day

B.I.D. = from the Latin means *bis in diem*, two times a day

19. Shira Shūla is covered in chapter 32, *Headache*, starting on page 269.

pain. Send the person to the hospital, as that patient needs a smooth muscle relaxant and intravenous flushing to assist in passing the kidney stone.

For management of vāta udara shūla, internally give:
Triphalā Guggulu    300 mg, 1 tablet TID
Hingvastak Chūrna  ½ teaspoon BID with warm water

Or make a tea using:
1 teaspoon Ginger
½ teaspoon Cinnamon
Pinch of Clove
Pinch of Rock Salt

Keep the colon clean by nightly giving:
½ teaspoon gandharva harītakī with warm water

***Pitta Udara Shūla.*** If the pain is accompanied by nausea, vomiting, or peptic ulcer and the patient says food relieves the pain, the cause may be pitta.

Internally give the following mixture, ½ teaspoon TID after food:
Shatāvarī              500 mg
Shankha Bhasma   200 mg
Kāma Dudhā        200 mg

At night give:
Sat Isabgol       ½ teaspoon in 1 cup of water

Suggest a pitta soothing diet. Licorice tea with equal proportions of cumin, coriander and fennel is also soothing.

Many times pitta pain is accompanied by nausea and vomiting. For nausea, add jatamāmsi 300 mg to the above formula. Or quickly drink the following to relieve gas, improve digestion and soothe pitta pain:
1 cup warm water
¼ teaspoon baking soda
Pinch of salt
Juice of ¼ lime

***Kapha Udara Shūla.*** Kapha pain is generally due to āma and the person feels dull with a sense of heaviness.

Internally give:
Lasunadi Vati        200 mg, 1 tablet twice a day after food
Or Shanka Vati     200 mg, 1 tablet once a day

If there is no āma, don't use shanka vati, because it is stronger than lasunadi vati.

At night give:
1 teaspoon bibhītakī with warm water

Once the kapha pain has subsided, induce vamana, but don't do vamana while there is pain.

In generalized abdominal pain, apply the appropriate paste around the belly button. For vāta, use ½ teaspoon dashamūla powder or ½ teaspoon garlic powder mixed with a little water. For kapha, use ½ teaspoon punarnavā powder and then sprinkle asafoetida powder on this paste.

## Parshva Shūla

Parshva shūla is pain in the sides of the chest, which is pleuritic pain. The patient has pain toward the end of each inspiration, along with shallow breathing and worsening of pain during the act of coughing, sneezing or yawning. Many times there is referred pain in the supraclavicle area around the C3 and C4 vertebrae, because of involvement of the phrenic nerve, which is connected to the pleura. If there is irritation of the pleura, there may initially be pain due to inflammation or vāta aggravation. Then if either pitta-type of inflammatory exudate or kapha-type of transudate accumulates in the pleural space, the pain is relieved. There may also be referred pain at the top of the shoulder, especially on the right side. Pain in this area suggests diaphragmatic pleuritis.

Pleuritic pain can be caused by vāta, pitta or kapha. The vāta type is called dry pleurisy and the pitta type is pleuritis, where the inflamed surfaces of the pleura rub against each other. Kapha creates pleurisy with effusion, with diminished movement on the involved side and a prominent sternal mastoid on the opposite side. With this kapha type of pleuritic pain, one must also consider the possibility of pneumonia.

## Management of Parshva Shūla

*Vāta Pārshva Shūla.* Internally give the following mixture, ½ teaspoon TID after food:

| | |
|---|---|
| Dashamūla | 500 mg |
| Mustā | 400 mg |
| Pushkaramūla | 300 mg |

If there is muscular pain, add yogarāja guggulu 200 mg to the above formula.

Apply a castor oil pack to the site of pain.

*Pitta Pārshva Shūla.* If there is inflammation, use the following mixture, ½ teaspoon TID after food:

| | |
|---|---|
| Gudūchī | 400 mg |
| Kāma Dudhā | 200 mg |
| Mustā | 300 mg |
| Pushkaramūla | 300 mg |

*Kapha Pārshva Shūla.* For the dull ache of kapha pleuritic pain use the following mixture, ½ teaspoon TID after food:

| | |
|---|---|
| Punarnavā | 500 mg |
| Tālīsādi | 300 mg |
| Tankana (Borax) | 200 mg |
| Mustā | 200 mg |
| Pushkaramūla | 300 mg |

## Parināma Shūla

Parināma shūla is pain created during the process of digestion. The entire gastrointestinal tract is divided into six areas relating to the six stages of digestion. The first stage is sweet and kledaka kapha is secreted in the upper part of the stomach. During the next hour, as the food passes into the middle part of the stomach, the sour taste is activated, created by *pāchaka pitta*. Then during the third hour, the food enters the duodenum and the salty taste is predominant. This is followed by the pungent and bitter stages in the small intestine and the astringent stage in the colon, which is governed by vāta dosha. The early stages of digestion are governed by kapha, while the middle stages are controlled by pitta.

It is important to know how long it is after taking food that the pain appears. Then the doshic cause can be identified. If there is an ulcer, its location can also be determined by how soon after eating the pain begins. To ascertain this, the stomach is divided into thirds.

If the ulcer is in the upper third, it is due to depleted kledaka kapha and will create pain within one hour, during the sweet phase of digestion. If the pain appears within two hours, the ulcer is in the middle curvature of the stomach and is due to pitta during the sour phase of digestion. An ulcer at this location may be caused by the over secretion of hydrochloric acid. Pain within three hours, which occurs during the salty phase of digestion in the lower portion of the stomach and the duodenum, is due to pitta dosha. In the pyloric area, the enzymes are more alkaline and they try to regulate the acidity. If these alkaline enzymes are produced in excess, the ulcer will occur in the lower third of the stomach or the duodenum. We have to treat pitta in all three locations, but there is a secondary doshic involvement. The stomach is kapha, the small intestine is pitta and the colon is vāta. If the ulcer is in the upper portion, there is not enough kledaka kapha. If the location is in the middle section, there is too much pāchaka pitta. In the lower pyloric area, *prāna vāta* is involved in the disease process.

An ulcer may be a complication of parināma shūla, but parināma shūla doesn't just mean ulcer. Therefore, don't immediately jump to the conclusion that the pain is due to an ulcer. Acute pain in the stomach could be due to gastritis or food poisoning, which can aggravate pitta dosha. Or the person may have gone from doctor to doctor with no cause found for the pain. In that type of parināma shūla, the stomach pulse will generally reveal a kapha pulse and the pain will not respond to antacid treatments. This kapha pain is always present within the first hour of eating and the pain is dull, often with slight mucoid nausea. This condition can lead to cancer of the stomach, so always inquire about past history and present symptoms.

## Management of Parināma Shūla

*Āma Parināma Shūla and Kapha Parinā Shūla.* Pain will occur within an hour of taking food. The nature of the pain is heavy and dull and the quality of kledaka kapha is disturbed. Internally give:

Pāchak Vati, 1 pill of 200 mg. This will burn āma and take care of the pain.

If Pāchak Vati is not available use:
Ajvain          300 mg

Raw Sugar        300 mg

***Pitta Parināma Shūla.*** Pain occurs about two hours after eating. Internally, give the following mixture, ½ teaspoon TID, in the middle of the meal:

Shatāvarī        500 mg
Kāma Dudhā     200 mg
Moti Bhasma     200 mg
Yashthi Madhu  300 mg

At night give ½ teaspoon avipattikar churna, which contains nishottara. Do not give triphalā.

***Vāta Parināma Shūla.*** Pain occurs three hours after food. Internally give the following mixture, ½ teaspoon TID before food:

Dashamūla            500 mg
Hingvastak Chūrna  200 mg
Shankha Bhasma     200 mg

At night give ½ teaspoon harītakī an hour before sleep, which is a specific remedy for high vāta in the abdomen.

## Anna Drava Shūla

Anna drava shūla means pain during the process of liquefaction of food, which is experienced while the food is still in the stomach. After chewing and swallowing the food, it enters into the stomach where kledaka kapha is secreted through the stomach wall and churning of the food breaks it up into smaller and smaller pieces. The food at this stage is called anna drava. In cases of low jāthara agni, there will be production of āma within the stomach. Āma and increased kledaka kapha suppress pāchaka pitta, which is hydrochloric acid, leaving insufficient agni to digest the food. The resultant undigested food further adds to the āma. When food is in the process of liquefaction (anna drava), this āma sticks to the stomach wall, which prevents absorption and creates pain in the stomach. As long as food is present in the stomach, there will be pain. The pain is due to hypochlorhydria, or diminished hydrochloric acid; hence, taking hydrochloric acid can help these people. This hypochlorhydric pain may indicate a pre-cancerous condition, so it should be taken seriously.

Internally give the following mixture, ½ teaspoon TID after food:
Ajvain           200 mg
Citric Acid      5 mg
Chitrak          300 mg
Punarnavā        400 mg
In addition, take one tablet of hydrochloric acid after food to maintain optimal acidity.

## Hrid Shūla or Hricchūla

Hrid shūla is pseudo-cardiac pain. Due to fermentation of food in the stomach, gases are created in the fundus of the stomach. Those gases back up and can create pain in the precordium. This pseudo-cardiac pain is not involved with the functioning of the heart, but rather with the digestive process. It has a specific cause and must be treated accordingly.

Internally give the following mixture, ½ teaspoon TID after food:

| | |
|---|---|
| Arjuna | 300 mg |
| Shringa Bhasma | 200 mg |
| Hingvastak Chūrna | 200 mg |
| Avipattikar | 400 mg |

# Chapter 5                    Pain

Chapter 6

# The Concept of Cancer in Ayurveda

Fall 2005, Volume 18, Number 2

## Tumors and Tissue Irregularities

IN AYURVEDIC LITERATURE, a detailed description is given of various types of tumors. Terms such as *gulma, granthi, utseda* and *arbuda* are used for specific tumor conditions.

A growth, enlargement or cluster is called gulma, which is specifically used to indicate a tumor. Gulma is a benign tumor that has defined borders. There are many types of gulma. For instance, *rakta gulma* means a fibroid tumor, or even a fatty tumor. *Māmsa gulma* is a tumor arising from the muscle tissue. *Vāta gulma* refers to diverticulosis or accumulated gases in the colon. It creates localized bunching, which moves from one part of the abdomen to another.

Granthi is the name given to a glandular tumor. *Rasa granthi* is a lymphoid tissue tumor arising from the lymphatic system (rasa dhātu). *Meda granthi* means lipoma, which takes place in meda dhātu, in the fatty tissue. *Jatru granthi* means a thyroid tumor, while *yakrut granthi* is a tumor arising from the liver or gall bladder and *kloma granthi* is a tumor of the pancreas.

The Sanskrit word utseda means bulging, referring to any kind of localized bulging underneath the tissue.

Finally, arbuda is a malignant tumor or cancerous growth. That means an uncontrolled growth of abnormal tissues, due to low dhātu agni, which is related to damaged nucleic acid within the healthy tissues—either locally or spread throughout the body. Arbuda can occur in the breast, prostate, lungs, colon or elsewhere in the body. The description of arbuda in Ayurvedic literature gives us a detailed picture of malignant tumors or cancer.

### Cellular Dynamics

According to Ayurveda, the cancer disease process happens at the subtle cellular level, called *ati anu srotas*. Agni is metabolic activity and there are thirteen main types of agni. Jāthara agni is the gastric fire, which governs gross digestion, absorption, assimilation and transformation of food into micro chyle. *Bhūta agni* is present in the liver and governs subtle molecular digestion of food into the five elements: Ether, Air, Fire, Water and Earth. It is this molecular digestion that is affected by arbuda. Every tissue also has its own agni component, called dhātu agni, which refers to the enzymes and amino acids that govern tissue nutrition and cellular metabolic activity. The seven dhātus (tissues) are rasa (plasma), rakta (blood), māmsa (muscle), meda (fat or lipids), asthi (bones and cartilage), majjā (bone marrow and nerve tissue), and shukra (male reproductive) or ārtava (female reproductive tissue).

At the cellular level, each cell is a center of awareness, a conscious microscopic life. Every cell has cellular integrity and governs its own metabolic activity. There is a flow of communication from one cell to another, which is called prāna. Tejas is responsible for cellular metabolic activity and ojas governs immunity. These three (prāna, tejas, ojas) are the factors that control reproduction of arbuda at the cellular level.

Arbuda has its own tejas and it can produce new blood vessels (sirā) as part of the process of angiogenesis. Arbuda also has its own perverted prāna, which absorbs nutrients. It can produce agni (enzymes) and, with the help of prāna, it can invade the circulatory system and find a place to grow. Arbuda can also stimulate its own proteins to grow and multiply. It demands increased metabolic output; as a result, there is often severe weight loss in the patient.

### The Role of Ahamkāra

Why does a normal, healthy, life-maintaining cell become so crazy? That is a key point. According to Sankhya's philosophy of creation, *Purusha* is the conscious principle and *Prakruti* is primordial matter and creative potential. The first expression of Prakruti is *Mahat,* which is intelligence. Next comes *ahamkāra,* the 'I' former. Ahamkāra is a central energy field that is present in every substance, and it maintains that thing's form, shape, color, and consistency. For the past millions of years, mango seeds have never forgotten to produce mango trees, mango flowers, and mango fruits. The ahamkāra (or 'I' former) of the mango governs the specific forms of the tree, flower and fruit that are produced from the seed.

Ahamkāra is the energy that is responsible for the creation of all forms and the specific arrangement of their molecules. If we look at the human body, at the time of fertilization, a single sperm fertilizes a single ovum and mitotic division happens. Each cell is divided into two and continues multiplying to eventually create the beautiful form of a human mammal. What is true with the human being is also true in the rest of the animal and plant kingdoms. This philosophy of creation is applied at the cellular level. Every cell has definite form and functions, and the structure of the cell is maintained by cellular ahamkāra. Therefore white blood cells have a certain form, red blood cells have a typical form, the platelets and multiple nucleated muscle cells have specific forms, and so forth. These are all maintained by ahamkāra.

Ahamkāra can be called self-esteem. We all have this self, ego, 'I' or me. We all have consciousness, but it is the consciousness of millions and trillions of selves. Ahamkāra is the collective consciousness of trillions of cell bodies. There is some deep connection between ahamkāra at the gross physical level and at the cellular level. Disturbed ahamkāra can create a severe distortion of the physical body and individual identity. If someone doesn't have self-esteem and self-respect, that person may become depressed or have an inferiority complex, and he or she will become sad and miserable. That will slowly affect the immune system and the person's metabolism, distorting the whole psychosomatic identity.

---

## Arbuda Pūrva Rūpa: Warning Signs of Cancer

Cancer is a silent enemy in the beginning, with few signs and symptoms. The following is a list of the prodromal signs and symptoms of arbuda or cancer.

*Malāvashtambha* means repeated chronic constipation or absolute constipation. Changes in bowel habits are quite common after age 65, but if such a person does not have a bowel movement even after taking triphalā, one should think about cancer of the rectum as a possibility. It is helpful to do a colonoscopy just to rule out cancer.

*Mūtra krichra* means a change in bladder habits, repeated urethritis, or cystitis.

*Rakta gama* means bleeding. Say children are playing and a child who receives a pinch to the skin suddenly develops a balloon-like hematoma; that is an early sign of cancer. Rakta gama are bleeding disorders. One can rule out cancer when there are repeated attacks of bleeding from the nose, the ear, the vagina or the rectum.

*Srava* is a foul smelling discharge from a wound.

*Kāthinya granthi* means thickening of a tumor.

*Avipāka* is chronic indigestion, which is another preliminary symptom (pūrva rūpa) of cancer.

*Sakashtha anna pravesha* means difficulty in swallowing. If a person feels like they have swallowed some food but it is stuck near the heart area, and especially if such a person is elderly, one can think about the possibility of cancer and encourage the person to have it checked out.

*Tīvra kāsa* is a nagging cough that doesn't respond to cough syrups. A nagging cough can be due to cancer of the lungs.

*Svāra bheda* means hoarseness of voice. A hoarse voice is due to dryness of the vocal cords and it is an important sign of cancer that is due to depletion of ojas. This may indicate a malignant tumor in the vocal cords, or a tumor elsewhere in the body. It is more common in the case of someone with a history of smoking. However it can also be a sign of pandu, which means anemia. In that case, the person looks fair and has low energy levels.

*Arbuda granthi* is a hard nodular mass. This is another pūrva rūpa that can occur in a person who has developed cancer.

*Deha laghutā* means extreme, severe weight loss. It is another warning sign of cancer.

---

The same thing is true at the cellular level. Each cell has its own self-esteem and self-importance and, if the cell membrane is clogged with āma, there is poor communication. Such a cell is an isolated cell that becomes lonely. A lonely cell starts to act independently, producing its own enzymes and its own agni. That cell goes on growing independently and, as a result, it becomes malignant. These arbuda cells have a distorted self and hyperactive metabolism, demanding more metabolic output and attacking their neighboring cells. They convert neighboring cells into cancerous cells.

Not every disease noticeably undergoes the standard process of samprāpti (pathogenesis) in its ordinary sequence. The cellular factors and pathological changes that occur in cancer may not appear to follow this process, yet they do. At the cellular level, there is defective tejas, which can be responsible for radical changes in cellular metabolic activity. This results in production of metabolic waste, creating cellular āma. This cellular āma covers the cell membrane, then it affects the defensive mechanism (ojas) and metabolic activity (tejas), and as a result there is a disturbance in the flow of intelligence (prāna) from one cell to another. Prāna, tejas, and ojas lose their functional integrity.

### Prognosis

A prognosis for cancer depends upon both the type of cancer and the stage of the disease. The type of tumor is important in this regard and understanding this can save a life. Cancers in rasa and meda dhātus are easier to treat, whereas the deeper tissues are harder to treat. Similarly, the prognosis will usually be better if there is early diagnosis, but most people ignore the warning signs and don't go to the doctor. As a result, the disease starts to spread, sometimes rapidly, and the prognosis is poor.

Warts and moles can become cancerous, if they start to be irritated. Hoarseness of voice (*svāra bheda*) and a nagging cough are warning symptoms for cancer and they may be specifically related to cancer of the trachea and lungs. Thickening of a lump in the breast can indicate breast cancer. Esophageal cancer can produce difficulty swallowing, while stomach cancer may manifest as low appetite, poor digestion and hypochlorhydria (extremely low stomach acidity). Colon cancer can lead to constipation, while cancer of the uterus may lead to profuse bleeding. Note that any sore wound that doesn't heal can be malignant. If cancer is detected in its late stages, it is bound to create a bad prognosis.

### Prevention of Cancer

Prevention is an important part of the Ayurvedic approach to arbuda. In the case of lung cancer in particular, it is most important to avoid the causative factors, such as smoking tobacco and exposure to asbestos and chemicals. It is also important for someone to regularly perform a self-examination of the body, with regard to early identification of possible cancer symptoms. This should include women examining their breasts and men checking their testicles. If there is a hard lump, immediately rush to the doctor. Don't wait for it to spread; just find out whether or not it is malignant.

## Arbuda Vyādhi Vinischaya: Diagnosis of Cancer

There are various ways by which Ayurveda can diagnose arbuda. First, prakruti-vikruti parīkshā is used, which means physical and pathological examination.

Second, the practitioner uses *ashtavidhā parīkshā,* which is the eight-fold examination process. This is comprised of assessing the *nādī* (pulse), *mutram* (urine), mala (wastes), *jihva* (tongue), *shabda* (voice), *sparsha* (palpation), *drig* (eyes) and *ākruti* (bodily form). All these ashtavidhā parīkshāna should be done in order to thoroughly diagnose the problem. An expert Ayurvedic physician should assess the prakruti by reading the pulse and also find out the vikruti and any weak organs.

Third is *srotas parīkshā,* the examination of the bodily channels. A srotas examination is a systemic examination of every channel. *Prāna vaha srotas* (the respiratory system), *anna vaha srotas* (digestive system) and *udaka vaha srotas* (the water metabolism system) are the first three important srotāmsi to be examined. The seven *dhātu srotas*—rasa, rakta, māmsa, meda, asthi, majjā and shukra or ārtava—and the three excretory channels of mala, *mūtra* and *sveda* (sweat) *vaha srotas* are also thoroughly assessed.

The fourth diagnostic tool used for arbuda is *granthi parīkshā,* which is examination of any abnormal growth. It may be a growth under the skin, the subcutaneous tissue, fatty tissue, muscle tissue, bone tissue, or nerve tissue, and this category also includes examination of the lymph glands. If one feels a tumor, one should feel whether it is palpable, movable, or fixed. Generally fixed tumors belong to māmsa and asthi dhātus, whereas a mobile tumor may be in the subcutaneous tissue or fatty tissue.

The fifth diagnostic technique is *vividha parīkshā,* which is a series of tests. In modern medicine, this includes X-ray, ultrasound, magnetic resonance imaging (MRI), cytological examination, and lab tests. In the past, they depended upon ashtavidhā parīkshā, the eight-fold examination, and the diagnostic skills were totally based upon the ability of perception of the physician.

## Arbuda Rupani: Signs and Symptoms of Cancer

Once cancerous growth occurs, it produces various signs and symptoms that in Sanskrit are called *arbuda rupani*. The following are the most common signs and symptoms of arbuda.

*Rujā* (pain). A cancer patient has pain as a persistent symptom, because a cancerous tumor is irritating. There is no pain without the involvement of vāta dosha. In cancer, prāna vāta at the cellular level is constantly irritated and causes persistent pain.

*Daurbalya* (weakness). There is extreme fatigue and weakness, because ojas is depleted and the person's metabolism is affected. The healthy tissues start to suffer from lack of nutrition. Whatever nutrients the person takes in are absorbed by the cancerous cells. Even if the person takes a tonic, with rasāyana herbs such as shatāvarī, ashvagandhā and brahmī, it feeds the cancerous cells, because these have a greedy demand for nutrients. Cancerous cells suck the nutrients faster than healthy cells, leaving the healthy cells to starve. That is why a cancer patient has weakness.

*Alpa poshanam or Kuposhanam* (malnutrition). A cancer patient often shows a deficiency of iron, calcium, magnesium, vitamin $B_{12}$ and folic acid. The reason is the same as above: most of the nutrients are absorbed by the malignant cells.

*Balakshaya* (extreme fatigue). This is due to defective agni, because healthy agni governs the biological strength of a human being. A malignant growth affects both cellular agni and dhātu agni, and it results in fatigue.

*Asthi Bhagnatā* (bone fractures). This symptom is due to malabsorption and malnutrition. This may lead to a spontaneous medical fracture or there may be a malignant tumor arising from within the bone. At the edge of the tumor, the bone tissue may become weak and that can lead to a fracture of the bone.

*Pakshavadha* (paralysis). Stroke-like paralysis is a complication of cancer and it commonly happens in cases of a cancerous tumor in the brain. A space-occupying tumor in the motor area of the brain can paralyze the opposite side of the body.

*Arbudam Prasaratvam.* Means cancer spreads and starts to metastasize. This metastasizing nature of cancer is due to pitta and rakta. *"Pittam tu sveda raktayo"* means pitta is present in sweat (sveda) and blood (rakta), so the cancerous cells spread throughout the plasma and blood stream, the lymphatic system and, in the case of skin cancer, they can even spread through the sweat.

# Arbuda Chikitsā: Management of Cancer in Ayurveda

The Ayurvedic approach to cancer is fundamental and radical. There is no standard treatment. The treatment varies from person to person. An Ayurvedic physician has to pay complete attention to the prakruti and vikruti of the patient, to determine which doshas are involved. It is also important to find out what dhātus and organs are affected. Based upon that understanding, one can then deal with arbuda by means of snehana, svedana and panchakarma, using specific cleansing measures for each dosha. Typically, vamana (emesis) is used for kapha, virechana (purgation) for pitta, and basti (enema) for vāta.

Cancer care should be provided by a team of experts and your Ayurvedic physician should have great skill and experience in treating cancer, so that all aspects can be covered. Ayurveda has many treatment protocols that can be chosen according to the specific symptoms, including the following:

- *Shalya tantra* refers to surgically removing a tumor.
- *Sroto rodha* relates to clearing the obstruction of the vital pathways, which can be done either surgically or medically.
- *Shalya majjā* refers to cutting the nerves that carry the pain. This is actually a symptomatic form of treatment but when there is constant pain, a cancer patient may wish to commit suicide. This is sad and painful, so cutting the nerves results in that person being free from pain.
- Another type of protocol is *vyādhi pratyanika chikitsā,* which is specific treatment according to the specific disease. In modern medicine, chemotherapy, and radiation therapy have great value if done early enough. In Ayurveda, there is no chemotherapy or radiation therapy, but there is herbal therapy.
- Lastly, rasāyana or Ayurvedic immunotherapy is used to enable the patient's body to produce a substance that resists the growth of cancer. This is done through the use of naturally occurring substances that increase the activity of the immune system to increase ojas. The body's failure to detect and destroy the abnormal cancer cells is due to low ojas; in general management, we have to protect the patient's ojas.

## Ayurveda Management following Chemotherapy, Radiation, and Surgery

Ayurveda can also be used to alleviate the side effects of chemotherapy and radiation therapy. Radiation therapy creates anorexia, nausea and hair loss, while chemotherapy causes the same symptoms, plus bone marrow suppression, anemia and low grade fever. For example, in cases of low grade fever, Ayurveda uses laghu mālinī vasanta or mahā tikta ghrita, while for anemia; either mandūra bhasma or abhrak bhasma is used. For bone marrow suppression, Ayurveda also suggests the use of brahmī oil or shatāvarī ghee, bhringarāja oil for hair loss, and shankha bhasma and kāma dudhā for nausea.

The list below contains the main categories of therapies that are used in Ayurveda for the management of cancer patients who have undergone any of the therapies that are commonly used in modern medicine.

- Snehana (oleation therapy) is a useful treatment for this purpose. To choose the appropriate oil for snehana, look at the person's prakruti and vikruti. If vāta, one can use sesame oil or a medicated oil such as dashamūla oil or balā oil. For pitta, use sunflower or coconut oil, or any bitter oil. For kapha types, mustard, corn or sesame oil is a good choice. Neem oil is particularly good for snehana for pitta and kapha as it is both antipyretic and antiviral. Tumbī oil, also known as dāruharidrā, is also effective as an antipyretic and antipruritic. Guñjā is a detoxifier and it helps to grow the hair.

- Svedana (sudation therapy) is used for post-medical situations. For vāta types, it is best to use nirgundī essential oil in the steam treatment; for pitta people, sandalwood essential oil is good; and for kapha, lemon-scented eucalyptus essential oil can be added to the steam.

- *Shodana* (detoxification program) is generally used following cancer treatment. If there is absolute constipation, one should administer basti (medicated enema). For pitta kinds of rashes, one can give mild virechana (purgation). If there is mucus formation and other kapha disorders, vamana (emesis) therapy may be given.

- *Shamana* (palliative therapy) is based upon pacifying the dosha in its site. Dosha pratyanika means a treatment that is pacifying to the dosha, *vyādhi pratyanika* is specific to the disease, and *dhātu pratyanika* means specific to the dhātu.

- Rasāyana (rejuvenation therapy) is important to use after *shodana* or *shamana chikitsā,* so that the immune system is strengthened. Certain herbs and other powerful rejuvenative substances are given for this purpose.

- *Lepana* (application of paste) is generally used to take care of localized pain. Common examples for the kind of pain found in arbuda are kāñchanār lepa, which is antiviral and reduces tumors; varuna lepa, which is anti-inflammatory; punarnavā lepa, which reduces swelling; and sandalwood and turmeric lepa.

## Herbal Adjuvants

Herbs that are frequently used in a shodana detoxification program for arbuda are chitrak, katukā, and neem. Chitrak, with pungent and bitter tastes, heating *vīrya* (potency) and pungent *vipāka* (post-digestive effect), is a digestive herb that kindles agni and detoxifies āma. Katukā, which is known as kutki, has bitter and pungent rasa, cooling vīrya and pungent vipāka, is antipyretic, kindles gastric fire and aids in the scraping of abnormal tissue. Neem is bitter, cooling and pungent in vipāka. It is antiviral, antipyretic and also detoxifies āma.

Herbs used in shamana include gudūchī, guggulu, jatamāmsi, and tagara. Gudūchī is bitter and astringent in rasa, with a heating vīrya and pungent vipāka. It is anti-pyretic, an immune booster and a blood cleanser. Guggulu is bitter and pungent, heating and has a pungent vipāka. It scrapes āma and fat from the body, purifies the blood, and is a lymphatic cleanser and rejuvenative tonic.

Jatamāmsi and tagara are widely used as painkillers during arbuda. Jatamāmsi is bitter, astringent and sweet in taste, cooling in vīrya and with a sweet vipāka. It is antipruritic, antipyretic, analgesic and a tranquilizer. Tagara is astringent, heating and it has a pungent vipāka. It is a tranquilizer, analgesic and sedative.

For *rasāyana chikitsā,* which boosts the immune system, the herbal jam compound called chyavānaprāsh is widely used. Chyavānaprāsh contains various rejuvenative herbs, such as ashvagandhā, balā and vidārī. Ashvagandhā is bitter and astringent in rasa, has a heating vīrya and a sweet vipāka, and it is a rejuvenator for vāta and kapha, although it may overly stimulate pitta dosha. Balā is sweet, cooling and has a sweet vipāka, and it is tridoshic. Balā provides energy, vigor and vitality. Vidārī is sweet and bitter, cooling, and with a sweat vipāka, and it increases strength and stamina. Other common rasāyanas are pippalī rasāyana and punarnavā rasāyana. Pippalī is pungent in taste, heating in vīrya and sweet in vipāka. It is known for its antiviral and rejuvenating actions and it is generally good for pulmonary dysfunctions. Punarnavā is sweet and bitter, heating with a pungent vipāka. It is diuretic and it reduces tumors and is a rejuvenative tonic.

Herbs used in *lepana chikitsā,* which is the topical application of pastes, include kāñchanār, varuna and haridrā. Kāñchanār is astringent, cooling, and has a pungent vipāka. It is antiviral and reduces tumors. Varuna is sweet, bitter and astringent in taste, heating in vīrya and has a pungent vipāka. It reduces swelling and is anti-inflammatory. Haridrā is bitter, astringent and pungent in taste, heating in vīrya with a pungent vipāka. It is beautiful in reducing tumor.

## Conclusion

Students of Ayurveda should know the dynamics of arbuda and pay attention to the three doshas, seven dhātus and three malas, and their involvement in the pathogenesis of this disease. Based upon the individual samprāpti (pathogenesis), the treatment plan will change. That is why there is no standard treatment for cancer in Ayurveda. What is statistically common in a thousand people is the standard according to modern society, whereas Ayurveda gives emphasis to the individual and says that one cannot judge that person based upon statistical data. By virtue of this unique approach, some cases of arbuda, along with the complications of both the cancer and the related treatments, can be effectively treated with Ayurveda.

## Arbuda Nidāna: The Etiology of Cancer

References in the ancient text, *Mādhava Nidānam,* give us the etiological factors that are still, today, the true causes of arbuda. This gives us a complete picture of the etiological factors that can lead to cancer.

*Ātapa seva* means overexposure to solar radiation, and in this case refers to ultraviolet light in particular. Overexposure to ultraviolet radiation may disturb tejas at the cellular level.

*Vidāhāni annapānāni* is another cause of arbuda. *Vidāhi* means burning and irritating, *anna* is food and *pana* is drinks. This refers to a cause of cancer being food, drinks, and other substances that have irritating or burning properties. This includes alcohol, marijuana, tobacco, and many other carcinogenic chemicals and substances.

Another cause is *tīkshnāni aushadhāni,* which means sharp or penetrating cytotoxic drugs.

A fourth factor is cellular *āma,* which is toxic metabolic waste at the cellular level.

*Viruddha āhāra* means incompatible food, such as a pitta person eating too much hot, spicy food, or a vāta person eating too many beans or raw vegetables, or a kapha person consuming excessive amounts of dairy products and hydrophilic substances. These foods may be incompatible to someone's prakruti and also to the person's vikruti.

*Viruddha vihāra* means wrong lifestyle and this is another important etiological factor in the production of cancer.

Next, the *Mādhava Nidānam* says *bīja dosha* is a cause of arbuda. *Bīja* means seed and it refers to genetic predisposition. If someone's father died of cancer of the colon and his grandfather also died of the same type of cancer, it indicates an increased likelihood that the person himself may develop colon cancer. In a certain family, there may be racial or genetic factors that predispose them to a particular type of arbuda and this is called bīja dosha.

*Sūkshma krumi* means invisible parasites or micro-organisms in the blood that provoke arbuda. Perhaps there may even be a cancer virus.

*Vyavasāya* means occupational hazards and exposure to toxic substances. There are certain carcinogens or 'arbudogens,' if I may call them that, that are important substances in the etiology of cancer. Tobacco, asbestos, radioactive substances and any irritant substances that aggravate are examples of this category. People working in chemical factories, mines or asbestos factories may develop arbuda. Exposure to contactants also falls into this category.

*Mano vedana* means psychological and emotional factors, such as unresolved grief, sadness and other emotions, which can be called stress. If a person has intense grief, sadness, sorrow, stress and so forth, it may lead to arbuda. It is true that if a woman loses her loved one during middle age, she is more likely to get breast cancer or uterine cancer.

*Vārdhakya* refers to old people (over age 65), who are more prone to cancer of the prostate and colon.

*Paryāvartanam* means pollution. A polluted environment, maybe due to cars emitting carbon monoxide, can poison the air or water. Polluted water, air and food are all factors that can lead to arbuda. Pollution is a factor that is difficult for the individual to difficult to control, especially in third world countries.

# Chapter 7

# Thyroid Disorders

Winter 2011, Volume 24, Number 3

Here we discuss various thyroid disorders with special reference to Ayurveda. The thyroid gland is called jatru granthi. Jatru means the collarbone and upper part of the breastbone, and granthi means gland. Hence, jatru granthi means the gland above the breastbone, which is the thyroid.

The thyroid is located at the root of the throat on either side of the trachea, at the level of the third and fourth tracheal rings. It weighs between 20 to 25 grams in an adult and the left lobe is a little smaller than the right lobe. It is a highly vascular,[20] ductless gland that moves upwards upon swallowing.

The thyroid produces three major hormones: thyroxine (T4) and triiodothyronine (T3), as well as calcitonin. Calcitonin helps to regulate calcium levels in the blood. The gland also produces thyroglobulin (Tg), an iodinated glycoprotein that helps produce the three thyroid hormones. The production of thyroid hormones is regulated by the pituitary gland, which releases thyroid-stimulating hormone (TSH) to stimulate production of T3 and T4.

The thyroid gland accumulates inorganic iodine, which is necessary for the production of thyroid hormones (*jatru agni*). When there is a lack of dietary iodine, it affects the production of thyroid hormones, resulting in the cells of the thyroid gland becoming enlarged in an attempt to acquire more iodine. This produces goiter, which appears as a swelling at the front of the throat. Consumption of excess calcium can also cause this condition.

The ocean is the basic source of iodine, so salt, seaweed, and fish have relatively high levels of iodine. In the United States, the soil of the Great Lakes region is the most iodine deficient, while in Europe the mountainous Alps region has low iodine levels. A lack of iodine in the soil, along with usage of non-iodized salt, directly results in a higher incidence of goiter.

---

20. Highly vascular means it contains a lot of blood vessels.

The stomach is the seat of jāthara agni (gastric fire), which governs digestion, absorption, and assimilation of foodstuff in the gastrointestinal (GI) tract. The liver is the seat of bhūta agni, and liver enzymes are a component of bhūta agni that act via the thyroid. Bhūta agni governs mineral metabolism and this has an important role in the functioning of the thyroid gland. Dhātu agni governs further molecular digestion and transformation of the organic elements of food and water into the biological components of bodily cells.

Jatru agni is the bridge between bhūta agni and dhātu agni. According to an Ayurvedic sūtra, if *agni* is increased then the *dhātus* are decreased, whereas if agni is low, there will be undue production of raw tissue which leads to excess tissue growth.

## Metabolism

The thyroid governs a number of important metabolic functions. During normal activity, the thyroid accelerates energy consumption and increases oxygen consumption of all tissues. Therefore, when the thyroid is affected, the person feels fatigued.

Its second metabolic function is governance of carbohydrate metabolism, including assimilation and absorption of glucose from the intestines. Glycogen is a storage unit for glucose. When blood glucose levels drop, glycogen is broken down so that glucose can be released into the bloodstream to fuel bodily processes. The thyroid mobilizes glycogen from the liver and heart in the process of glycogenesis (biosynthesis of glycogen). If this function is affected, it can cause diabetes. Consequently, diabetes and hypothyroidism go together.

Thirdly, the thyroid governs heart rate. Excessive thyroid functioning (hyperthyroidism) can increase the heart rate (tachycardia), while insufficient thyroid activity (hypothyroidism) may decrease the heart rate (bradycardia). The thyroid also governs a number of other metabolic functions.

### Goiter

The thyroid gland is highly vascular and thyroid cells are compact. When there is a lack of iodine and/or other factors, the cells of the gland undergo hyperplasia (enlargement), causing the gland to become swollen in the front of the throat. The thyroid will look slightly swollen before full-blown goiter happens.

Goiter usually causes the thyroid to become overactive, and symptoms of excess vāta and pitta can be observed. This condition is called hyperthyroidism (see Hyperthyroidism below). Goiter can also be caused by Hashimoto's thyroiditis (a form of hypothyroidism) and other medical conditions.

Goiter may be toxic or non-toxic. The whole thyroid gland may become enlarged without much toxicity, in which case the condition is called diffused goiter. This is common in Grave's disease and is found more often in younger subjects.

On the other hand, when the thyroid is enlarged accompanied by excessive production of thyroid hormones, due to over-activity of the gland or because of excessive dosages of thyroid hormone, thyrotoxicosis can occur. This can lead to toxic multinodular goiter, which is found more commonly in older people. In this condition, excessive thyroid hormones act as a kind of toxin, so the bodily tissues react against them by producing thyrotoxicosis, which is a form of hyperthyroidism.

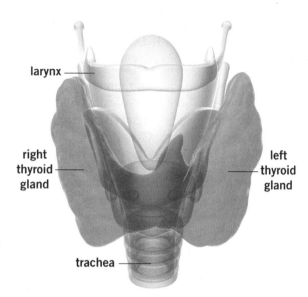

## Hyperthyroidism

When the thyroid gland becomes overactive, it produces excessive amounts of T3 and/ or T4 hormones and is called hyperthyroidism. This condition results in symptoms of increased vāta and pitta doshas. The vāta symptoms include nervousness, anxiety, palpitations, tachycardia (rapid heart rate), tremors, bulging of the eyeballs (exophthalmos), and deviation of the trachea if there is unilateral enlargement of the gland. Pitta symptoms include excessive hunger, heat intolerance, excessive sweating, high blood pressure, irritability and emotional disturbance, and menstrual changes. There will be an increased metabolic rate and weight loss, and the person will become easily fatigued. The thyroid gland may become enlarged.

In hyperthyroidism, the conversion of food into energy is so accelerated that the person has no energy. There is low glucose tolerance, so blood sugar levels are increased. The skin becomes soft, moist, and flushed. The increased iodine levels in the blood cause cholesterol levels to drop. This indicates liver functions are depressed. The heart rate increases up to 140 beats per minute. The muscles are fatigued and there may be tremors. An EEG shows abnormal alpha waves. There will be an increased need for vitamins, due to the increased basal metabolic rate.

Because of increased dhātu agni, the dhātus get depleted. This can result in skeletal disorders such as osteoporosis. Calcium deficiency can be a key factor in the development of osteoporosis. Hyperthyroidism can also cause infertility.

Patients with hyperthyroidism are unable to sit still and they often wear lightweight clothing even on cold days. Even though the person has a strong appetite, there is remarkable weight loss. Finally, a particular symptom of increased thyroid function is lid lag, which occurs when the person closes the eyes and the upper eyelid does not meet with the lower eyelid.

Times of hormonal change are when a person is most prone to hyperthyroidism and goiter. For many women, this is the perimenopausal period, during their 30s, 40s, and 50s.

In the majority of patients with hyperthyroidism, the thyroid gland is either profusely hyperactive, which is called Grave's disease, or the gland consists of multiple nodules with inactive areas within the gland.

Grave's disease is an autoimmune disorder that results in excessive production of thyroid hormones. There is a typical orange peel texture of the skin and Grave's ophthalmopathy (bulging eyes and associated symptoms), as well as many of the common symptoms of hyperthyroidism. Generally, a patient with Grave's disease is in the pitta age (particularly 30 to 50 years). It is more common in women than in men.

Another cause of hyperthyroidism is toxic multinodular goiter, which is more common in older patients and not found in children. This condition usually begins with a simple goiter, which leads to formation of nodules in the gland. This ultimately leads to increased production of thyroid hormones and the symptoms of hyperthyroidism. There are many other possible causes of hyperthyroidism, but only a tiny percentage of hyperthyroid cases are due to excessive TSH production by the pituitary gland.

Note that an overactive gland may become hypoactive later and, because of this, the person may gain weight and suffer from fatigue and depression. These are kapha symptoms. Hypothyroidism exhibits more kapha symptoms, whereas hyperthyroidism has more vāta and pitta symptoms.

## Signs and Symptoms for Hyperthyroidism

- Fast metabolism
- Nervousness and anxiety
- Heart palpitations
- Tachycardia (rapid heart rate)
- Tremors
- Bulging of the eyeballs (exophthalmos)
- Excessive hunger
- Heat intolerance
- Excessive sweating
- High blood pressure
- Restlessness and Irritability
- Menstrual changes
- Weight loss
- Fatigue
- Enlarged thyroid gland
- Increased blood sugar levels
- Soft, moist, and flushed skin
- Low cholesterol
- Muscle fatigue
- Osteoporosis
- Infertility
- Eyelid lag

## Ayurvedic Protocol for Hyperthyroidism

*Herbal formula.* Take ½ teaspoon of this mixture, two times per day, with two tablespoons of aloe vera gel.

Dashamūla 500 mg (for tremors, palpitations, dyspnea and muscle fatigue)
Ashvagandhā 400 mg (to maintain muscle tone and coordination)
Arjuna 300 mg (for palpitations and cardiac symptoms)
Pushkaramūla 300 mg (acts like a beta-blocker to slow down the heart rate)
Gulvel sattva 300 mg (anti-inflammatory and anti-diuretic)
Kāñchanār guggulu 200 mg (anti-goiter)
Kāma dudhā 200 mg (anti-inflammatory)

### Other Remedies

- One teaspoon of bhumi āmalakī nightly at bedtime.
- Brahmī ghee nasya is also recommended to calm down any thyroid storm and pacify tremors and overstimulation of the nervous system.
- Apply punarnavā lepa (paste) to the gland to reduce swelling and myxedema.
- Apply kukkutanakhi lepa (paste) to the gland to block excessive hormone release.
- Shītalī prānāyāma – start with seven rounds in one session and increase up to seventeen at a time. This will help to cool down pitta and increase heat tolerance.

If you have hyperthyroidism, rock salt is better than sea salt and kelp is also good, as it contains a natural form of iodine. Iodine is also present in samshamana vati, a traditional Ayurvedic remedy. Nowadays, health food stores carry iodine; dilute one drop in an ounce of water and take every other day. Iodine supplements should not be taken daily.

Modern medicine uses radioactive iodine to kill the thyroid in severe cases of hyperthyroidism, and then they remove the thyroid. We can suggest that someone with hyperthyroidism can follow the above Ayurvedic protocol for at least six months and see how things go. If the condition does not respond, the person can then follow the modern route if they wish. Either way, the individual should consult an endocrinologist.

### Hypothyroidism

Hypothyroidism is an underactive thyroid gland that produces insufficient thyroid hormones. It is caused by a disorder of the thyroid gland or occasionally by a disorder of the pituitary gland or hypothalamus. Iodine deficiency is the most common etiological factor, but there are many other possible causes. If congenital, this condition can result in cretinism (stunted growth). Children born after only six or so months in the womb may develop *vāmanatvā* (cretinism), resulting in deformed bones and stunted growth.

Hereditary factors play an important role in hypothyroidism and women are affected more often than men. During pregnancy, the thyroid can become imbalanced because of hormonal changes. Psychological trauma or surgical trauma can also lead to hypothyroidism as can unresolved, repressed emotions such as sorrow or grief.

Because hypothyroidism is a condition of low agni, there is undue production of raw tissue or fat. However, the skin will look dry, rough, and wrinkled, because the low basal metabolism rate causes *meda* (fat) to be pushed into the deep tissues. Even the skin of a child with hypothyroidism looks dry and rough. The mala of meda is *sveda,* and there will be a lack of sweat, resulting in dry skin. Note that in order for someone to sweat, there must be a sufficiently high metabolism. The face will look bloated with thick lips. This is especially true in the case of children. There will be an enlarged tongue (macroglossia), large stomach (gastromegaly), and possibly enlargement of the heart (cardiomegaly).

Hypothyroidism can go together with myxedema, which produces thickened, dry skin, swollen lips, and reduced mental activity. However, this does not mean that every hypo-thyroid patient will get myxedema. Myxedema can change someone's personality and the person may seem depressed. Frank (clinically evident) psychosis is sometimes called myxedema madness, and is found in some people with hypothyroidism.

In hypothyroidism, blood iodine levels are low, and there is decreased excretion of creatine. Because they are synthesized by the thyroid gland, vitamins A and K accumulate under the skin and the person's skin looks pale yellow.

Hypothyroidism can cause increased cholesterol and remove calcium and phosphate from the bones, leading to osteoporosis. It can also cause abdominal or plural effusion, extremely low appetite and low blood sugar, and tingling and numbness of the hands and feet with loss of the sense of touch (paresthesia), which can lead to carpel tunnel syndrome. This is due to kapha blocking vāta.

Chronic thyroid inflammation can lead to hypothyroidism, due to deficiency of TSH. Hashimoto's thyroiditis, an autoimmune disease, can also lead to hypothyroidism because of decreased TSH.

## Signs and Symptoms of Hypothyroidism

- Slow metabolism
- Undue growth of tissues, leading to obesity
- Enlarged stomach
- Thick lips and tongue
- Patient is easily exhausted
- Low immunity
- Pale skin and thickening of the skin (myxedema)
- Intolerance of cold
- Recurrent infections
- Dry skin and dry hair
- Puffiness of face and hands
- Slow mental activity
- Slow pulse rate
- Dryness in the vagina
- Premature orgasm
- Menstrual disorders
- Tingling and numbness in the fingers
- Carpal tunnel syndrome
- Sadness, depression, feelings of worthlessness
- Loss of concentration and poor memory
- Lethargy

- Deafness, due to weakened nerves
- Muscle pain from decreased muscle tone and power
- Sluggish reflexes
- Angina pain and low heart rate, with irregular EKG pattern
- Constipation due to āma, because of low agni
- Husky voice because of double chin
- Protruding tongue
- In children, lack of interest and slow growth
- In infants, umbilical hernia

Make sure that the forest is not missed for the trees. The key symptoms are slowness, dry skin and puffy face, sluggish reflexes, slow heart rate and, in case of children, poor academic performance.

# Ayurvedic Protocol for Hypothyroidism

*Herbal formula.* Give ½ teaspoon of this mixture three times daily.

Punarnavā 500 mg (a mild diuretic, it reverses excessive tissue growth)
Triphala guggulu 200 mg (stimulates thyroid functions and removes toxins)
Kutki 200 mg (helps to eliminate excess fat)
Chitrak 200 mg (kindles agni, especially jatru agni and dhātu agni)

## Other Remedies

- 200 mg each of ārogya vardhinī and chandraprabhā, twice daily.
- 200 mg each of brahmī, jatamāmsi, and shankha pushpī to improve concentration, memory, and intelligence.
- 200 mg smriti sagar ras once daily to aid concentration.
- 1 teaspoon of brahmī prash twice daily as a general nervine tonic.
- Vacha nasya, which is good for a husky voice.
- Bhastrikā, kapāla bhāti, ujjāyi, and anuloma-viloma prāṇāyāma are all good for improving thyroid functioning.
- If there is constipation, give ½ teaspoon of triphala at bedtime with water.
- If the person is anemic, use 200 mg of abhrak bhasma or loha bhasma.
- If the heart rate is slow, use 10 drops (approximately 1 ml) of gold water twice daily to increase cardiac output.
- If the tongue is enlarged and protruded, apply ½ teaspoon each of vacha and honey to the tongue and let the child lick it.

The protocol for hypothyroidism in modern medicine is to put the patient on hormone supplementation, using extracts from animal or synthetic hormones. The person is usually told to take lifelong hormonal therapy. Ayurveda can help to manage the symptoms of a thyroid disease and treat the causes of the disorder, so the person should follow the Ayurvedic protocol for at least six months, as well as consult an endocrinologist.

## Table 2: Comparison of Key Symptoms

| Hyperthyroidism | Hypothyroidism |
|---|---|
| Possibly goiter | No goiter |
| High agni & increased metabolic rate | Low agni & decreased metabolic rate |
| Protruding eyes | No exophthalmos |
| High blood pressure | Low blood pressure |
| High blood sugar | Low blood sugar |
| Can lead to overgrowth of bones | Can lead to undergrowth of bones |
| Low cholesterol | High cholesterol |
| More pitta and vāta symptoms | More kapha symptoms |
| Anxiety | Depression |
| Tachycardia | Bradycardia |
| Hyperkinetic personality | Asthenic personality |

## Chapter 8

# Autoimmune Disorders

Summer 2015, Volume 28, Number 1

AUTOIMMUNE DISORDERS are those in which the immune system produces auto-antibodies to an endogenous antigen[21], with consequent injury to the bodily tissue (*dhātu*).

Within the intracellular space, every cell has its own components of ojas, tejas, and prāna. Ojas maintains cellular immunity. Tejas maintains cellular metabolic activity, selectivity, and intelligence. Prāna is the flow of communication within and between cells.

When agni is low, digestion is not at par. The āhāra rasa (micro chyle) is unprocessed, forming āma (toxicity). This āma travels with the chyle to the deeper cellular level, where it alters the functioning of tejas, which affects cellular intelligence. Then the bodily cells do not recognize each other, so their immune systems start to destroy their neighboring cells. Normally, tejas allows each cell to recognize that another cell is a muscle cell or a lung cell or whatever. This is important for the harmonious functioning of the immune system. This function is disturbed when tejas is affected by āma.

This can be explained by modern medicine through the concept of antigens. An antigen is a substance that causes the immune system to produce antibodies against it. It can be a bacterium, virus, chemical, or other foreign substance. Alternatively, it could be formed inside the body, as in the case of āma such as bacterial toxins, in which case it is called an autoantigen.

The word antigen is interesting. "Anti" means against, while "gen" means "to produce", as in "generate". So, these antigens could be a foreign protein, such as an oligosaccharide, or an unprocessed protein on the surface of the cell that identifies the type of the cell, such as whether it is a skin cell, a kidney cell, or so forth.

An antibody, which is also called an immunoglobulin, is a Y shaped protein produced in response to a specific antigen. It identifies and neutralizes the foreign bodies.

21. Antigen that is produced from within the cell as part of normal cell metabolism or when the cell is infected by bacteria or viruses.

A specific chemical interaction occurs between the antibodies, produced by the B cells of the white blood cells, and the antigen. There is a cytotoxic response, with an increase in monocytes and lymphocytes. This is a subtle cellular war between antigen and antibody. It protects the body from bacteria, viruses and so forth, and it can also be the factor responsible for autoimmune disease.

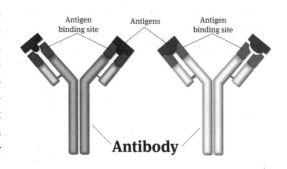

There are several types of antibodies and antigens and each antibody is capable of binding only to specific antigens. This specificity of binding is due to the particular chemical constituents of each antibody. For instance, a certain antibody is only able to bind a specific type of bacteria.

The antigen-antibody reaction happens through a chain of qualities, which are the different amino acid sequences. The amino acids reflect the twenty *gunas* (qualities) that are the basic principles of Ayurveda.

Normally, antibodies alone do not produce disease, unless they combine with an antigen. However, in autoimmune disease, autoantibodies react against their own tissues.

An autoimmune disorder occurs when cellular āma covers the tejas molecules and affects cellular intelligence. The healthy cells then send a signal to the neighboring cells, which are covered in āma, but there is no response. The healthy cell then sends a signal to the B-lymphocytes to produce antibodies to destroy the neighboring cell. This is the root cause of autoimmune disease according to Ayurveda.

Even aging is due to antibodies attacking and destroying the normal cells, which causes wrinkling of the skin, hair loss, and aging. Aging is *dhātu kshaya* (depletion of the tissue), where the bodily ojas is destroyed by tejas. Some people age fast, especially *vāta* individuals. Vāta is dry, light, cold, and mobile, so the body naturally demands more ojas to protect from vāta dosha. If there is depleted ojas and impaired agni, then aging occurs faster.

## Etiological Factors (Causes)

Many things can become etiological factors of autoimmune disease. Long-lingering infection can produce āma. *Vāta* or *pitta prakruti,* eating a vāta and/or pitta-provoking diet, with *vishama* or *tīkshna agni* can all lead to the production of āma. That is why emphasis is given to a dosha-balancing diet and lifestyle.

Infection may cause a strong immune response that results in a reaction against some of the body's own normal tissue.

Many times, autoimmune disease is triggered by drug exposure. This creates inflammation, irritation, and destruction, so we have to pacify pitta dosha. Some people have a history of using immune suppressant drugs, such as steroids, adrenaline-related drugs, antihistamines, or anti-inflammatory agents. These are cytotoxic and develop antitumor agents, which often results in tumors. Drugs such as methyldopa also alter a person's immunological response.

Sperm antibodies from a vasectomy can alter the immune response, because ojas is produced as a by-product of shukra dhātu.

Genetic factors play an important role in autoimmune diseases. Autoimmune disease is transmitted from generation to generation, as we carry the cellular memory of autoimmune dysfunction within our bodily cells.

In Ayurvedic terms, we carry the genetic molecules of vāta, pitta, and *kapha* in our unique genetic code. This *dosha prakruti* normally corresponds to the ratio of prāna, tejas, and ojas (respectively). Due to certain genetic factors, which cause a defective structural arrangement of the genes, some people have overactive tejas, producing a genetic change that may lead to autoimmune disorders.

Overactive tejas can burn ojas and attack the neighboring cells. Or systemic āma can cover the cell membrane and affect cellular communication (prāna), so that a healthy cell does not recognize its neighboring cells. The antibodies that attack the neighboring cells are specialized tejas molecules.

There are many similar qualities between tejas and vāta as well as between tejas and pitta dosha. Tejas is light, subtle, and dry. Vāta is also light, subtle, and dry. As a result, when vāta is increased by its light, subtle, and dry qualities, it can trigger those attributes of tejas. Pitta dosha also shares certain attributes with tejas. These are the light, hot, and sharp qualities.

That is why vāta and pitta people are particularly prone to autoimmune disorders. In particular, any individual with overpowering tejas is predisposed to autoimmune disease. Depending upon the specific disease process, vāta or pitta may be more involved.

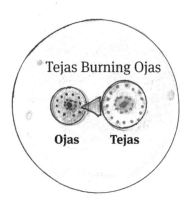

Tejas Burning Ojas

Ojas    Tejas

So most autoimmune disorders are due to tejas burning ojas. On a doshic level, that corresponds to pitta overpowering kapha and it involves a disturbance of agni. If we pour hot water on the digestive fire (agni), the fire goes out and āma is produced.

## Samprāpti (Pathogenesis)

Ayurveda says that āma is the root cause of all disease. Āma is due to vishama agni, tīkshna agni, or *manda agni*. Manda agni āma creates kapha disorders because it produces kaphagenic āma. Likewise, tīkshna agni creates pitta disorders because of its sharp quality.

Systemic āma is formed in the GI tract and then pushed into the general circulation, from where it goes into the dhātus. There, it affects the dhātu agni and bhūta agni in the liver, along with *pīlu agni* in the cell membranes and *pithara agni* in the nuclei of the related cells. This microcytic āma covers the cell membrane, so the immune system doesn't recognize the cell as part of "itself".

There is a lack of cellular communication. The neighboring cells send a signal, but due to the āma, there is no response or communication. As a result, the healthy cell sends a biochemical message to the B-lymphocytes to produce antibodies and try to destroy the neighboring cell. The immune system reacts against some of its own tissue and produces antibodies due to tejas. In autoimmune disorders, tejas burns ojas.

This simple mechanism happens at the cellular level in autoimmune diseases. It produces inflammation, degeneration, wasting of the bodily tissues, and many other symptoms. Depending upon the khavaigunya (weak areas), autoimmune disease can occur in any of the tissues.

### Signs and Symptoms

Generally, antiglobulin antibodies (rheumatoid factor) can be detected in blood tests.

A typical person with an autoimmune disorder is a bright, brilliant pitta person, with prematurely grey hair (and for men, a receding hairline). He or she is often a profoundly intelligent, professional person, success-oriented, with a competitive, Type A personality. These people show high tejas tendency, and are prone to get tejas burning ojas, which can result in autoimmune disease.

## Examples of Autoimmune Disorders

*Rheumatoid Arthritis* – long-lingering systemic āma is pushed into the synovial membrane, resulting in some cells of the synovial membrane being covered by micro āma. Therefore, the immune system does not recognize the other cells of the synovial membrane and they try to destroy them.

*Hashimoto's Thyroiditis* – Initial inflammation of the thyroid then destruction and fibrosis of the gland, leading to hypothyroidism.

*Graves' Disease* – a disorder of the thyroid gland with excessive production of TSH (thyroid stimulating hormone). Produces enlargement of the thyroid gland and may cause ocular conditions.

*Systemic Lupus Erythematosus* – this attacks multiple organs.

*Myasthenia Gravis* (muscular weakness) – a neuromuscular disorder in which there is fluctuating weakness of voluntary muscle groups, the muscles lose their tone, power and coordination, and the facial muscles are pulled down because of gravity. Vāta is high in the neuromuscular cleft.

*Hemolytic Anemia* – tejas burns ojas, and tejas starts destroying the cell membrane of red blood cells before the end of their normal 120-day life cycle. This disintegration of red blood cells is called hemolysis, which produces large amounts of *rañjaka pitta* that overloads the liver, causing the person to get hemolytic jaundice. Symptoms include fatigue and weakness.

# Examples of Autoimmune Disorders

*Pernicious Anemia* – a serious blood disorder where red blood cells are destroyed because of an autoimmune response. The red blood cells are big in size but small in number. There is impaired uptake of vitamin $B_{12}$ due to lack of gastric intrinsic factor, a rañjaka pitta disorder. Symptoms include a smooth, red tongue with depapillated surface.

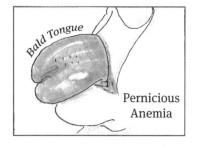

*Aplastic Anemia* – tejas burns ojas in the hematopoietic system, inhibiting red blood cell formation. There is total absence of red blood cell formation.

*Glomerulonephritis* – the immune systems starts to destroy the glomeruli, which can lead to kidney disease.

*Addison's Disease* – there is a gradual progressive failure of the adrenal glands and insufficient production of steroid hormones. The person develops adrenal fatigue and postural hypotension.

*Celiac Disease* – autoimmune inflammatory changes happen within the intestinal villi and this produces gluten intolerance. Gliadin acts as an antigen, forming an immune complex in the intestinal mucosa, producing antibodies and aggravation of killer lymphocytes, which damage the villi.

*Crohn's Disease* – regional ileitis or enteritis, in which there is inflammation in the ileum, which can spread through the layers of the gut, producing thickening or hardening of the intestinal wall tissues. There is diarrhea (4 to 6 bowel movements per day), colic pain in the right side of the abdomen, and weight loss.

*Chronic Fatigue Syndrome* – There is incapacitating fatigue that rest does not relieve. Associated with decreased concentration, irritability, insomnia, swollen lymph nodes, and low-grade fever. Genetic predisposition and hormonal imbalance can be factors. High tejas in the liver burns ojas, and the liver is usually enlarged and palpable. This can begin as an autoimmune disorder or Epstein-Barr virus can lead to immunological dysfunction.

*Chronic Hepatitis B and C* can be an autoimmune disorder where tejas is burning ojas and destroys hepatic parenchyma.

*Multiple Sclerosis* – The immune system destroys the protective covering of the nerves, resulting in lack of muscle coordination, muscle spasms, and fatigue. These people often show a history of optic neuritis with double vision.

*Alopecia Areata* – localized or generalized hair loss on the scalp or elsewhere on the body. Patches can vary in size. It is due to tejas is burning ojas at the roots of the hairs, caused by high pitta in asthi dhātu.

*Amyloidosis* – a rare disease in which a protein is not processed (*dhātu āma*) leads to ankle swelling, severe fatigue and weakness, tingling and numbness of hands and feet, carpel tunnel syndrome, diarrhea with blood alternating with constipation, irregular heartbeat, difficulty swallowing and enlarged tongue. It can lead to life-threatening organ failure and there is no cure.

*Ankylosing Spondylitis* – āma in the joints can cause chronic inflammatory changes within the lumbosacral area.

*Pancreatitis* – is due to high pitta and āma in the pancreas, causing reduction in insulin production. It can lead to Type 2 diabetes.

*Optic Neuritis or Sympathetic Ophthalmia* – occurs where tissues inside of the eye are injured and they release toxins into the bloodstream. The tissue is recognized as a foreign body and antibodies attack, which is tejas attacking ojas. This causes irritation, inflammation, injury and destruction, and it can produce double vision and even blindness. It often leads to multiple sclerosis.

*Fibromyalgia and Fibromyositis* – inflammation of connective tissue of the muscles causes musculoskeletal aches, spasm and pain in the neck, shoulders, back and buttocks. Causes are exposure to cold and damp, non-articular muscular rheumatism, and certain occupations. There are trigger points that are particular tender spots.

*Raynaud's Disease* (vasculitis) – the immune system can destroy the lining of the blood vessels, creating inflammation of the blood vessels (vasculitis), which is also called Raynaud's syndrome. Peripheral circulation becomes poor, the fingertips turn purple and cold, and the fingernails look blue. It can lead to scleroderma.

Raynaud's Syndrome

*Scleroderma* – a systemic autoimmune skin disease that produces hardening and tightening of the skin, which can affect the internal organs. It commonly affects the skin of the hands, arms and face, producing thick, hard pigmented skin patches. Raynaud's Disease can lead to scleroderma.

*Urticaria and Contact Dermatitis* – some people wear a metal bracelet and the bodily sweat reacts with the metal and creates a reaction, leading to contact dermatitis. Likewise, sunlight can produce a unique antibody reaction in some people.

## General Treatment Protocol

There are so many autoimmune conditions, depending upon which dhātu or srotas the tejas is burning ojas. The root cause is the same—the only difference is the location.

When dealing with autoimmune disease, the Ayurvedic practitioner should take a thorough medical history, including a family history. Do a comprehensive clinical examination and find out the person's prakruti and vikruti. Through *darshana* (observation), sparshana (palpation) and *prashna* (questioning), decide which organs and systems are affected.

Try to detect the exact etiological factors, so the patient can avoid the cause(s). Also understand the samprāpti, including dosha gati (direction of the doshas) and *vyādhi mārga* (disease pathway). Discover which dosha, dhātu and srotas (bodily channel) are mainly involved, and whether it is a *sāma* (with āma) or *nirāma* (without āma) condition. Through this thorough investigation, we can create a proper treatment protocol.

The treatment plan (chikitsā) should incorporate dīpana (kindles digestive fire), pāchana (neutralizes āma), shodana (cleansing therapies) and shaman (palliation therapies), including herbal remedies and other treatments. The specific protocol varies according to the particular autoimmune disease that is present.

In all cases, one should give a *dosha pratyanika*[22] to pacify the aggravated dosha, *dhātu pratyanika* to treat the affected dhātu, and *sroto pratyanika* for the affected srotas.

Firstly, one must do shamana chikitsā. For example, in many autoimmune diseases, we have to treat pitta dosha and balance tejas. A good generalized herbal formula for those conditions is:

Shatāvarī 500 mg (reduces pitta)
Gulvel sattva 400 mg (anti-inflammatory)
Kaishore guggulu 300 mg (tissue restorative that detoxifies hematopoietic and skeleton-muscular systems and controls antibody production)
Kāma dudhā 200 mg (anti-inflammatory)
Moti bhasma 200 mg (tissue restorative, subtle cellular micro-anti-inflammatory, neutralizes auto-antibodies)
This mixture should be given three times daily with tikta ghrita or maha tikta ghrita, a type of medicated ghee that protects ojas and is anti-inflammatory.

Note that this formula is useful for many autoimmune conditions, but will not be appropriate for some other autoimmune disorders.

One should also give virechana each day, to pacify pitta dosha. This is the main line of shodana for high tejas. It creates a vacuum within the cells of the villi, so they suck excess pitta and tejas molecules back into the intestines, from where they can be eliminated. The patient should take 1 teaspoon of āmalakī, bhumi āmalakī, or nishottara at bedtime.

If there is a rash, we can use 200 mg each of:

Neem (antiviral)
Manjisthā (anti-inflammatory)
Turmeric (antipruritic and antibacterial)
These same herbs can also be applied topically as a *lepa* (paste).

The following herbal medicated wines (*āsavas/arishtas*) can be beneficial:

Maha manjisthadi kvātha (blood cleanser)
Kumārī āsava number 1 (hepato-detoxifier)
Rakta shuddhi kadha (hematopoietic rebuilder)
Nimbadi tailam (antiviral and inflammatory)

Each autoimmune disease requires a specific treatment protocol. The Autoimmune Disorder Remedies starting on page 79 are a bird's eye view of some common autoimmune diseases. All herbal formulas should be given three times daily unless otherwise stated.

---

22. An herb, food, or treatment that has an affinity for a particular dosha, dhātu, or srotas.

Rheumatoid arthritis is covered in detail in "Rheumatoid Arthritis (Āma Vāta)" on page 254. We will now examine four autoimmune disorders in some detail.

## Hashimoto's Thyroiditis

The pituitary gland regulates the production of the thyroid-stimulating hormone (TSH). When secretion of this hormone is decreased, it can cause this autoimmune disease.

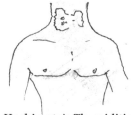

Hashimoto's Thyroiditis slowly destroys the thyroid gland. The initial acute inflammation of the thyroid gland is the expression of excess pitta dosha. As the disease progresses, the thyroid gland function diminishes and becomes hypothyroidism.

Hashimoto's Thyroiditis

Hypothyroidism

Common symptoms include:

- Weight gain
- Easily exhausted
- Pale skin
- Dry skin
- Puffy face
- Feels cold; intolerance of cold weather
- Depression
- Sluggish mental activity
- Vague pain; joint and muscle pain
- Constipation
- Menstrual disorders
- Deafness
- Loss of concentration and poor memory (especially in elderly)
- Low libido
- Enlarged thyroid (goiter)

See Remedies on page 79 for herbal remedies and other management options.

## Grave's Disease

This is an autoimmune disease of the thyroid gland that results in the increased production of thyroid hormone. It is the most common cause of hyperthyroidism.

Common symptoms include:

- Rapid heartbeat (tachycardia) and palpitations
- Unexplained weight loss, due to increased conversion of food into energy
- Excessive hunger
- Tiredness and fatigue
- Severe nervousness
- Generalized hyperactivity
- Tremors
- Excessive sweating
- Heat intolerance

- Increased body temperature
- Loose stools
- Insomnia
- Emotional instability
- Altered menstrual cycle
- Infertility
- Muscle weakness and muscle fatigue
- Bulging eyes (exophthalmoses) because of increased retrobulbar fat
- Lid lag
- Skin is warm and moist
- Itching on the legs and feet
- Enlarged thyroid gland (goiter) is common

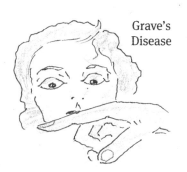

Grave's Disease

There is tīkshna agni, with sharp appetite and increased food intake. Even though the person eats a large amount of food, that food is burned quickly and the tissues are not properly nourished, resulting in weight loss.

In this condition, there is excessive production of thyroxin, enlarged thyroid gland, increased basal metabolic rate, and anxiety. The skin is warm, flushed, moist, and soft. The person is easily fatigued and is prone to osteoporosis due to excess loss of calcium and phosphorus from the bones. There is commonly high blood sugar, due to the hormonal imbalance.

The iodine levels in the blood are increased and there is usually low cholesterol, depressed liver functions, muscle tremors, and tremors to the outstretched tongue. Finally, there is lid lag, which means the person's eyelids don't cover the eyes. These are all symptoms of excess vāta and pitta.

## Treatment Protocol

Modern medicine uses beta blockers are given to treat some of the symptoms of Grave's Disease. Radioactive iodine is used to kill the goiter. However, radioactive iodine will also damage the thyroid gland, so in Ayurveda we use punarnavā lepa applied topically to the thyroid gland. We can also apply tikta ghrita or maha tikta ghrita topically to the thyroid area.

A good general herbal remedy that addresses both the excess vāta and pitta for this condition is:

Dashamūla 500 mg
Ashvagandhā 400 mg
Arjuna 300 mg
Pushkaramūla 200 mg (acts like a beta blocker)
Gulvel sattva 200 mg
Kānchanār guggulu 200 mg (for goiter)
Kāma dudhā 200 mg (for hot, flushed skin and heat intolerance)
Give this mixture three times daily after meals.

To regulate thyroid gland activity:

Ashvagandhā 500 mg
Balā 400 mg
Vidārī 300 mg
Kaishore guggulu 200 mg
Brahmī ghee is helpful for anxiety; 1 teaspoon three times daily.

Shītalī and shītkāri prāṇāyāma are recommended to calm and cool down the person. The best forms of prāṇāyāma therapy for thyroid goiter are bhrāmarī, ujjāyi and anuloma-viloma.

For lid lag, give one drop of castor oil in each eye at bedtime. For sweating, just give one tablespoon of onion juice. One can use onion juice, kaishore guggulu, and arjuna to regulate the heart rate. Alternatively, 300 mg ātmaguptā with onion juice will also regulate heart activity.

For tremors, use:

Ātmaguptā 300 mg
Kaishore guggulu 300 mg
Arjuna 200 mg
This mixture can be given three times daily.

For localized treatment of goiter, we can apply punarnavā lepa, kukutanaki lepa, tikta ghrita, or maha tikta ghrita.

Give daily nasya using vacha tailam. Also 1 teaspoon of bhumi āmalakī nightly.

## Systemic Lupus Erythematosus

Lupus is a widespread autoimmune inflammatory disorder where blood vessels, connective tissue, joints, skin, and various organs such as the heart, lungs, liver, intestines, and kidneys are affected. It is a chronic disease that is caused by aggravated *bhrājaka pitta*.

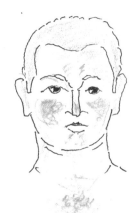

Lupus primarily affects the skin and connective tissue of the joints and muscles. There is a red rash with a butterfly appearance on the face, neck and other parts of the body, which first appears when there is exposure to sunlight.

There is often pain in the joints, intermittent fever, fatigue and visible damage of the blood vessel to the kidney.

Systemic Lupus

## Treatment Protocol for Lupus

Lupus is treated with the anti-malarial drug quinine, which is extremely bitter. Ayurveda uses mahasudarshan, as it is also a very bitter compound.

Modern medicine also uses the hormone cortisol to suppress the symptoms. The Ayurvedic protocol is to reduce pitta, balance tejas, and boost ojas. A good herbal formula is given on page 80 along with other management options.

## Myasthenia Gravis

Myasthenia gravis is an uncommon disease of the nerves and muscles that causes great fatigue and muscular weakness. It is due to tejas burning ojas in the neuromuscular cleft. Myasthenia gravis is a slow, progressive condition that affects adult women from around age 25 and men from 40 years of age.

This neuromuscular disorder is caused by a lack of acetylcholine, which is one of the key neurotransmitters. The muscles become weak and fatigued, especially the facial muscles. The person often gets double vision, the mouth and lips become pendular as can the jaw, and there is drooping of the cheeks and lower eyelids. The patient easily becomes irritable. There is often thymus gland involvement, with excessive growth of the gland or a tumor of the thymus.

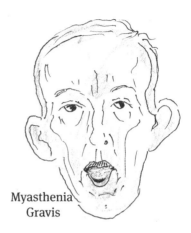
Myasthenia Gravis

See **Autoimmune Disorder Remedies** below for herbal remedies and other management options.

## Types of Agni

**Manda Agni** – Slow metabolism and poor digestion, related to increased kapha, leads to kapha disorders

**Tīkshna Agni** – Sharp metabolism and quick digestion, related to increased pitta, leads to pitta disorders

**Vishama Agni** – Irregular metabolism and fluctuating digestion, related to increased vāta, leads to vāta disorders

**Sāma Agni** – Balanced metabolism and optimal digestion, brings balanced doshas

# Autoimmune Disorder Remedies

### Rheumatoid Arthritis
Simhanad guggulu 300 mg
Āma pachak vati 200 mg
Yogarāja guggulu 200 mg

1 teaspoon castor oil mixed with 1 cup of hot ginger tea.

Topically, apply a green paste of bacha nāga, dhattūra, and tentu.

Also topically apply visha garbha tailam for sāma (with toxins) conditions, or mahānārāyana oil for nirāma disorders.

### Chronic Fatigue Syndrome
Ashvagandhā 500 mg
Balā 400 mg
Vidārī 300 mg
Shatāvarī 300 mg
Kāma dudhā 200 mg

This mixture with a small cup of almond milk.

If liver is palpable, add 200 mg kutki.

1 teaspoon bhumi āmalakī nightly.

4 teaspoons of kumārī āsava #1 with equal water after lunch and dinner.

Almonds

## Lupus Erythematosus
Shatāvarī 500 mg
Mahasudarshan 400 mg
Gudūchī 300 mg
Kāma dudhā 200 mg
Moti bhasma 200 mg

This mixture is given three times daily with 2 teaspoons of tikta ghrita (or 2 tablespoons of aloe vera gel).

Mahasudarshan kadha can also be given.

1 teaspoon āmalakī at night.

## Pernicious Anemia
Gulvel sattva 200 mg
Abhrak bhasma 200 mg
Mahayogarāja guggulu 200 mg
Tapyadi loha or Loha bhasma 200 mg
Take this with tikta ghrita

Give Vitamin B$_{12}$. Person should eat carrots, beets, spinach.

4 teaspoons of kumārī āsava #1 with equal water after lunch and dinner.

## Aplastic Anemia
Navjivan rasa 200 mg
Lauha bhasma 200 mg
Gomutra harītakī 200 mg
Abhrak bhasma 200 mg

Take this formula with shatāvarī ghee or tikta ghrita.

1 teaspoon bhumi āmalakī nightly.

4 teaspoons of kumārī āsava #1 with equal water after lunch and dinner.

## Celiac Disease
Dashamūla 500 mg
Rasa parpati 200 mg
Chitrak 200 mg
Kāma dudhā 200 mg

1 teaspoon Sat isabgol nightly.

## Myasthenia Gravis
Shatāvarī 500 mg
Dashamūla 400 mg
Ashvagandhā 400 mg
Balā 300 mg
Vidārī 200 mg
Yogarāja guggulu 200 mg

1 teaspoon gandharva harītakī nightly with warm water.

Snehana (application of oil) by massaging with balā tailam.

Svedana (sweating therapy).

Nasya (nasal application) with vacha oil.

## Hemolytic Anemia
Shatāvarī 500 mg
Gudūchī 300 mg
Lotus 200 mg
Moti bhasma 200 mg
Abhrak bhasma 200 mg
Mustā 200 mg

Take this mixture with tikta ghrita or pomegranate juice.

Pomegranate is good to eat or drink pomegranate juice.

## Glomerular Nephritis
Punarnavā 500 mg
Gokshura 300 mg
Shilājit 200 mg
Gudūchī 200 mg
Mūtrala 200 mg

Ginger (fresh juice) and jaggery nasya: 3 to 5 drops

1 teaspoon triphala nightly.

## Crohn's Disease
Shatāvarī 500 mg
Gudūchī 300 mg
Kutaja 200 mg
Bilva 200 mg
Pañchāmrit parpati 200 mg

1 teaspoon Sat isabgol nightly.

## Addison's Disease

Punarnavā 500 mg
Gokshura 300 mg
Yashthi madhu 200 mg
Shardunikā 200 mg
Neem 200 mg
Turmeric 200 mg

1 teaspoon triphala nightly.

## Grave's Disease

See section on Grave's Disease page 76 for some specific remedies.

## Amyloidosis

There is immunoglobulin malformation that results in abnormal protein deposits in vital organs, such as the heart, kidneys and central nervous system. Therefore, the treatment protocol varies according to the organs involved.

## Hepatitis B and C

Shatāvarī 500 mg
Gudūchī 300 mg
Kutki 200 mg
Neem 200 mg
Shankha pushpī 200 mg

1 teaspoon triphala nightly.

4 teaspoons of kumārī āsava #1 with equal water after lunch and dinner.

## Alopecia Areata

Shatāvarī 500 mg
Gudūchī 300 mg
Bhringarāja 200 mg
Brahmī 200 mg
Shankha pushpī 200 mg

1 teaspoon bhumi āmalakī nightly.

Apply maha bhringarāja tailam topically on the scalp.

4 teaspoons of kumārī āsava #1 with equal water after lunch and dinner.

## Hashimoto's Thyroiditis

During an acute disorder:
Shatāvarī 500 mg
Gudūchī 400 mg
Kāma dudhā 300 mg
Kaishore guggulu 200 mg
Later on in chronic conditions:
Punarnavā 500 mg
Chitrak 200 mg
Kutki 200 mg
Sarasvatī 200 mg
Kaishore guggulu 200 mg

Brahmī prash for memory (or brahmī).

If there is inflammatory swelling, use sandalwood and turmeric paste.

If enlarged thyroid (goiter), use kānchanār guggulu 200 mg.

For localized treatment of goiter, apply kukutanaki lepa or punarnavā lepa.

1 teaspoon bhumi āmalakī nightly.

## Multiple Sclerosis

Dashamūla 500 mg
Gudūchī 300 mg
Yogarāja guggulu 300 mg
Kaishore guggulu 200 mg

Mahānārāyana oil for massage.

Netra basti with plain ghee if history of optic neuritis.

1 teaspoon triphala nightly.

4 teaspoons of dashamūla arishta with equal water after lunch and dinner.

## Ankylosing Spondylitis

Dashamūla 500 mg
Ashvagandhā 400 mg
Yogarāja guggulu 300 mg
Mustā 300 mg
Tagara 200 mg

Topically, apply mahānārāyana oil.

Dashamūla tea basti.

4 teaspoons each of dashamūla arishta and maharasnadi kvātha with equal amount of water after lunch and dinner.

## Pancreatitis
Shatāvarī 500 mg
Gudūchī 300 mg
Kāma dudhā 200 mg
Neem 200 mg
Turmeric 200 mg
Shardunikā 200 mg

1 teaspoon bhumi āmalakī nightly.

## Fibromyalgia and Fibromyositis
Dashamūla 500 mg
Shatāvarī 400 mg
Gudūchī 300 mg
Kāma dudhā 200 mg
Kaishore guggulu 200 mg
Yogarāja guggulu 200 mg

4 teaspoons dashamūla arishta with equal amount of water after lunch and dinner.

Topically, massage with mahānārāyana oil.

## Scleroderma
Shatāvarī 500 mg
Gudūchī 400 mg
Kaishore guggulu 300 mg
Manjisthā 200 mg

1 teaspoon triphala nightly.

Topically apply chandan balā lakshadi tailam.

## Optic Neuritis
Netra basti with plain ghee, once or twice weekly.
Shatāvarī 500 mg
Gulvel sattva 300 mg
Kaishore guggulu 200 mg
Kāma dudhā 200 mg

1 teaspoon āmalakī nightly.

## Raynaud's Disease
Dashamūla 500 mg
Gulvel sattva 400 mg
Manjisthā 300 mg
Neem 200 mg
Turmeric 200 mg
Kaishore guggulu 200 mg

1 teaspoon bhumi āmalakī nightly.

Topically, massage with mahānārāyana oil.

## Urticaria and Contact Dermatitis
Shatāvarī 500 mg
Gulvel sattva 400 mg
Manjisthā 300 mg
Neem 200 mg
Kāma dudhā 200 mg

1 teaspoon triphala nightly.

Topically apply 50-50 mixture of coconut oil and castor oil.

Rub internal white part of cantaloupe (eat orange part).

Apply cilantro pulp topically. Also take cilantro juice orally.

**NOTE:** All herbal formulas should be given ½ teaspoon with warm water, three times daily unless otherwise stated.

# Chapter 9

# The Ayurvedic Perspective on Diabetes
## Prameha

Winter 2001, Volume 14, Number 3 and Spring 2002, Volume 14, Number

*Prameha* (WHICH MEANS PROFUSE URINATION), *prakrushta meha,* and *prakarshena meha* are names indicating a dysfunction in mūtra vaha srotas (the urinary system) and *ambu vaha srotas* (the water carrying channels). In this chapter, we will discuss prameha as diabetes syndrome and its associated disorders.

In prameha, there is a disturbance in ambu vaha srotas, mūtra vaha srotas, rasa vaha srotas, rakta vaha srotas and medo vaha srotas. The *kloma* (pancreas), *tālu* (palate) and choroid plexuses are all connected to ambu vaha srotas and are all affected by prameha. *Medo vaha srotas* (the channel of fatty tissue) and *rasa-rakta vaha srotas* (lymph and blood carrying channels) are affected by prameha due to their affinity for the water element. In fact, any system or tissue in the body that is associated with water will be affected.

It is very important to understand that Ayurveda sees prameha not as one disease, but as a multifaceted syndrome with various, complex metabolic disorders. Prameha describes a syndrome of varied symptoms and complications related to or causing diabetes. It includes the prodromal symptoms and disease conditions of diabetes mellitus types one and two and diabetes insipidus. However, it is important that we understand the doshas and systems involved, not just the modern medical definition of this disease.

The Ayurvedic picture is based on the concept that all dhātus (tissues) have a normal level of kleda (moisture or liquid). One function of kleda is to maintain the body's water-electrolyte balance. It also nourishes and lubricates all tissues. It is associated with kledaka kapha in the stomach and, in the prasara (spreading) stage of prameha, kledaka kapha *Samprapti* overflows from the gastrointestinal (GI) tract and enters the rasa dhātu (blood plasma). This kledaka kapha disturbs the kleda present in all dhātus. The function of urine is to remove excess liquids, so when kleda is increased, urination is also increased, called polyuria. Hence, prameha, or prakrushta meha, indicates this profuse urination.

Polyuria may be present in other conditions, such as hysteria, renal disorders, hyperparathyroidism (which may lead to hypercalcemia and then polyuria), or potassium deple-

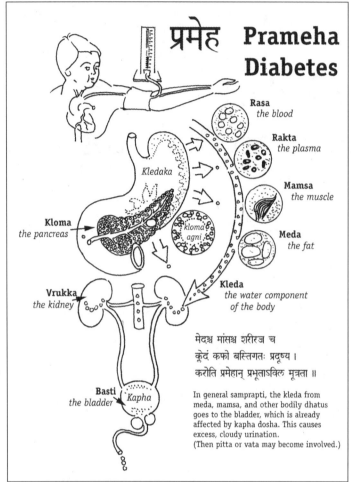

**प्रमेह Prameha**
**Diabetes**

**Rasa**
*the blood*

**Rakta**
*the plasma*

**Mamsa**
*the muscle*

**Meda**
*the fat*

**Kleda**
*the water component*
*of the body*

*Kledaka*

**Kloma**
*the pancreas*

*kloma agni*

**Vrukka**
*the kidney*

**Basti**
*the bladder*　*Kapha*

मेदश्च मांसश्च शरीरज च
क्लेदं कफो बस्तिगतः प्रदूष्य ।
करोति प्रमेहान् प्रभूताऽविल मूत्रता ॥

In general samprapti, the kleda from
meda, mamsa, and other bodily dhatus
goes to the bladder, which is already
affected by kapha dosha. This causes
excess, cloudy urination.
(Then pitta or vata may become involved.)

tion, which is a kidney disorder. Due to these etiological factors, one or more of the doshas increases, leading to progression of the diabetic disease process.

The first three stages of any disease are called sanchaya (accumulation), prakopa (provocation) and prasara (spreading). High blood sugar is described in Ayurveda as increased kapha in the prasara stage of disease, affecting the *rasa-rakta dhātus* (circulatory and lymphatic systems). The increased kledaka from the dhātus starts leaking via the digestive system, through the kidneys and into the bladder, causing the prodromal signs and symptoms of diabetes. These are called pūrva rūpa and occur after the dosha enters the third stage of the disease process.

During this period, the person commonly accumulates tartar on the teeth and notices that they have to go to the dentist more frequently to clean the teeth. Generally there is sticky sweat, even after a bath, and an increase in khamala (nasal crust, ear wax, sebaceous secretions and smegma). There is excess urination, nocturnal urination and when one is passing the last drops of urine, the urinary sphincter muscles constrict and create goose bumps. It is common for the person to have a sweet taste in the mouth and for the breath to smell like vinegar. Charaka says that these are all early or prodromal signs and symptoms of prameha.

The general samprāpti (pathogenesis) of prameha almost always begins with increased kapha, as seen in most of the signs and symptoms. Later, vāta and pitta can enter the picture, because prameha is a complex syndrome that can involve all three doshas.

## Causes of Prameha

Prameha is most often due to hyperglycemia (increased blood sugar) caused by diminished insulin production by the kloma (pancreas). It is a chronic endocrine disorder that affects the metabolism of carbohydrates, proteins and fats as well as the water-electrolyte balance. It can cause functional and structural changes in the bodily cells, creating complications of the eyes, kidneys, nervous system and other organs.

Some other causes of prameha are:

- It may be a secondary condition to pancreatitis, which is a pitta disorder. Viral infections such as mumps or staphylococcal infections can create pancreatitis.
- Heredity plays an important role in the predisposition to destruction of beta cells in the pancreas. This can cause pancreatitis or neoplasm or tumor of the pancreas, leading to diabetes.
- A tumor of the pancreas, which is a pitta-kapha condition.
- Autoimmune dysfunctions, whereby tejas burns ojas and antibodies affect the pancreas.
- Obesity, which is almost always associated with non-insulin-dependent diabetes. This is a metabolic disorder of kapha dosha.
- Diet, emotional overeating, and excess consumption of sugar.
- Pregnancy. During pregnancy there is an excessive demand for insulin and if the pancreas cannot provide that insulin, it becomes stressed. This can lead to gestational diabetes, a type of diabetes mellitus. Also, there is a natural physiological increase in kapha dosha because kapha is responsible for the creation of the new baby and placenta. This increased kapha can inhibit the pancreatic function, which can also lead to gestational diabetes.
- Liver diseases, including hepatitis and cirrhotic changes, can lead to portal hypertension and affect the pancreatic function, resulting in diabetes.
- Corticosteroid therapy is an iatrogenic (drug- induced) cause of diabetes. Steroidal hormones are kapha-provoking and steroid toxicity often creates underactive thyroid, water retention, hypertension (high blood pressure) and obesity. It also compromises kidney functions and causes 'moon face,' which results in a swollen and fatty appearance of the face.

The famous Ayurvedic author, *Mādhava*, says that worry, anxiety, fear, and anger are all connected to cerebral kloma and these can affect glandular functions, leading to prameha.

## Types of Diabetes

The modern definition of diabetes differentiates two main types, mellitus and insipidus. Diabetes insipidus, at least in the beginning, is an imbalance of the diuretic hormone vasopressin. It is rare and occurs most often in young people.

Diabetes mellitus is a metabolic disorder characterized by increased blood sugar and passing of sugar in the urine, due to a dysfunction of *kloma* (pancreas) *agni*. It is classified as either insulin-dependent diabetes (IDD) or non-insulin-dependent diabetes (NIDD). Insulin-dependent diabetes is type I diabetes mellitus and is also known as juvenile-onset diabetes, because it generally

---

**PURVA RUPA OF PRAMEHA**

**(Prodromal Signs and Symptoms)**

- Excess tartar on teeth
- Burning hands and feet
- Excess thirst
- Frequent, excess urination
- Nocturnal urination
- Goosebumps during and after passing the last drops of urine
- Sweet, sticky saliva
- Acetone-like smell to the breath
- Sticky sweat and increased kha mala (nasal crust, earwax, etc.)
- Pulse becomes slow and sluggish; the stomach pulse shows a kapha spike

begins prior to 30 years of age. The cells of the islets of Langerhans in the pancreas are unable to produce enough insulin and the person usually requires external sources of insulin for the rest of his or her life.

Non-insulin-dependent diabetes is type II diabetes mellitus. It is the most common form of diabetes and is found throughout the world, but especially amongst <u>affluent</u> people and therefore in Western countries. Type II mellitus is also known as late-onset or adult-onset diabetes, because it usually begins from age 40 to 50 or above. It can also occur in pregnancy. Women are more prone to this condition, especially obese women and those who have had many pregnancies.

Many of the signs and symptoms of type II diabetes relate closely to the various kapha types of prameha mentioned in Ayurveda. In this condition the functions of the pancreas are affected by fat clogging the cell membranes. These pancreatic cells then become <u>resistant to insulin</u>, resulting in the body not being able to process sugar. Unlike type I diabetes mellitus, type II does not require insulin injections. Promoting the pancreatic functions and controlling blood sugar, primarily through diet and lifestyle, can treat it.

> **RUPA OF PRAMEHA**
> **(Cardinal Signs and Symptoms)**
>
> - Polyuria (excessive urination) – the person may pass 10 to 20 liters of urine per day
> - Low specific gravity of the urine
> - Polydipsia (excessive thirst)
> - Fatigue
> - Disturbed water-electrolyte balance
> - Potassium depletion, which leads to kidney
> - malfunction
> - Hyper-parathyroidism
> - Excess water consumption, which inhibits anti-diuretic hormone and leads to water toxicity and low agni. Note: A vāta or pitta person typically needs 5 to 10 glasses of water per day, whereas a kapha person may require less than this.

In diabetes mellitus, the Earth and Water elements are not properly digested, leading to excess sugar in the urine and blood. These are known as hyperglycemia (high blood sugar) and glycosuria (excess glucose or sugar in urine). Sushruta calls the condition *rakta sharkarā,* which means high blood sugar.

## Ayurvedic Classification of Prameha

There are <u>twenty</u> types of prameha identified by Ayurveda, which correspond to the various signs and symptoms found in diabetes syndrome. Diabetes is included in prameha, but prameha is more than diabetes. We can say that all 20 types of prameha may end up within one of the Western classifications of diabetes. Alternatively, we can state that the 20 types of prameha can be seen as different stages or conditions that may lead to one of these types of diabetes.

Prameha is a metabolic disorder of agni, the energy of transformation. The stomach is the seat of jāthara agni, which is the central bodily fire; the liver the seat of bhūta agni; the pancreas has *kloma agni;* and each dhātu (tissue) has its own agni. When there is a dysfunction of these agnis, especially kloma agni, the carbohydrate metabolism is disturbed.

Ayurveda classifies prameha according to the primary dosha involved. There are ten kapha, six pitta, and four vāta types related to this complex syndrome.

- Kapha Prameha — 10 types; relatively easy to cure; non-insulin-dependent
- Pitta Prameha — 6 types; difficult to cure; may be insulin-dependent
- Vāta Prameha — 4 types; incurable or very difficult to treat; insulin-dependent

In kapha type of prameha, kledaka kapha slows down agni so that the kleda goes partly unprocessed into rasa dhātu. Rasa, rakta, meda and shukra dhātus are all involved in kapha prameha. In pitta type, rakta is the major dhātu affected. In vāta prameha, all dhātus can be involved, but complications involve mainly majjā, as in diabetic neuropathy.

We will now examine these twenty types according to the signs and symptoms and appropriate treatments for each.

## Ten Kapha Types of Prameha

These kapha types of prameha fall into the category of type II (non-insulin-dependent) diabetes mellitus, or may be a precursor to that disease. These conditions commonly begin with low meda dhātu agni, which can cause obesity and other kapha disorders.

1. **Ikshu meha:** digestive or alimentary glycosuria. Ikshu means sugarcane juice and the urine looks cloudy like sugarcane juice. This condition is due to weak jāthara agni and kloma agni. The person eats too many sweet substances and the GI tract gets overloaded with sugar. Kleda is then unprocessed, which creates the glycosuria.

The function of urine is to carry kleda and there is functional integrity between urine and kleda. Kleda from the stomach and pancreas add to the quantity of urine, producing excessive urination, which makes the person feel tired and also leads to constipation. It is necessary to increase agni and eliminate toxins, so a good formula is:

| | |
|---|---|
| Gudūchī | 300 mg |
| Neem | 300 mg |
| Tumeric | 200 mg |
| Chitrak | 200 mg |
| Trikatu | 200 mg |

Take ½ tsp TID with warm water.

> T.I.D. = from the Latin means *ter in diem*, three times a day

2. **Sitā meha:** sita means rock candy. This type of prameha can be compared to renal glycosuria, which means the presence of sugar in the urine. It is a kidney dysfunction due to depleted agni of the glomeruli. Apāna vāyu governs glomeruli filtration, which maintains the concentration of urine. Because of disturbed apāna the glomeruli permeability increases, which is responsible for leaking kleda and causing renal glycosuria. This causes the urine to become more diluted, so the person passes cool, clear, water-like urine that feels like frozen water and looks like rock candy dissolved in water. Diagnostically, you will find the kidney pulse is weak. Sitameha can be helped by taking the following formula:

| | |
|---|---|
| Punarnavā | 500 mg |
| Gokshura | 400 mg |

Gudūchī          300 mg
Shilājit          300 mg
Take ½ tsp TID with warm water.
Also useful is chandraprabhā, one tablet daily.

**3. Udaka meha:** <u>diabetes insipidus</u>. This is due to a dysfunction in the posterior pituitary gland that produces the anti-diuretic hormones arginine and vasopressin, which constrict the blood vessels of the glomeruli in order to prevent the elimination of excess water. There is polyuria (excessive urination) and polydipsia (excess thirst). The urine looks like water and excess water retention can cause water toxicity. This slows agni and lowers kidney energy.

This condition occurs mostly in young people. It begins with disturbed kledaka kapha, leading to over-secretion of kleda into the rasa dhātu, which is the prasara stage of this disease. This can affect *tarpaka kapha* in the posterior pituitary, causing <u>inadequate secretions of vasopressin and anti- diuretic hormone</u>. This in turn results in excess kapha and kleda going into the kidneys, which creates polyuria (excess urination) and other symptoms. Remember that prameha means profuse urination.

Diabetes insipidus may be due to a growth hormone disorder such as acromegaly (gigantism), pituitary tumor, excess ACTH hormone, excess thyroid hormones that affect carbohydrate metabolism, diminished glomeruli threshold in the kidneys, or diminished production of anti-diuretic hormone. It might also be due to vāta pushing pitta in the majjā dhātu, which can manifest as encephalitis, basal meningitis, syphilis, or a trauma (cerebral concussion, compression, or contusion). These disturb the functioning of tarpaka kapha and become kapha prameha.

This posterior pituitary dysfunction, which causes the inadequate secretion of vasopressin, happens in young people at a kapha age. <u>Anti-diuretic hormones</u> can be compared to tarpaka kapha, because of their cold and stable qualities. For this condition, we can use the following formula to promote secretions of anti-diuretic hormone:

Parijata          300 mg
Mustā          300 mg
Vanga Bhasma   50 mg
Arka Patra (calatropis)  1 drop
Take ½ tsp TID with cumin, coriander, and fennel (CCF) tea.

Yashthi madhu (licorice), the herbal compound tikta, and cumin, coriander and fennel tea also promote the secretion of vasopressin and maintain the glomeruli function.

**4. Pistha meha:** phosphate urea. Pishta means refined white flour and the urine looks cloudy and pale, like a mixture of water and flour. The urine is alkaline and the phosphate molecules start to leak through the glomeruli filtration system in the kidneys, which can lead to renal calculi. This condition may be associated with diabetes.

Chandraprabhā 300 mg
Dāruharidrā     300 mg (a special kind of turmeric)
Shilājit          200 mg
Take ½ tsp TID with warm water.

5. **Shukra meha:** shukra is the male reproductive tissue (semen). Kleda from shukra dhātu passes through a weak prostate gland and sperm starts leaking into the urine, which is called spermatorrhea. This predisposes one to diabetes and is part of the prodromal symptoms that develop about six months before diabetes. There is a biochemical dysfunction of *ashthīlā agni,* the enzymes that maintain the functions of the prostate. Spermatorrhea may be due to gonorrhea, syphilis, trauma, excess sexual activity, anxiety, fear of sex and excessive or forceful masturbation, which can all deplete shukra agni and weaken the prostatic sphincters. The person can also get constipation, pass mucus in the stools and strain to pass urine or feces. The condition may also be associated with amoebiasis.

We can use certain herbs to improve the prostate tone and control the spermaturia:

Ātma Guptā    300 mg (kapikacchū)
Shilājit    300 mg
Cardamom    200 mg
Asafoetida    100 mg
Take ½ tsp TID with warm water or guñjā tea.

Guñjā (*Abrus precatorius*) is a plant with small, tamarind-like leaves. It enhances the tone of the prostate and helps to prevent semen from leaking. The leaves can be made into a tea by boiling with water or milk. Use as an anupāna (a carrier or vehicle).

Note that ātmaguptā works on the male reproductive and nervous systems and is indicated for Parkinson's Disease.

6. **Lālā meha:** *lālā* means drool, and lālā meha means that the person's urine becomes thick like saliva. This is also called prostate urea, because it occurs when a man passes stringy, prostatic secretions in the urine and gets spasms and goose bumps. There is also leakage of prostatic secretions during the day, which indicates that he could become diabetic. It is common in males from about age 55 on. The same type of thing can also occur in women, but instead of prostatic secretions they have profuse secretions from the Bartholin's glands that can mix with the urine. Additionally, the vagina becomes overly lubricated.

Tulsi    300 mg
Turmeric    300 mg
Pātthā    300 mg
Agaru    200 mg
Shilājit    200 mg
Take ½ tsp TID with warm water.

Men can also do a daily massage over the prostate region.

7. **Sikata meha:** *sikata* means sand, so sikata meha means lithuria or crystalluria. The urine has a crystalline dust or coarse sand made up of phosphates, calcium, uric acid, or oxalate crystals. A person with lithuria may become diabetic. The glomeruli allow these crystals to pass through the urine, so the condition is associated with kidney stones. When the person passes kidney stones he feels great pain from the loin to the groin. If a baby boy

cries incessantly and pulls the penis while peeing, consider the possibility of urinary stones. A female gets a radiating pain from the loin to the labia (renal colic), indicating it may be kidney stones.

If the stone is just silently sitting in the kidney, it will create a typical tenderness in the renal angle. At the time of passing the stone, when it is coming through the urethra, or even coming through the ureter into the bladder, it is extremely painful. In sikata meha, the person passes broken down stones that look like gravel. When a baby with this condition passes urine, you can see the stain of minerals (yellow for oxalate, white for phosphate).

For this condition we can use:

| | |
|---|---|
| Punarnavā | 500 mg |
| Gokshura | 400 mg |
| Chitrak | 200 mg |

Take ½ tsp TID with warm water.

Also give kidney bean flowers, steeped in warm water, which are a good astringent. Alternatively take cumin, coriander and fennel tea.

8. **Shanaih meha:** this means increased frequency of urination. The person has frequent urination during both day and night, because they cannot completely evacuate the bladder due to an obstruction. This may be due to enlarged prostate, stricture of the urethra, or kidney stones. It is also necessary to rule out benign prostatic hyperplasia. The bladder loses its tone, so when the person goes to bed it stretches and creates the desire for urination, but the blockage doesn't allow urine to easily pass.

For frequent, profuse urination we use catechu (khadira), which is astringent and helps to control urination. If there is a blockage of the urethra, which is generally a secondary complication to syphilitic urethritis, surgical intervention is needed. If it is a prostate problem, one must treat the prostate. A good formula is:

| | |
|---|---|
| Arka Pushpa | 200 mg |
| Vanga bhasma (tin ash) | 200 mg |

Take ½ tsp TID with warm water.

9. **Sāndra meha:** turbid urine. The urine looks turbid and dense because of protein. When the nephron lining is compromised, there is a tendency to get urinary tract infections. Sugar is the best medium for bacteria to grow, so the excess sugar in the system combined with the disturbed nephron lining will cause the patient to lose his or her natural resistance. That is why diabetic people are prone to infection. The person also passes minerals into the urine.

For this condition we use the juice of fresh saptaparnī, a bitter, seven-leaf plant that is one of the ingredients of mahāsudarshan.

| | |
|---|---|
| Saptaparnī | 300 mg |
| Shilājit | 300 mg |
| Gokshura | 300 mg |

Take ½ tsp TID with warm water.

**10. Surā meha:** *surā* means alcohol and surā meha is acetone urea. This condition exists when a person passes acetone without consumption of alcohol. The urine smells like alcohol and ferments.

| | |
|---|---|
| Kutki | 300 mg |
| Tikta | 300 mg |
| Chitrak | 200 mg |

Take ½ tsp TID with aloe vera.

These are the ten types of kapha prameha. The following can also be associated with kapha prameha:

***Lāsikā meha or phena meha.*** Albumin urea. When passing urine there is lots of foam, which indicates a change in the specific gravity. The urine looks like carbonated water or beer. This is due to albumin and the person passes protein in the urine, due to kidney infection, pre-diabetes, a high protein diet, or toxemia in pregnancy. It can lead to nephrotic syndrome. A good formula is:

*Albuminurea*

| | |
|---|---|
| Punarnavā | 500 mg |
| Gokshura | 300 mg |
| Triphalā | 200 mg |
| Shilājit | 200 mg |

Take ½ tsp TID with warm water.

For all types of kapha prameha, a kapha pacifying diet and small sized meals is recommended. Take 1 teaspoon of triphalā each night at bedtime. Do regular exercise and also yoga, including spinal twist, bow, boat, bridge, and peacock poses. (see yoga poses in Appendix page 450)

## Table 3: Etiological Factors of Prameha

| Primary | Secondary |
|---|---|
| Kapha-provoking diet – especially excess sugar consumption | Viral infection |
| Obesity | Pregnancy – excess demand for insulin |
| Sedentary lifestyle | Thyroid gland disorder – excess production of thyroid hormones |
| High cholesterol and high triglycerides | Pituitary gland disorder relating to ACTH or growth hormone |
| Emotional overeating | Pituitary tumor |
| Stress | Liver diseases – hepatitis, cirrhosis, etc. |
| Genetic predisposition | Encephalitis |
| Pancreatic disorder: pancreatitis is pitta, tumor is kapha | Basal meningitis |
| Auto-immune disorder | Syphilis |
| | Corticosteroid therapy |
| | Diminished glomerular threshold |
| | Physical or psychological trauma |

This covers the principle kapha-related prameha conditions, which are non-insulin-dependent and relatively easy to treat. Next, we will discuss the pitta and vāta-dominant disturbances, both of which are more difficult to treat. This is according to the Ayurvedic concept of prameha as it relates to the western syndrome of diabetes.

## Six Pitta Types of Prameha

In these six pitta types of prameha, the pancreas may or may not be directly involved, depending on whether the person has a khavaigunya (weak space). Management of the doshas can control the metabolic imbalance if there is not pancreatic involvement, so for these six types of prameha, pitta must be pacified. The moment the pancreas is severely affected, the person can develop type I diabetes mellitus, which is primarily a vāta type of prameha. Once this happens, the person needs to severely limit the intake of sweet foods and support the pancreas, as well as manage the doshas.

In pitta prameha, it is common to have complications such as diabetic neuropathy, diabetic retinopathy and diabetic nephropathy. Patients are prone to repeated infections, boils, abscesses and other inflammatory disorders. The six pitta prameha follow.

1.  **Kshara meha:** alkalinuria. *Kshara* means salt, which is alkaline, and here the urine becomes alkaline. Acids can burn, but a substance that is alkaline may also cause inflammation, because it fosters infection. There are two types of pitta: *sāma pitta,* which is pitta with āma (toxins) and is acidic; and *nirāma pitta,* which is pitta without āma and is alkaline. Hence, alkalinuria is related to nirāma pitta and is common when there is a liver dysfunction. Bile is alkaline, so if a patient has excess bile passing through the urine, it too becomes alkaline. This condition is also known as non-specific urethritis and is treated with āmalakī. Āmalakī is acidic, so it neutralizes the alkali. Take ½ teaspoon TID with hot water.

2.  **Amla meha:** aciduria. *Amla* meha means aciduria, where the urine becomes acidic, and it is the opposite of kshara meha. For this, use bibhītakī or harītakī. Or if you're not sure which, just use triphalā and it will bring balance. This condition can also be helped by:

    | | |
    |---|---|
    | Shatāvarī | 500 mg |
    | Gulvel sattva | 300 mg |
    | Kāma dudhā | 200 mg |

    Take ½ tsp TID with warm water.

3.  **Nila meha:** *nila* means indigo, and here the urine looks purple-blue, which is known as urocyanosis or indicanuria. It is a sign of congestive heart failure and happens because of central cyanosis. In chronic congestive heart failure, the heart fails to fully pump blood out of the chamber and there is stagnation of venous blood, so the visceral organs look cyanotic. If you look at the tongue it is purple-blue and in this case even the urine looks purple or indigo. The person passes unoxidated blood cells in the urine. To test the color, put the urine in a glass jar or vial and hold it up to the light. This is a serious condition that is due to a chronic pitta disorder. However, another cause of indigo urine is iron toxicity. If the liver doesn't process iron efficiently, it can be stored in the liver. Liver disease is a serious complication of diabetes, as are vascular and heart problems.

The best herb for both causes of nilameha is kutki (also called katukā), because it enhances iron metabolism and scrapes excess cholesterol from the arteries. For iron chelation, katukā is the herb of choice. For both these you can give 200 mg TID. A good formula is:

Kutki (Katukā)  200 mg
Neem          200 mg
Raktachandana  200 mg (red sandalwood)
Turmeric       200 mg
Take ½ tsp TID with warm water.

4.  **Rakta meha:** hematuria, which occurs when the person passes blood in the urine. It may be due to oxalic acid crystals, or a hemorrhage into the kidneys. First, rule out all other causes for hematuria, such as stricture of the urethra, kidney stones, or polyps. If these causes are eliminated and the person still passes some red blood cells in the urine, it means that he or she is likely to develop pitta type of diabetes. For this condition we use hemostatic herbs.

Gudūchī      300 mg (or gulvel sattva)
Manjisthā    300 mg
Arjuna       300 mg
Karanja      300 mg
Take ½ tsp TID with warm water.

5.  **Manjisthā meha:** *manjishthā* means red, so this is red urine or hemoglobinuria. The person passes microscopic oxygenated red blood cells in the urine. This means that disintegration of red blood cells has already happened.

Manjisthā    300 mg
Chandana     300 mg (white sandalwood)
Ushīra       300 mg
Take ½ tsp TID with warm water.

6.  **Haridrā meha:** haridrā means turmeric, and in this type of prameha the urine looks dark yellow, the color of turmeric. It can be caused by bilirubinuria, chronic hepatitis, or cancer of the liver. One of the causes of diabetes is a liver dysfunction. The liver doesn't process carbohydrates and there is an overproduction of bilirubin that passes through the urine, so the person has dark colored urine, called haridrā meha. The best medicine for this condition is:

Shankha pushpī 400 mg
Tulsi        300 mg
Kutki        200 mg
Bilva        200 mg
Take ½ tsp TID with aloe vera gel.

For all these pitta types of prameha, a pitta pacifying diet and regular meals is recommended. Regular exercise and yoga is good, along with a teaspoon of triphalā at bedtime.

Triphalā is particularly helpful for pitta prameha because it balances the acid-alkaline balance (pH) of the urine and removes toxicity from the bladder. If it causes excessive urination at night, it may be an indication of low glomerular threshold in the kidneys, which can predispose the person to diabetes or reflect a family history of diabetes.

## Four Vāta Types of Prameha

These four vāta types of prameha can fall into the category of type I (insulin-dependent) diabetes mellitus, or may be a precursor to that disease. They are the most difficult to treat and some texts even list them as incurable. However there is much we can do to help these conditions.

1. **Vasa meha:** *vasa* means subcutaneous fat, so this is lipiduria. The person passes lipids in the urine, which show as oily droplets. It is a severe disorder of the fat metabolism that is often seen in the later stages of type I diabetes mellitus. The individual loses fat so rapidly that there can be severe emaciation and extremely dry skin. There is often high cholesterol, fatty diarrhea and fatty degenerative changes in the liver.

It is caused by disturbed *apāna vāta,* which allows lipid molecules to leak through the glomeruli and Bowman's capsule, resulting in either lipiduria or heavy proteinuria.

The treatment needs to strongly pacify vāta dosha:

| | |
|---|---|
| Dashamūla | 500 mg |
| Ashvagandhā | 500 mg |
| Katukā | 300 mg |
| Agni mantha | 200 mg |

Take ½ tsp TID with warm water.

2. **Sarpi meha:** *sarpi* means ghee. This condition is known as chyluria and it is a disorder of rasa dhātu. Chyle is the end product of digested food and the precursor of all bodily tissues. It is a milk-like alkaline substance containing lymphatic secretions that normally flow through the blood stream. In this condition, the astringent phase of digestion that happens in the colon is disturbed, creating vāta aggravation due to the dry, light and rough qualities of astringent taste. Disturbance of apāna vāta affects the pelvic organs and rasa and rakta dhātus. The glomerular threshold is also so disturbed that, instead of filtering kleda, it also filters chyle. This results in the person passing chyle into the urine, which can lead to emaciation.

In this disorder, vyāna vāta is disturbed and the chyle is pushed through the glomeruli of the kidneys, which makes the urine look like liquefied ghee. Note that in vasa meha, the urine appears to contain oil droplets, but here the whole urine looks like ghee.

A good formula is:

| | |
|---|---|
| Balā | 500 mg |
| Pātthā | 300 mg |
| Katukā | 300 mg |
| Hing | 200 mg |
| Kutaja | 200 mg |
| Kushtha | 200 mg |

Take ½ tsp TID with warm water.

DM

**3.   Madhu meha:** the person gets a sweet taste in the mouth, which later becomes sour, then salty, pungent, bitter and ultimately astringent. That indicates a very serious condition. Initially, the sweet taste from āhāra rasa (the food precursor of the tissues) cannot be converted into *sthāyi rasa dhātu* (fully processed plasma), so that dhātu becomes depleted. Sweet is the most nourishing taste and also the heaviest to digest, so it is the first to be unprocessed. Eventually even astringent, the final taste in the sequence, cannot be digested. At this point, agni has weakened to the extent that it cannot digest any of the tastes. Hence, the rasa dhātu becomes very depleted causing severe emaciation and all seven dhātus can also be affected in this way. This condition can then turn into type I diabetes mellitus.

Madhu meha means sweet urine, which is called glycosuria. There is also hyperglycemia (high blood sugar levels), due to diminished effectiveness of insulin. It is an endocrine disorder that affects carbohydrate, fat and protein metabolism, plus the water-electrolyte balance in the body. However the glomerular threshold is not directly affected. Madhu meha is a chronic condition that generally involves all three doshas, but ends up being a predominantly vāta imbalance. Insufficient insulin can be confirmed by a vāta spike on the pancreas pulse, which is found at the site of the spleen pulse.

It is a difficult condition to treat, but certain herbs do help. Shardunikā regulates carbohydrate and sugar metabolism and thereby helps to control blood sugar levels. Karela is bitter gourd (or bitter melon) and it is most effective for madhu meha. Vasant kusumakar contains purified gold, silver, pearl and mercury ash, so it is not allowed in the United States. However in India, most patients with type I diabetes mellitus take one pill daily to regulate blood sugar, so they do not require insulin.

| | |
|---|---|
| Shardunikā | 200 mg (or Gurmar or Madhuharini) |
| Bitter Gourd | 200 mg |
| Neem | 200 mg |
| Turmeric | 200 mg |

Take ½ tsp TID with warm water.

Also: Vasant Kusumakar 200 mg once daily

**4.   Hasta meha:** *hasta* means elephant. The patient passes astringent urine and has incontinence. There is extreme polyuria, with gushing of urine like an elephant. The best formula is:

| | |
|---|---|
| Palash | 300 mg |
| Kapittha | 200 mg |
| Arjuna | 300 mg |
| Vangeshvara | 200 mg (contains vanga bhasma, along with other ingredients)[23] |

Take ½ tsp TID with warm water.

---

23. A tin-lead oxide compound. This is of the types known as a rasa shastra product, alchemical combinations that usually include metals, some of which are considered toxic in their raw forms.

For all four vāta types of prameha, a vāta pacifying diet with regular, small meals is recommended. Gentle exercise, such as yoga, and basti (medicated enema) can also be helpful, as can taking a teaspoon of triphalā at bedtime each night. If it causes excess urination during the night, the triphalā can be soaked overnight and drunk the following morning. Overall, treatments for vāta prameha can generally only alleviate the symptoms, because vāta prameha is extremely difficult to cure.

## Summary of Treatments for Prameha

These are the twenty major categories of prameha and we have to treat each one according to the doshas involved. Herbs, or insulin if necessary, can regulate blood sugar, but there needs to be a holistic treatment program to treat this syndrome. That usually includes proper diet, daily exercise, yoga, hygienic measures, an appropriate lifestyle and pancha-karma cleansing, all according to the individual's constitution and the particular type of prameha.

It is also necessary to rebalance agni (metabolic fire) to regulate carbohydrate, fat and protein metabolism, and restore the water-electrolyte balance. Kapha types need to focus on controlling their weight and treat any edema. Pitta types must be vigilant about preventing infection and acidosis and should be particularly careful about cuts and abrasions. Vāta types should have a nourishing diet and not overdo things. Finally, anyone with prameha should keep a close watch on associated conditions such as glucose levels in the urine, hyperglycemia, high blood pressure, bacterial infections, blurring vision, glaucoma, cataracts, insulin shock, and diabetic nephropathy.

Prameha is a metabolic disorder, but if you manage the doshas you can control the pathogenesis. Find out the person's prakruti, vikruti, and the organs involved. When making an herbal formula, keep in mind that it has to be dosha pratyanika (specific to the doshas involved), vyādhi pratyanika (specific to the disease), and *dhātu poshaka* (supportive to the tissues).

Physical exercise is very important for improving circulation, glucose utilization, and agni. Diabetes patients can take part in athletics and high-level activities, although insulin-dependent diabetics should not do intense exercise.

Yoga postures can also help, particularly the camel, cobra, boat, bow and peacock poses. (see yoga poses in Appendix page 450) Ujjāyi prānāyāma, *udara bandha* (abdominal lock), *nauli* (an abdominal intestinal movement that massages the pancreas), and alternate nostril breathing with retention of the in-breath are all effective for most types of diabetes. These should all be learned from an experienced yoga instructor and done gently.

Doing panchakarma for five or seven days a week can help prameha conditions immensely. In panchakarma, the client receives snehana (oleation) and svedana (sweating therapy), which help to bring the doshas stuck in the tissues back to the gastrointestinal tract. If it is vāta type of prameha, do basti (medicated enema); for pitta type, virechana (purgation); and for kapha type, do vamana (vomiting therapy). Vamana can be very helpful in certain kinds of kapha prameha, especially diabetes insipidus. The uvula is connected to the pineal gland, so if you drink a cup of licorice tea and then rub the tongue to create a gag reflex, this induces vomiting, thereby releasing vasopressin and anti-diuretic hormones from the posterior pituitary.

One of the therapies used in panchakarma is shirodhāra. It consists of pouring a constant flow of warm oil onto the forehead area, on the third eye. Use a mix of base oil and jatamāmsi oil for vāta, brahmī oil for pitta or vacha oil for kapha. Pouring these medicated oils onto the forehead creates a situation where the head is surrounded by warm oil, which is similar to a baby being surrounded by the amniotic fluid inside the mother's womb. This calms the nervous system and helps to rebalance the doshas. Shirodhāra directly helps patients of diabetes insipidus by acting on the cerebral kloma to rebalance the hormones.

When the body receives oil during abhyanga massage and shirodhāra, the oil penetrates through the skin and into the fascia and affects the nerve endings, stimulating the secretion of hormones, neurotransmitters and neurological peptides, including acetylcholine and serotonin. Neurotransmitters are the functional integration of tarpaka kapha, *sādhaka pitta* and prāna vāta. These subtypes of the doshas are responsible for maintaining optimal neurological and cerebral functions and play an important role in hormonal balance. Oil massage can improve communication in the nervous and glandular systems, thereby helping to address the cause of prameha. Shirodhāra also regulates the hormonal balance in the body.

After panchakarma, Ayurveda recommends rasāyana, or rejuvenation therapy. There are a number of good rejuvenative tonics for the pancreas, including shilājit, kutki, neem, gokshura, and karela (bitter gourd). In India, they make a cup out of wood from the jambul tree, put water in it overnight and then drink that water to regulate blood sugar. Licorice and manjishthā are two herbs that have a diuretic action, which is useful for kapha type of prameha. Note that although licorice is very sweet, it does not increase blood sugar.

Ayurveda believes that our bodily cells carry the memory of our parents' and grandparents' illnesses. This includes our glandular and nervous systems, which are part of majjā dhātu and therefore heavily involved in prameha. By treating majjā dhātu in the ways we have described, we can address these underlying genetic factors and manage diabetes.

Prameha or diabetes often has associated emotional factors, such as psychological trauma, abuse, depression, or deep-seated grief and sadness. Diabetes and depression often go together. If we manage the doshic imbalance that is responsible for these factors, there will be a radical improvement in the condition, both physically and mentally. Diabetes is often a chronic disorder, yet the patient can live a long, happy life.

# Chapter 10

# Celiac Disease with Reference to Grahani Roga

Spring 2009, Volume 21, Number 4

CELIAC DISEASE (ALSO CALLED CELIAC SPRUE) is a chronic intestinal malabsorption disorder. It is caused by intolerance to foods that are rich in gluten, or more specifically to gliadin and gliadin-like protein fractions in wheat, rye, barley and possibly oats. Most people call these gliadin and gliadin-like proteins gluten.

The word sprue comes from the Dutch word 'spruw,' which means mouth blisters. These were highlighted by the Dutch physician Vincent Ketelaer as a noticeable symptom of celiac disorders in 1669, almost three centuries before a reaction to gluten was found to be the cause of celiac disease. Note that tropical sprue is an infectious disease, due to bacterial infection. It is different from celiac disease and gluten sensitivity.

Ayurveda categorizes this disorder as being due to an imbalance of agni. Celiac disease falls under *grahani roga,* because *grahani* is the name for the small intestine. Grahani is the container, while agni is the content. If one is affected, the other is also bound to be disturbed.

The functional unit of the small intestine is the villus. The intestinal villi hold food molecules during the digestive process. If agni is strong, the villi are strong and healthy. They maintain their tone, coordination, and rhythmic movement, and correctly perform their actions in the process of digestion, absorption, and assimilation.

When there is agni imbalance, the functioning of the villi are affected and the person can get either gluten enteropathy or non-tropical celiac sprue. Any food substances that are heavy, fatty, and gross can suppress agni. Gluten is gross, heavy, sticky, dull, and oily in nature, so it can cause low agni and result in the production of āma.

According to Ayurveda, cellular agni maintains cellular intelligence and selectivity. In cases of a chronic agni disorder, the bodily cells lose their intelligence, which affects their selectivity. These cells react to gliadin molecules as if they are a bacteria or virus.

Gliadin acts as an antigen. To fight with this antigen, the cells of the intestinal mucous membrane produce antibodies, creating an immune reaction. The aggregation of killer T lymphocytes attacks the neighboring mucous membrane, causing mucosal damage and loss of some of the villi. This leads to poor assimilation and malabsorption of foodstuff. The affected person typically has low iron levels, malabsorption of fat-soluble vitamins A, D, E and K, and possibly dehydration. If gluten is removed from the diet, the patient's health can show noticeable improvement.

After someone with celiac disease eats wheat or another gluten-containing grain, the food enters the small intestine and, once it reaches the jejunum, antibodies in the intestinal wall are stimulated. These antibodies destroy the villi. This is one theory behind celiac disease.

The other theory is that due to a chronic agni imbalance, the undigested gluten acts like a toxin (āma). This āma clogs the channels of the villi and creates a thick coating of toxic matter over the intestinal mucosa, resulting in malabsorption.

Irritable bowel syndrome (IBS) is another form of grahani roga, producing abdominal pain when passing stools as well as bloating, gas, abdominal distension, mucous in stools, and episodes of alternating diarrhea and constipation. More women are affected by this condition than men and there is no weight loss. In IBS, the symptoms disappear when the patient is asleep. This is partly because IBS is sometimes related to a history of sexual or physical abuse. In sprue syndrome or celiac disease, there is usually weight loss and the symptoms are always present.

## Diagnosis

Various tests can be performed to determine if someone has celiac disease. A biopsy has historically been the main diagnostic tool. Blood tests taken after eating wheat or other gluten foods can reveal if there is a reaction to gluten as well as whether there are low levels of minerals, vitamins and other nutrients. However, not everyone with gluten intolerance has celiac disease.

The only way to tell if you have celiac sprue is through biopsy and laboratory tests. It is important to rule out other causes of nutritional deficiencies, so consult with a gastroenterologist if you want an accurate analysis.

Ayurveda uses examination of the intestinal pulse to discern whether someone has celiac disease or gluten sensitivity. If the intestinal pulse is extremely feeble, it may mean celiac disease; whereas if it is strong, it can indicate food sensitivity.

Celiac disease has hereditary factors. In certain families, the family members carry a low agni disorder from one generation to another. The affected children may be born with a khavaigunya (defective space) in the small intestine. In such cases, these individuals can often develop gluten sensitivity and may have a genetic predisposition to celiac disease.

## Diagnosis

People with northwestern European ancestry are most often affected by celiac disease. It equally affects men and women. Ayurveda says that pitta and kapha types mainly get this disorder: either pitta predominant and kapha secondary, or kapha predominant and pitta secondary.

In terms of vikruti, celiac disease can involve all three doshas. Either increased vāta suppresses agni by its cold quality, aggravated pitta disturbs agni due to its liquid quality, or increased kapha suppresses agni by its heavy and dull qualities.

In vāta celiac disease, there is more atrophy of the villi, causing pain, bloating, gas, and hyper-peristalsis. The person commonly feels fear and anxiety, and suffers from insomnia. Pitta type of celiac disease causes significant inflammation, leading to burning, pulling, and sucking sensations in the intestines. It often produces rashes, urticaria, and irritability. Kapha celiac disease features clogged and hypertrophied villi, smooth intestinal walls and bulky, pale, fatty stools (steatorrhea). The person may have feelings of heaviness, dullness, sleepiness, and depression. This Ayurvedic symptomatology gives us a clear picture of the various types of celiac disorder.

**Children.** The general signs and symptoms of celiac disease can begin in children during infancy, when the child starts to eat cereals or other foods with gluten. The affected baby or child does not thrive and may cry after eating because of painful gas and bloating. The baby may pass pale, foul-smelling, bulky stools and he or she might have abdominal distension.

Malabsorption of iron and other minerals can cause to the child to look pale. Poor protein absorption can result in edema (swelling). The child will be underweight, with stunted growth and little fat on the body, and there may be bony deformity. These babies don't sleep soundly and awaken at night crying, due to abdominal gas.

Children tend to develop celiac symptoms during the fourth to sixth month after eating cereals. If there is a family history of celiac disease, one has to take great care with the children's diet. Be very careful about feeding gluten-containing foods to these children. A gluten-free, anti-doshic diet should be given at the first sign of symptoms. Basmati rice and mung dal kitchari are great alternatives to the gluten-containing grains.

**Adults.** In adults, the signs and symptoms are similar to those in children. Common symptoms include:

- Bulky, fatty, foul-smelling stools that sink
- Weight loss
- Diarrhea
- Malnutrition (vitamin and mineral deficiency)
- Paleness
- Anemia
- Fatigue
- Headaches
- Aches and pains in the bones
- Epigastric fullness or abdominal distension
- Mouth blisters

- Burping
- Pricking pain
- Tingling sensations or numbness in the hands or feet
- Untimely cessation of menstruation
- Mood changes
- Atrophy of the intestinal villi
- A biopsy will show no villi or damaged villi, and a disorganized network of blood vessels.

## Management by Following a Gluten-Free Diet

The treatments for celiac disease can also be used to manage other gluten intolerance disorders. The main line of management is a gluten-free diet.

This means no wheat, rye, or barley, and possibly also no oats. Refer to a dietician for a full list of foods to avoid. It includes no hamburgers, hot dogs, or sausages, which often contain gluten fillers. The person should also avoid candy bars, baked goods, ice cream, and canned foods, because these contain ingredients that slow down agni.

Eat a healthy diet that is relatively high in calories and protein and low in fat. Most celiac patients do not digest fat very well. Ghee is an exception because it kindles agni, promotes ojas, and calms down immune reactions.

The best foods are basmati rice, mung dal, quinoa, blue corn, millet, and buckwheat as well as vegetables such as broccoli, asparagus, zucchini, lettuce, sprouts, leafy greens, Jerusalem artichoke, bitter melon, gourd, and banana flower. The best fruits are berries and pomegranate. Avoid dairy products other than ghee and *takra* (buttermilk). End each meal with a glass of takra with a pinch of cumin powder.

The Ayurvedic approach to management of celiac disease is basic, fundamental, and radical. Determine the client's prakruti and vikruti, i.e., which dosha is out of balance. Then give dīpana and pāchana chikitsā to kindle agni and eliminate āma. For dīpana, give trikatu (ginger, black pepper, long pepper). Then as pāchana, give the person chitrak, fennel, cumin, and takra (buttermilk).

**For vāta-type sprue syndrome**

| | |
|---|---|
| Dashamūla | 500 mg |
| Ashvagandhā | 400 mg |
| Trikatu | 200 mg |
| Sanjīvanī | 200 mg[24] (to digest āma and fat in the stools) |

Give ½ teaspoon of this mixture TID with warm water.

Additionally, one teaspoon of ashvagandhā ghee should be taken during each meal.

Finally, the person can take ½ teaspoon of sat isabgol with a cup of warm water at night.

---

24. Can substitute kutaja (*Holarrhena antidysenterica*).

**For pitta-type sprue syndrome**

| | |
|---|---|
| Shatāvarī | 500 mg |
| Gulvel Sattva | 400 mg |
| Kāma dudhā | 200 mg |
| Kutaja | 200 mg, when there is diarrhea |

Give ½ teaspoon of this mixture TID with 1/3 cup of cranberry juice.

T.I.D. = from the Latin means *ter in diem*, three times a day

Take one teaspoon of shatāvarī ghee or bitter ghee (tikta grihta) during each meal.

**For kapha-type sprue syndrome**

| | |
|---|---|
| Punarnavā | 500 mg |
| Yashthi madhu (licorice) | 300 mg |
| Trikatu | 200 mg |
| Chitrak | 200 mg |

Give ½ teaspoon of this mixture TID with honey and/or hot water.

The person should also take one teaspoon of licorice ghee or bitter ghee (tikta grihta) during each meal.

# General Management

For all celiac or sprue patients, an herbal tea made of equal parts of coriander, cumin, fennel, khus, ginger, and bilva is effective as dīpana and pāchana. This is called *dhanyaka-dhi kashayam* and it is useful for kindling agni.

Once the sprue symptoms are under control, the person should undertake panchakarma treatment. Vamana is good for kapha type of sprue syndrome, virechana for pitta type of celiac disorder, and basti for vāta type.

Get plenty of rest by going to bed early. Avoid heavy exercise, such as weightlifting and jogging, as this will further aggravate vāta. Yoga is very beneficial, including camel, cow, cobra, boat, bow and bridge poses as well as leg lifts. (see yoga poses in Appendix page 450) Anuloma-viloma, kapāla bhāti, and ujjāyi prānāyāma are also helpful when done under the guidance of an expert.

In old people particularly, grahani can be very difficult to cure, and it can lead to complications. Common complications that result from celiac disease or severe gluten intolerance include:

* Vāta type: malabsorption, weight loss, irritable bowel syndrome, degenerative arthritis
* Pitta type: rashes and skin disorders, gout
* Kapha type: diabetes, edema, steatorrhea and multiple lipoma

In severe cases, corticosteroid drugs are recommended to reduce inflammation and manage the symptoms. However, these medicines can produce many adverse side effects. Ayurveda traditionally recommended the use of licorice or licorice ghee as an alternative to synthetic steroid therapy.

## Prognosis

Celiac disease can be helped by dietary therapy that is further supported by herbal programs, panchakarma, and rasāyana. The best rasāyana for grahani is parpati, a medical preparation of mercury and sulphur as well as various herbs. However, these compounds are not allowed in the West.

This ailment is usually completely treatable through an Ayurvedic protocol. The prognosis is good for most patients, especially if young, with only a few exceptions. Recovery can be dramatic in children, whereas in severe, chronic cases, a complete return to normal intestinal functions can take months or years. Then again, it may never fully resolve in some cases. Success in treatment depends upon restoring the strength of the person's agni.

# Chapter 11

# An Ayurvedic Perspective on Allergies
## Asātmya

Summer 2002, Volume 15, Number 1

ALLERGY AND INTOLERANCE are explained in the Ayurvedic literature as the concept of *asātmya*. *"Aushadha anna viharanam upayogam sukhavaham sahi satmyam"* is an ancient Ayurvedic phrase saying that *sātmya* is when a person's doshas accept and adjust to medicines, dietary, and environmental changes. Sātmya means tolerance. Asātmya, or intolerance, is when one or more doshas do not accept these things and they react, often as an allergy. Intolerance and allergy are conditions of hypersensitivity, a reaction of one or more doshas to a causative factor. The root cause is imbalanced agni.

Sātmya is natural tissue tolerance, or specific immune response. The two most significant factors determining one's resistance to infection and allergy are agni (metabolic fire) and the specific qualities of a person's prakruti. Agni maintains our natural resistance and immunity by producing balanced ojas, tejas, and prāna, which destroy or neutralize any invaders. Certain specific immune responses may produce unpleasant and sometimes very severe hypersensitivity (allergic reactions). The substance (either food or medicine) may be eaten, inhaled, or brought into contact with the skin and cause the individual to develop a reaction or allergy.

Each dhātu agni in the human body regulates the physiological functions of its particular tissue. The elemental components of cells—ether, air, fire, water, earth—govern the structural aspects of the cells, while their derivative doshas—vāta, pitta, kapha—organize and govern the functional activities of the cells and intercellular communication.

When bacteria or toxic substances invade the tissues, prāna promotes the secretion of ojas and tejas in the cells. These three subtle energies move to the affected region and either destroy the bacteria or neutralize the toxins with the help of the respective dhātu agni. Ojas is the essence of all tissues and it plays a primary role in maintaining immunity. It is derived from kapha molecules, but it functions along with tejas and prāna. If the dhātu agni is inadequate, the invading substance may damage the cells and produce toxic material, called āma. This āma affects the doshas according to the characteristics of the invading substance and the individual's constitution.

Each of the three doshas interacts with āma to produce local or general reactions of a vāta, pitta, or kapha nature. The substances that produce these reactions are called allergens. The form an allergy takes depends upon the specific type of allergen and the aggravated dosha (vāta, pitta, or kapha).

Circulating throughout the body in the bloodstream are molecules of vāta, pitta and kapha, proportionate to the ratio of the doshas in a person's prakruti and vikruti. An allergen may be absorbed into the bloodstream and come into contact with these doshic molecules. If *rasa* or *rakta agni* is low, the doshas will react to the allergen, depending upon the strength and qualities of the allergen. This is called *dosha rūpa,* which is the doshic reaction of the allergy.

The factors that determine whether or not there is an allergic reaction and its severity are:

- Prakruti dosha (the amount of any dosha at conception)
- Vikruti dosha (current state of a dosha)
- Dhātu agni
- Quantity of allergen that enters the body

An important point is that the dosha rūpa of a prakruti dosha will create a mild allergic reaction, while the dosha rūpa of vikruti doshas creates severe allergic reactions. For instance, suppose two people have weak rasa dhātu agni and they get exposed to a moderate amount of kapha-type pollen. If person A has balanced kapha, he or she will have no reaction or only a mild reaction to the allergen. If person B has high kapha, he or she will have a much more severe reaction, possibly even going into anaphylactic shock if exposed to a large quantity of the substance.

- It is the production of toxins (āma) due to poor agni that causes an allergy. There are four types of āma that can be produced:
  1. *Rasa āma* – from unprocessed āhāra rasa
  2. *Mala āma* – from improper elimination
  3. *Āma dosha* – from imbalanced doshas in the $3_{rd}$ stage of pathogenesis onwards
  4. *Mano āma* – mental toxins from unprocessed, unresolved, and suppressed emotions. It is due to low sādhaka agni and it reduces clarity.

All occur only if there is low agni in that particular process. Hence, if there is *dosha dushti* (qualitative disturbance of a dosha) but strong agni, there will be no āma, just nirāma (no āma) doshic disturbance.

Note that a person with strong and robust dhātu agni will generally not have an allergic reaction at all, even if there is vikruti dosha. The only exception is if the person is exposed to a huge amount of the particular allergen and it overwhelms the dhātu agni.

## The Role of the Thymus and Spleen in Asātmya

Agni is the first protective barrier against allergens. When foreign organisms or allergens invade the tissues, the bodily cells often respond by releasing substances that cause local blood vessels to dilate and become more permeable. The cell membrane actually secretes an irritant chemical substance that is toxic to the body, a type of āma. This is due to low agni in those particular cells.

These substances that are released are a manifestation of tejas. As they are produced, the tissues become reddened, leaking excess fluids into the interstitial space due to the local reaction of pitta. The swelling produced by pitta is an allergic, inflammatory reaction that is a protective barrier to delay the spread of the invading allergen or microorganism into other tissues.

At the same time, ojas liberates more kapha molecules at the site of the lesion. Thus, ojas and tejas act together to detoxify the foreign substances that enter the tissues through the lungs or intestinal tract. In this defense mechanism, the thymus and spleen play an important role.

The thymus is a soft, bi-lobed gland located in the chest in front of the heart, behind the upper part of the sternum and just above the pericardium. In Ayurvedic texts, this gland is called jatru granthi. It is a predominately kapha gland, located in the kapha site of the chest and is relatively large in children during kapha age. After puberty, it tends to decrease in size and in adult years it may be quite small. The agni of this gland helps to produce ojas, which includes T-lymphocytes that either destroy a bacteria or virus or neutralize toxins. Weakness of this gland may be one of the causes of allergies and can be detected as low energy at the pericardial pulse level.

> **THE ROLE OF OJAS IN ASATMYA**
>
> | | |
> |---|---|
> | Ojovisramsa | Mild allergies |
> | Ojovyapata | Moderate allergies |
> | Ojokshaya | Severe allergies |
>
> Allergy is the great effort of ojas to reach the heart. In ojo visramsa, a normal amount of allergen only causes a mild reaction, whereas in ojo kshaya the same amount of the allergenic substance can cause a more severe reaction. However even in ojo visramsa, a very strong allergen may not allow the processed ojas to stabilize in the heart. This causes very severe allergies and even anaphylactic shock. Hence the emphasis in Ayurveda to protect ojas at all costs. This is accomplished through proper lifestyle and appropriate use of rasāyana.

The spleen, an organ made up largely of lymphoid tissue and located in the upper left portion of the abdominal cavity, is called *plīhā* in Sanskrit. Its role is to remove bacteria from the blood. The spleen lies beneath the diaphragm and a little behind the stomach. It is the root of rakta vaha srotas (the hematopoietic system) and is filled with rakta (blood) and rañjaka pitta. It acts as a blood reservoir and stores and filters blood.

Embryologically, the spleen produces red blood cells, but in an adult that function is transferred to the bone marrow. The subtle molecules of rañjaka pitta present in the spleen destroy foreign particles and microorganisms. A defective spleen can cause depleted immunity and such individuals may be prone to allergies.

## Assessment of Asātmya (Allergies and Intolerances)

Atopic allergy is defined as a tendency for hypersensitivity to a specific allergen that is inherited as part of the person's genetic predisposition. This khavaigunya (weak or defective space) can also be due to childhood trauma and suppressed or unresolved emotional issues accumulated into the organs.

Repressed emotions—such as anxiety, fear, or anger—produce stress. This stimulates the secretion of toxins in the body. Repressed fear, anxiety, and insecurity aggravate vāta dosha. Repressed anger, hate, and envy aggravate pitta dosha. Repressed greed, possessiveness, and attachment aggravate kapha dosha. Meditation, breathing exercises (prānāyāma), and stress management are particularly effective in minimizing allergies due to repressed emotions.

Ayurveda places emphasis upon clinical observation of the signs and symptoms of allergy. The pulse, tongue, nails, skin, heart and lung sounds and other bodily systems are examined thoroughly. The prior health of the individual as well as the family history must be taken into account along with the present problem. The person is carefully observed in order to assess prakruti (constitution) and vikruti (the doshic imbalance, which in this case is the type of allergy).

Vāta type of allergy is due to vishama agni (irregular digestion), causing gas, bloating, distention, discomfort, and breathlessness. It may create headaches, arthritic changes, sciatica, or hemorrhoids. Pitta type is due to tīkshna agni (sharp digestion), which causes sudden symptoms such as stomach ache, diarrhea, nausea, vomiting, hives, rashes, urticaria, eczema, or psoriasis. Kapha type of allergy is due to manda agni (slow digestion) and results in hay fever, cold, congestion, cough, wheezing, or asthma.

## Chikitsā (Treatment)

_Nidāna parivarjanam_ means to avoid the cause. If we know the most common allergens, we should teach the client how to identify them and thereby eliminate the causative factors. These can include household sprays and cleaners, fabrics, animals, and foods. However, depending upon the specific nature of the allergic reaction, this may not always be possible. Hence, a comprehensive approach to treatment along doshic lines is needed.

Modern medicine treats allergies with antihistamines and steroids, but this is best used to handle acute emergencies. Certain Ayurvedic herbs contain natural antihistamines and steroids. These include ashvagandhā, shatāvarī, and licorice (yashthi madhu), which are good for vāta, pitta, and kapha respectively as well as aloe vera, cilantro, hibiscus, and tikta ghee.

The Ayurvedic approach falls under two categories of chikitsā:
- Shamana – palliative therapy for acute phase of allergies
- Shodana – detoxification program (including panchakarma) to remove doshic causes of allergies. Panchakarma is only done once the acute symptoms are under control.

## Panchakarma and Allergies

Vāta from the colon, pitta from the small intestines and kapha from the stomach, can all undergo accumulation, provocation, and then spread (prasara). During the prasara stage, the dosha moves into the rasa and rakta dhātus. Longstanding, lingering doshas in rasa-rakta cause sensitivity to allergens.

By doing snehana (oleation), svedana (sudation), and massage according to the doshic type, the dosha moves back from rasa and rakta dhātus to its site. One can see this clinically and feel it in the pulse. Once the dosha has returned home, it can be eliminated by panchakarma (the five actions):

* Basti (medicated enema) for vāta
* Virechana (purgation) for pitta
* Vamana (therapeutic vomiting therapy) for kapha
* Rakta moksha (blood-letting) for blood cleansing
* Nasya (nasal administration) to remove the residual doshas

During this process, the person eats a cleansing mono-diet such as kitchari and drinks herbal teas in accordance with his or her constitution. Panchakarma should be carried out under the supervision of an experienced Ayurvedic physician or technician. It helps to detoxify the body and build the resistance of the tissues by gradually rebalancing agni. Panchakarma is also very helpful in stress management and accelerates the natural healing processes.

Panchakarma helps to eradicate the internal causes of allergies, so that there will not be any future recurrence. A proper rasāyana according to the person's prakruti and vikruti is also important following panchakarma.

### Rejuvenation Program (Rasāyana)

Ayurveda teaches the art of rebuilding and revitalizing tissues through proper lifestyle, diet, herbs, yoga, and meditation. When a subject is suffering from allergies, it is said to be the weeping cry of the tissues to change one's lifestyle, diet, and habits and thereby bring clarity and compassion to relationships. Allergy is nature's demand for physical, mental, and emotional cleansing through radical change.

Harītakī is a specific rasāyana for vāta type allergies, āmalakī for pitta allergies, and bibhītakī for kapha allergies. The combination of all three is called triphalā, which is balancing for all three doshas. Triphalā is a natural antioxidant that removes free radicals and helps to maintain doshic balance by detoxifying cells, thereby increasing longevity. It is a good cellular food and actually rejuvenates the cell.

## Management of Kapha Type of Allergies

Kapha allergy results in rhinitis, colds, cough, nasal congestion, wheezing, sneezing, asthma, or edema. The person is often sensitive to milk and dairy products, wheat, red meat, and other kapha aggravating foods. It is better to avoid these things and follow a kapha pacifying diet. Certain herbal teas, like ginger, cinnamon and coriander, are very effective to pacify kapha dosha. Regular kapha-reducing yoga postures and prānāyāma are also advisable.

Finally, an effective herbal formula to minimize kapha type of asātmya is:

Sitopalādi        500 mg
Mahāsudarshan 300 mg
Licorice           300 mg
Pippalī            200 mg
Abhrak bhasma      200 mg
Take ½ teaspoon with warm water after meals.

Note: Kapha type of allergy can also cause increased white blood cell count, which may be associated with worms. If there is krumi (worms) add Vidanga 200 mg and Shardunikā 200 mg.

## Management of Pitta Type of Allergies

Pitta allergies result in hives, rashes, urticaria, dermatitis, eczema, psoriasis, diarrhea, nausea, vomiting, headache, inflammatory responses, or even severe anaphylactic shock. When a person eats pitta-aggravating foods such as peanuts, strawberries, bananas, citrus fruit, cranberries, eggs, garlic, onion, hot spicy foods, pork, yogurt, and hard cheeses, pitta allergies can occur. Insect bites, strong sunlight and exposure to heat may also be causes of pitta allergies. Environmental chemical sensitivity also falls under pitta-type of allergy. Susceptible individuals should avoid these influences and follow a pitta pacifying diet.

In the case of recurrent allergic dermatitis, eczema, or psoriasis, Ayurveda suggests rakta moksha (bloodletting). It can be performed by either the application of leeches at the site of the lesion, or by aspirating approximately 100 cc of blood from the vein. This kind of bloodletting can improve the detoxifying function of the spleen, as more phagocytes (kapha cells) are attracted to the site of the lesion. At the same time, fresh ojas and tejas molecules are released by the cells to help neutralize the toxins. Rakta moksha is very effective in pitta individuals, but it should be done under the supervision of a medical doctor.

Pitta type of allergy symptoms may be associated with anger, hate, and irritability. To reduce these stressful factors, it is beneficial to practice shītalī prānāyāma *or chandra bhedana* (inhaling through the left nostril and exhaling through the right). Deep, quiet meditation can also accelerate the healing process. A useful herbal formula for pitta type of asātmya is:

| | |
|---|---|
| Shatāvarī | 500 mg |
| Gudūchī or Gulvel Sattva | 300 mg |
| Kāma dudhā | 200 mg |

Take ½ teaspoon with warm water or cilantro juice after meals.

Note: Severe allergies and even anaphylactic shock are more common in pitta individuals with pitta type of asātmya. If a severe allergic reaction occurs and the subject needs antihistamines or steroids, a medical doctor should be consulted immediately.

## Management of Vāta Type of Allergies

People having vāta type allergies may be sensitive to vāta aggravating foods such as night-shades (potato, tomato, eggplant), beans, and certain dry or bitter foods and herbs. After eating these substances, they have symptoms such as gas, bloating, headache, muscle spasms, palpitations, insomnia, and nightmares. Emotionally, people with *vāta asātmya* experience anxiety, fear and insecurity and they may become hyperactive. It is best to avoid all these causes and to eat vāta reducing foods and follow a vāta-pacifying lifestyle.

An effective herbal formula for vāta asātmya is:

| | |
|---|---|
| Dashamūla | 500 mg |
| Yogarāja Guggulu | 300 mg |

Triphalā Guggulu    300 mg
Trikatu             200 mg

Take ½ teaspoon with warm water after meals.

# Remedies for Specific Types of Allergies
## Skin Allergies (Hives, Rashes, and Urticaria)

These are all pitta disorders. One simple remedy is cilantro juice. Take a bunch of fresh cilantro (coriander leaf), chop it into pieces, put into a blender, add a couple of teaspoons of water, blend it, strain it through cheesecloth, and collect the fresh juice. One to two teaspoons of cilantro juice TID, will take care of hives and rashes. You can also apply the pulp onto the skin.

A second remedy is to drink coconut water, which is cooling to pitta. Alternatively, burn a dried coconut (not in the shell) so that it turns black. This tarry black carbon accumulated on the surface of the burnt coconut is the best medicine for rashes and urticaria. Apply topically.

Take bitter ghee (tikta ghrita) or just plain ghee. Add a pinch of black pepper and apply the mixture topically on the rash or urticaria.

You can mix equal parts of sandalwood and turmeric with just enough water to make a paste. Apply that paste to affected areas of the skin.

A cooling yoga exercise called the Moon Salutation is very helpful.

Watermelon has two uses for skin allergies: eat the red part of the melon, then rub the white part onto the skin.

Finally, a cool shower or bath can help to reduce aggravated pitta in the skin.

## Respiratory Allergies

In respiratory allergies, the agni of the respiratory tract (prāna vaha srotas) is depleted. The chest and sinuses are main seats of kapha, so kapha-type of respiratory allergies are more common. Examples are cold, congestion, cough, sneezing and wheezing.

For these types of allergies, use vacha (calamus root) oil nasya to remove the mucus. Once the mucus or kapha dosha from the lungs, throat and sinuses is clear, you can definitely control much of the respiratory allergy. For elimination of kapha, one should drink flax seed tea. At night boil one teaspoon of flax seeds in a cup of water and drink it, the tea along with the seeds. That will eliminate mucus and help the respiratory allergy.

In vāta-type of asthma or wheezing, udāna vāyu and *prāna vāyu* are affected and there is narrowing of the bronchial trees causing wheezing.

Another good remedy is to drink a cup of licorice tea with ten drops of mahānārāyana oil mixed in thoroughly. To make licorice tea, boil one teaspoon of licorice powder in a cup of water. Take one sip of this tea every ten minutes as needed. Also rub mahānārāyana oil on the chest and apply heat (such as a hot water bottle) to the chest.

Hay fever is a kapha or pitta disorder, where individuals are hypersensitive to pollen, dust, and debris. There are two types of hay fever.

| Spring Type Hay Fever (Kapha) | Summer Type Hay Fever (Pitta) |
|---|---|
| Allergy to airborne pollens such as oak, juniper, elm, hickory. Produces sinus congestion, watering of eyes, catarrh, and coryza.<br>  Punarnavā 400 mg<br>  Ginger 200 mg<br>  Turmeric 200 mg<br>  Pippalī 200 mg<br>Take ½ teaspoon of this mixture TID, plus<br>  vacha oil nasya (nasal drops) | Allergy to airborne pollens such as grasses, sorrel, hay, ragweed, house dust, combined with excess heat. Produces sinus congestion, inflammation of upper respiratory lining, headache, bronchitis.<br>  Kāma Dudhā 200 mg<br>  Gulvel Sattva 200 mg<br>  Sudarshan 200 mg<br>  Moti Bhasma 200 mg<br>Take ½ teaspoon of this mixture TID with aloe gel,<br>  plus ghee nasya. |

## Food Allergies and Intolerance

Generally food intolerance directly results from disturbed digestive fire (agni). In vāta people, agni commonly becomes irregular and creates intolerance to vāta-provoking foods such as beans, chickpeas, raw vegetables, and nightshades (potato, tomato, eggplant). These all aggravate vāta, causing gas, bloating, stomachache, abdominal discomfort, burping, breathlessness, and pains. You may use triphalā guggulu and trikatu 200 mg of each. Take ½ teaspoon of this mixture TID with warm water.

When pitta affects agni, there is strong appetite but poor digestion, causing intolerance to pitta foods such as sour fruit, citrus fruit, cheese, yogurt, fermented food, and hot spicy food. These things aggravate pitta and result in acid indigestion, heartburn, nausea, vomiting, diarrhea, hives, rashes, and urticaria. A good formula is:

Shatāvarī     500 mg
Gulvel Sattva   300 mg
Mahāsudarshan 200 mg
Kāma Dudhā   200 mg
Also see the remedies for hives, rashes, and urticaria.

> T.I.D. = from the Latin means *ter in diem*, three times a day

If kapha slows down agni, immediately after eating the stomach becomes heavy and the person feels dull, sluggish, and sleepy. There is excessive mucus and it can cause kapha disorders such as cold, congestion, cough, asthma, obesity, hypertension and diabetes.

## General Management of Allergies

Once the acute phase of allergy is over, one should treat agni to prevent future recurrence. For vishama and manda agni, use agni tundi 200 mg, chitrak 200 mg, and trikatu 100 mg. Take ½ teaspoon of this mixture TID with honey. If agni tundi is unavailable, use agni tea or ginger tea. For contactant allergies, apply tikta ghrita, sandalwood paste, neem oil, and cilantro pulp. For injectant allergies, treat according to the doshas.

*Important:* If one has serious complications, such as asthma, laryngeal edema causing breathlessness or choking, anaphylactic shock, severe rash, or urticaria, then prompt medical attention should be sought.

# Chapter 12

# Bronchial Asthma
## Shvāsa

Fall 1993, Volume 6, Number 2

IN THE ANCIENT Ayurvedic literature, *shvāsa* (asthma) is considered a kapha disorder; hence, it may start in the kapha time of life: childhood. Early onset asthma is more common in males having a kapha prakruti or vikruti and those with kapha-type allergies from external sources. The male reproductive tissue, shukra has many kapha characteristics. These individuals prone to early asthma may have allergic rhinitis (acute stuffy nose), kapha-type eczema, or a family history of such conditions.

Late onset asthma is more common in females. The female reproductive tissue, ārtava, has mostly pitta characteristics. This kind of asthma is not necessarily caused by external allergens, but is triggered by the intrinsic cause of high pitta. The cause of the high pitta may be a pitta-provoking diet, which can cause bronchial constriction and inflammatory reaction within the respiratory passage.

Allergic asthma is triggered by allergens such as pollen, house dust, feathers, animal hair, and fungal spores. Food allergies may also become aggravating factors in some individuals. Kapha increasing food, such as wheat and dairy, may stimulate bronchial congestion leading to asthma. Much less frequently, similar effects may be produced by ingested allergens derived from foods such as fish, eggs, nuts, and yeast.

A third category of asthma involves vāta aggravating substances such as dust, tobacco smoke, dry weather, and emotional stress like grief, sadness, and fear. This type of asthma can also be triggered by strenuous exertion, sexual activities, or exposure to cold air. Incompatible food combinations such as milk with banana, meat with dairy, or melons with grain can also provoke an attack. These causative factors inhibit agni (the gastric fire) by producing āma (toxins), which eventually enter the respiratory track and cause a constriction of the respiratory passages.

## Samprāpti (Pathogenesis)

The general pathogenesis of asthma starts in the stomach. Owing to the etiological factors, kledaka kapha undergoes accumulation and provocation, and during the spreading stage it moves into the lungs. Kapha is heavy, cold, slimy, and unctuous in nature while prāna vāta has dry, cold, rough, and active attributes. Within the lungs, kledaka kapha and prāna vāta intermix and alter each other's qualities in the respiratory passage. Due to the dry, rough qualities of vāta, the kledaka kapha becomes sticky and thick and adheres to the walls of the bronchi, causing narrowing of the bronchial tubes. This leads to breathlessness or an asthmatic attack. The prāna becomes stagnated within the alveoli, causing diminished air entry. Because the kapha is heavy, it accumulates at the bottom of the lungs. The person with this kind of asthma feels better in a sitting position where she/he can breathe through the less congested upper parts of the lung. When the person lies down, kledaka kapha moves to the middle and upper parts of the lungs, and causes congestion in the entire lung, leading to more obstruction and difficulty breathing. This is why a person with asthma sits propped up with pillows and often craves hot drinks during attacks. The cold attributes of kapha and vāta create this craving for heat. Though panchakarma is the main line of treatment for asthma, one has to understand the strength and the stage of asthmatic attack. Panchakarma should be done when the strength of the person is good and kapha is well-provoked in the stomach. Massage warm oil gently into the chest and give a pint or two of licorice tea (made from chopped licorice root, one teaspoon per cup of water) or a salt-water solution (one teaspoon to a pint of water) and induce vomiting to eliminate the kapha. This often provides instantaneous relief.

Individuals with low energy are not healthy enough for panchakarma during an attack, and they need a gentler approach. But if a person is strong and kapha is provoked in the stomach during an attack (if this is the case, one will feel heaviness in the stomach and have excess salivation and nausea), drinking sip-by-sip a cup of hot licorice tea with 5 to 10 drops of mahānārāyana oil is advisable. This mixture liquefies the kledaka kapha. And, although not the goal of this treatment, the tea may also induce vomiting and eliminate some of the kapha, relieving the spasm of the bronchial tree and calming down the prāna vāta. The person usually feels better immediately.

Taking a mixture of sitopalādi 500 mg, trikatu 200 mg, punarnavā 400 mg, and abhrak bhasma 200 mg with one teaspoon of honey TID can be beneficial. This formula eliminates

**Shvāsa (bronchial asthma)** is characterized by sudden attacks of short, gasping breath accompanied by wheezing. This is due to narrowing of the bronchial tree caused by muscle spasms, mucosal swelling or thick, sticky secretions. The normal free movement of air is obstructed within the lungs. Gaseous exchange is hampered and the lungs get stagnated with carbon dioxide which causes undue stimulation of the respiratory center, profuse mucous secretion and an acute awareness of respiratory distress. During shallow expiration, air gets trapped in the lungs and can not be expelled, causing the breathlessness to be more marked. The narrowed bronchi can no longer allow the mucous to be cleared or thrown out by the act of coughing. In a severe, acute asthma attack the bronchi become obstructed by the accumulated tenacious secretion of mucous. This eventually leads to the sensation of tightness in the chest. Progressive alveolar hypo-ventilation (shallow breathing) results in a lack of sufficient oxygen in the blood, possibly culminating in cardiac arrest.

the pathogenesis of asthma from the stomach. Drinking a cup of flax seed tea at bedtime also eliminates the residual kapha from the stomach.

There is a specific management for each specific type of asthma in the Ayurvedic literature. To regulate the normal physiological functions of each srotas (channel), the human body utilizes a type of agni called *sroto agni*. In asthmatic conditions, the agni of prāna vaha srotas becomes low, which is why a person with asthma gets repeated attacks of wheezing and chest colds. In order to kindle this sroto agni, Ayurvedic literature suggests pippalī rasāyana (rejuvenative). Daily take 2 pinches of pippalī (long pepper) with a teaspoon of honey in the morning on an empty stomach. This will help to prevent future asthma attacks.

When the attack is over, the subject should follow the doshic regime properly, do *yoga āsanas,* prānāyāma, and get accurate advice from an experienced Ayurvedic physician.

# Chapter 13

# Urah Shūla
## Chest Pain

Spring 2005, Volume 17, Number 4

HERE WE PRESENT an understanding of the Ayurvedic approach to chest pain, called *urah shūla* in Sanskrit. However, before we study chest pain, we should understand the Ayurvedic concept of pain. *Shūla* means pain in the general sense, but there are synonyms that refer to specific types of pain. For instance, *rujā* means a dull aching pain, *vedana* is radiating pain, and *dukkha* is deep aching or excruciating pain. Pain may be a sign of infection, but there is also non-inflammatory pain, such as congestive pain, stagnation pain, and pain due to physical trauma or psychological factors.

A famous sūtra says: *'Nahi vāta drute shulam,'* which means there is no pain without disturbance of vāta dosha. Vāta is the active, dynamic force that is behind all psycho-physiological and pathological changes. One aspect of vāta dosha is prāna vāyu, which is the life force that governs inhalation and many subtle, mental functions. Udāna is the upward moving form of vāta that brings energy, vitality and memory, and regulates exhalation. Samāna is the subtype of vāta that creates appetite and directs the movements of the gastro-intestinal tract and the processes of digestion, absorption and assimilation of food-stuff. Apāna is located in the pelvic cavity and helps in the elimination of urine, feces and flatus. Finally, vyāna is the type of vāta that governs bodily circulation and movements of the joints. These five subtypes are different vectors of vāta dosha that bring changes in structure and function as related to the physiological activities of vāta. When vāta is *anuloma,* which means it has normal movement, it supports the bodily functions. However, if vāta gets blocked, it becomes *pratiloma* and this creates pain.

Both quantitative and qualitative changes of vāta dosha cause pain. Dry, light, cold, rough, subtle, mobile, clear, and astringent are the qualities of vāta. Any attribute that goes out of balance can create pain. For example, too much exposure to the dry quality can create pain. The opposite of dry is oily, so pain caused by excessive dryness can be decreased by an oil massage. Likewise, if vāta is exposed to extreme cold, that can also create pain. In such a case, the application of local heat will relieve that pain.

Pain is nothing but disturbed vāta dosha, but vāta can be disturbed by a blockage created by pitta, kapha, or āma (metabolic toxins). In all cases, the pain is due to vāta, but if pitta, kapha, or āma is involved, it can be categorized as pitta pain, kapha pain, or āma pain.

Vāta pain means no other dosha is primarily involved. It includes shifting, fluctuating, spasmodic, excruciating, or colicky pain. Vāta pain occurs more during dawn and dusk and it causes fear, anxiety, and insecurity. It is increased by movement and often relieved by the application of heat and oil as well as by rest.

Pitta pain is usually sharp and it can be burning, sucking, or pulling pain with tenderness, which is pain upon pressure. Pitta pain is present in cases of inflammation, ulceration, and even tissue perforation and it is more common during midday and midnight. For instance, a silent peptic ulcer may become violent at midnight. Pitta pain can create irritability, anger, and frustration, and it can be relieved by the application of a cold compress or cooling paste, such as sandalwood or khus.

Deep, dull aching indicates kapha-type of pain. A person can sleep with kapha pain, which manifests due to kapha disorders such as congestion, stagnation and swelling of the tissues. Dry massage, exercise, and other forms of movement can relieve kapha pain. Also helpful is the application of a dry paste, such as vacha powder or ginger powder.

When āma blocks vāta, it creates pain due to indigestion, constipation, and other forms of toxic build-up. Āma pain is aggravated during dawn and dusk, on cloudy days and when it snows. It is also increased by indigestion, constipation, and gas, whereas it can be relieved by fasting and by drinking hot herbal teas such as ginger, cinnamon, and cardamom with a pinch of rock salt. Dīpana and pāchana herbs, such as chitrak and trikatu, are helpful when there is pain due to āma.

## Pain and the Organs and Channels

Ayurveda talks a great deal about doshic pain, but pain is also related to the organs and bodily channels. One common area of pain is chest pain, which may be caused by any dosha and be related to any chest structure such as the heart, lungs, pleura, and intercostal muscles. I will discuss simple treatments for some of the disorders that cause chest pain. All herbal formulas listed below are recommended for use three times daily unless otherwise stated.

The first category of chest pain is pain related to disorders of the lungs and respiratory tract. Some chest pain worsens during inhalation, exhalation, coughing, sneezing, or yawning. This is related to the pleura. Pleuritic pain can be relieved by topical application of an herbal paste that will pacify the disturbed dosha.

Dry pleurisy (vāta) is best treated by the following formula:

| | |
|---|---|
| Dashamūla | 500 mg |
| Pushkaramūla | 400 mg |
| Tagara | 200 mg |

Local application of a turmeric poultice is also useful for dry pleurisy or even a poultice made of fine oatmeal cooked together with turmeric and mustard seeds. This gruel or porridge can be put on a clean cloth or handkerchief and applied topically.

Pitta type of pleuretic pain is pleuritis. It can be treated with:

| | |
|---|---|
| Shatāvarī | 500 mg |
| Gulvel Sattva | 400 mg |
| Pushkaramūla | 300 mg |
| Tagara | 200 mg |

If pleuritis is not treated effectively, it can become pleurisy with effusion, which is a kapha disorder. Mild pleuritic pain is usually accompanied by fever, breathlessness, and diminished air entry, and it can be confirmed by an x-ray. For treatment, give a mixture of:

| | |
|---|---|
| Sitopalādi | 500 mg |
| Punarnavā | 400 mg |
| Pushkaramūla | 200 mg |
| Abhrak Bhasma | 200 mg |

If the pain is severe and there is breathlessness, it is necessary to refer the patient for aspiration. However, the above formulation is suitable for general management of mild kapha-type pleuritic pain.

If there is pleural pain with high fever and tachycardia and the patient looks toxic, it indicates acute pneumonia. Don't treat that person at home. Refer them to a hospital because he or she will need antibiotics. When there is intercostal pain, diminished air entry, mouth breathing, and prominent sternocleiomastoid muscles, think about the possibility it is emphysema and advise the patient to seek expert advice. Finally, any time there is severe breathlessness, immediately send the person to a hospital for a full investigation.

The second category of chest pain is related to the chest wall, due to an injury, trauma, or physical hurt. If this is muscular pain, the intercostal muscles can become extremely painful. Intercostal muscular chest pain can be relieved by topical application of heat and the use of a lepa (paste), such as garlic paste or dashamūla paste. Alternatively, one can rub mahānārāyana oil onto the painful area. Additionally, the person can take shūlah' vati (analgesic compound) or shanka vati.

One relatively common injury that causes chest pain is a rib fracture, which gives rise to tenderness in that area and serial pain on breathing. With a fractured rib there will be a history of trauma and there is always a local tender spot. It may be either a recent fracture or an old fracture. If you press the sternum and the backbone together with two hands, the pain worsens with the pressure because the ruptured ends of the ribs actually rub together to create the pain. This is a simple but important clinical test for a fractured rib. Of course, you can also confirm the fracture with an x-ray. Strapping to immobilize the chest may be required for this condition.

During winter or in cold weather, costochondritis is a common cause of anterior pain in the second, third and fourth ribs, giving parasternal or retrosternal tenderness along the border of the sternum. This is a condition of *asthi gata vāta* and giving the following mixture can treat the pain:

| Kaishore Guggulu | 300 mg |
|---|---|
| Tagara | 200 mg |
| Pravāl Pañchāmrit | 200 mg |

Topically, one can apply dashanga lepa, darushatak lepa,[25] or mahānārāyana oil to the chest and place a hot water bottle on the area. This is a simple way to deal with costochondritis with parasternal tenderness.

When the chest is barrel-shaped with intercostal tenderness (along the intercostal muscles) and possibly retrosternal tenderness (behind the sternum) as well as diminished air entry, this is a book picture of emphysema, which is common in chronic smokers. One can give:

| Sitopalādi | 500 mg (for expectoration) |
|---|---|
| Tālīsādi | 400 mg (for decongestion) |
| Mahāsudarshan | 300 mg |
| Abhrak Bhasma | 200 mg |
| Pippalī | 200 mg |

Latākaranja lepa can also relieve the emphysema.

The next category of chest pain is pain in the lower right chest. This indicates an amoebic hepatic abscess, which is related to a liver abscess. Here, an ultrasound can rule out a liver disorder, such as hepatic abscess or cholecystitis. If an amoebic hepatic abscess is the cause, use a combination of Liv 52®, ārogya vardhini, and sūkshma triphalā. Sometimes the person has to be referred to a surgeon to open and drain the abscess.

If there is scarring from healed herpes, there may be post-herpetic pain. Even though the symptoms of herpes zoster have healed, it can leave reddish-brownish spots along the line of the intercostal nerve and cause chest pain. In that case, one has to use the following formula:

| Shatāvarī | 500 mg |
|---|---|
| Gudūchī or Gulvel Sattva | 300 mg |
| Tagara | 300 mg |
| Mahāsudarshan | 300 mg |
| Kāma Dudhā | 200 mg |

Additionally, one can apply a topical paste of sandalwood and turmeric, which are both pitta-soothing herbs.

Chest pain after a meal usually indicates indigestion and gas. However, it could be due to angina. (see cardiac conditions below)

Retrosternal pain that increases when swallowing food may be due to esophagitis or hiatus hernia. Esophagitis is a pitta disorder, so treat the condition with:

| Shatāvarī | 500 mg |
|---|---|
| Gulvel Sattva | 200 mg |

---

25. Contains, dāruharidrā, mustā, shunthi, red sandalwood, sandalwood, haridrā and other ingredients.

Shankha Bhasma        200 mg
Kāma Dudhā            200 mg

The same treatment can be used for hiatal hernia but you should also teach the client beneficial yoga exercises such as camel pose, cobra pose, and breathing with pressure on the epigastrium, so that the hernia pain is relieved during exhalation.

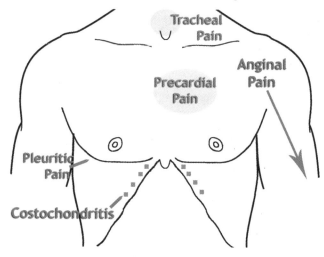

## Hrid Shūla (Cardiac Pain)

A number of disorders can be included in the final broad category of cardiac pain. A common form of cardiac pain is precardial pain (pain in front of heart area) that is usually centered a little to the left side of the chest. Pain may radiate down the left arm or up to the jaw.

If someone presents with cardiac pain, give first aid treatment as appropriate. If the cardiac pain is associated with sweating, restlessness, and falling blood pressure, one should suspect myocardial infarction. If it appears to be aggravated by exertion and relieved with rest, it is angina pain. If any cardiac pain does not subside, send the person to a doctor or hospital. One must take immediate action because a cardiac condition can damage the brain and the person may become unconscious.

Once any severe pain subsides or someone has taken care of an emergency, one can use this formula for cardiac chest pain:

Dashamūla          500 mg
Arjuna             300 mg
Abhrak Bhasma 200 mg
Shringa Bhasma 200 mg

The best paste is shringa shunthi lepa, which contains deer horn and dry ginger.

For anginal pain, Ayurvedic literature says to rub hema garbha and lakshmī vilas paste onto the tongue. Rub one hema garbha tablet on a sandstone in a circular motion for seven circles of about one-inch diameter, and then do the same for a lakshmī vilas tablet. Mix with just enough water to make a paste and rub it onto the person's tongue. That can immediately relieve angina pain.

Please note, chest pain that appears after a meal could be angina pain, it could be pain due to indigestion and gas, or it could even be cervical spondylosis. Pain in the neck area and jaw down to the chest, along with dizziness when the person looks up, indicates cervical spondylosis. When there is chest pain, a student of Ayurveda must bear in mind all these conditions. Do not take any chest pain lightly, as it may be an acute emergency.

In this chapter, we briefly examined the Ayurvedic understanding of pain and some common causes of chest pain. We also discussed some simple treatments that can be used to effectively ease the pain and manage the doshas, thereby treating the cause of the pain. This is beauty of Ayurvedic pain management.

**NOTE:** All herbal formulas should be given ½ teaspoon with warm water, three times daily unless otherwise stated.

## Table 4: Understanding Chest Pain

| Nature of Pain | Specific Symptoms | Condition |
|---|---|---|
| Retrosternal pain on left side (precardial pain) | Sweating, restlessness, falling blood pressure | Myocardial infarction |
| Retrosternal pain on left side, radiates down left arm or up to the jaw | Appears on exertion and reduces with rest | Angina |
| Severe unilateral chest pain while breathing, coughing, sneezing or yawning | Causes patient to support chest with palm; shallow breathing | Pleuritis |
| Pain when breathing, coughing, sneezing or yawning | Mild fever and breathlessness | Pleuritis with effusion |
| Pain when breathing, coughing, sneezing or yawning | High fever, tachycardia, toxins | Pneumonia |
| Intercostal pain | Diminished air entry, mouth breathing, and prominent sternocleidomastoid | Emphysema |
| Right side chest pain | Pain mainly in the lower right chest, tender liver | Amoebic hepatic abscess |
| Pain along margin of ribs | History of trauma | Rib fracture |
| Mid-sternal pain | Occurs when swallowing | Esophagitis or Hiatus hernia |
| Neck and jaw pain | Dizziness when looking upwards | Cervical spondylosis |

# Chapter 14

# The Heart

Fall 1996, Volume 9, Number 2

THE HEART IS a maternal muscular organ that contracts and relaxes regularly in order to receive and pump blood through the body. It is closely connected with thoughts, feelings and emotions and is the substratum of individual consciousness. The mental functions of love, devotion and intelligence are related to the heart. It is a vital organ, the abode of ojas and life. The Sanskrit word *hridayam* means the individual heart. Its three root syllables convey the meaning of the word quite significantly. *Hri* means to carry, to convey, to receive; *da* means to give, to donate and *yam* (pronounced yum) means to circulate or to distribute. The heart receives, donates and circulates blood and nutrients throughout the body.

The heart in the Ayurvedic literature is not only an anatomical organ but it includes the concepts of the heart *chakra,* represented by the cardiac plexus, and the heart as the seat of awareness, the substratum of consciousness and consequently the abode of mind. It is a maternal organ, as it is the site of ojas and prāna. It governs the functions of prāna vaha srotas—the system in the body for respiration and the flow

अर्थे दश महामूलाः समासक्ता महाफलाः।
महलार्थट्ट हदयं पर्यायै+च्यते बुधैः।
षडङ्गमङ्गं विज्ञानमिन्द्रियाण्यर्थपञ्चकम्।
आत्मा च सगुणट्टेतट्टिन्त्यं च द्यादि संट्टितम्।

*Ca. Su. 30, 3-4*

of intelligence—and rasa vaha srotas—the system in the body for nutrition and nourishment including blood plasma, the right chamber of the heart and the ten great vessels. The heart is the main reservoir of blood in the cardiovascular system and is essential in the distribution of rasa and rakta dhātus. In the heart, vyāna vāyu, sādhaka pitta, and *avalambaka kapha* express the feeling of self.

The sūtra above, from Charaka Samhita, is quite significant. In it Charak describes the six main parts of the body: the trunk, the four extremities, and the head. The center of these six divisions is the heart. The functional aspects of *buddhi* (intellect), *vijñānam* (specialized knowledge), and the senses are closely connected to the heart. In Sankhya's philosophy mahat is the principle of universal intelligence while, in Ayurveda, it is the individual's reasoning capacity or intellect, whose abode is the heart. Therefore, the heart is also called mahat.

Around the heart is a special membrane called the pericardium, which contains a fluid known as avalambaka kapha. Within the heart, a thin basement membrane, called the endocardium, secretes kapha to aid in the easy passage of blood nutrients throughout the body in order to protect and support all systemic kapha. Avalambaka kapha indirectly nourishes the doors of perceptions through the heart.

*serous fluid*

In the Charaka Samhita, the commentator goes on describing the heart as:

◆   a maternal organ
◆   the site of ojas
◆   the location of prāna
◆   the dwelling of vyāna
◆   the seat of sādhaka pitta
◆   the source of avalambaka kapha
◆   the root of rasa vaha srotas
◆   the beginning of prāna vaha srotas
◆   the reservoir of blood
◆   the center of consciousness
◆   the place of mind
◆   the seat of feelings and emotions
◆   the home of self

The ancient Vedic concept of heart is as a mystic lotus with twelve petals, each having its own seed sound, as shown in the picture on the cover. It is a seat of the god Shiva or Rudra. The heart is connected to the ten nādis, which are the five pairs of sensory pathways. These manifest psycho-physiologically as the five cognitive organs existing in pairs—two ears; two eyes; two nostrils; even the tongue is divided in half, the right and the left sides; and the tactile sense of the skin is also located on the right and left sides of the body. Anatomically, there are ten important blood vessels related to heart. The ten great vessels which carry the vital fluid ojas throughout the body are:

◆   the superior vena cava vein
◆   the inferior vena cava vein
◆   the aorta
◆   the right and left subclavian
◆   the right and left carotid artery
◆   the right and left brachial artery
◆   the coronary vessels

## Ojas and the Heart

These vessels carry ojas (the vital fluid) to individual dhātus (tissues) and to their respective cells to maintain the activities of life. On the subtle cellular level ojas acts as a fuel, where tejas transforms ojas into immunity in order to protect the life energy of cells, called prāna. The heat maintained by the heart acts as the radiant energy of tejas. The flow of life energy is prāna. Without this functional harmony between ojas, tejas, and prāna, the life of a creature is not possible.

The biological essence of all tissues is ojas, which is essential to male and female reproductive tissues. In each sperm and ovum, ojas, tejas, and prāna are present as the cell's basic essential material. These cellular principles are needed for fertilization and later they protect and help the growth of the fetus in the womb. Ojas coordinates the formation of the fetal heart during the third month of pregnancy. That is why the heart is considered the seat of ojas and ojas is the mother of the heart. As the pregnancy progresses, ojas continues to move back and forth from the mother's heart to the heart of fetus. Gradually, the baby begins to communicate to the mother through this flow of ojas. The child in the womb slowly expresses his or her likes and dislikes and this is reflected in the mother's cravings. Ayurveda says that it is quite important to satisfy the pregnant mother's desires at this time, because it will promote the baby's ojas, tejas, and prāna and help the child to develop a healthy heart. On the other hand, if the mother suppresses her cravings and doesn't satisfy her natural biological longings, it may affect the fetal heart and can cause congenital heart conditions.

There are two aspects of ojas. One is apara (raw and unprocessed) and other is para (processed and superfine). The processed and refined ojas is the sustainer of the life of a cell. If a living cell is removed from the body and put under a microscope, it will die in a minute or two because it does not receive ojas to maintain it's life functions. The life sustainer, para ojas, needs raw apara ojas to nourish it. That is why cells perish so quickly when removed from the body.

Superfine, processed ojas is the pure essence of all the tissues. It is formed in the body during the metabolic process. The ingested food undergoes the process of grosser digestion in the gastrointestinal tract due to gastric fire. Later, bhūta agni from the liver begins a more subtle process of digestion culminating in āhāra rasa, the food precursor for the tissues. This food precursor is the *maha phala,* referred to as the juicy fruit in the first line of the sūtra at the beginning of this article. The ten great vessels of the heart carry this maha phala, the fruit of food nutrients, into the six parts of the body—the head, trunk and four extremities. The fire component of individual tissues, called dhātu agni, creates the superfine ojas from the systemic raw ojas. This transformation is governed by the tejas of the individual cell and occurs during the further stages of cellular metabolism, called *pīlu pāka* and *pithara pāka.* The ultimate product of food nutrients after digestion, the pure essence, is ojas, which is a vital factor established in the heart.

## The Etiology of Heart Disorders

The Sanskrit word dhamanī is described in the sūtra as a pulsating, red-colored blood vessel—known today as an artery—that carries blood away from the heart. The word sirā is described as a non-pulsating, bluish-colored vein that carries blood toward the heart. The systemic ojas flows through arteries and veins with the help of vyāna vāyu and maintains the essential movement of life. Excessive worries, anxiety, and stress affect the normal flow of ojas. The ojas may be consumed too fast and weaken the heart. Ayurveda says that the causes of heart disease are overwork, excessive eating, overindulgence in sexual activities, intense grief, sadness, and biochemical stress. When the heart is stressed, ojas becomes depleted and gradually, or suddenly, an individual begins to have signs and symptoms of heart disease, depending upon the severity of the causative factors. Other pathological conditions such as obesity, diabetes, hypertension, and rheumatic conditions may affect the heart. Ayurveda talks about bacterial infections under *krumi hridroga* as one of the etiological factors of heart disease. Functional defects of rasa and rakta vaha srotas can be a major root cause. In spite of these elements, the constitutional doshic imbalance of vāta, pitta and/or kapha is the leading initial causative factor in heart conditions. Diet, lifestyle, genetic factors, and emotional reactions in daily relationships play an important role in many conditions of heart disease mentioned in Ayurvedic literature.

All symptoms can be classified according to vāta, pitta, and kapha. When vāta is predominant, there will be twisting pain, palpitation, breathlessness, and mental confusion. The individual experiences sleeplessness and doesn't tolerate loud noise. Anxiety, fear, and insecurity are the cardinal signs of imbalance in vāta subjects; while nausea, vomiting, fever, and syncope are due to pitta. The pitta individual may feel smoke-like heat in the heart and have profuse sweating and fever with dizzy spells. Increased kapha may be responsible for cough, swelling, dull pain and excess salivation. A sense of heaviness in the heart, anorexia, excessive sleep, and a cold and/or cough may manifest in kapha-type individuals. A sudden heart attack that comes and goes is vāta type. In connection with heart disease inflammation, fever and profuse sweating indicate a pitta type of heart condition. While slow, progressive congestive cardiac failure with edema belongs to kapha-type heart problems. Owing to the nature of causes, dual or triple symptoms may manifest. If the cause is worms, then the individual may get a throbbing, cutting pain in the heart with fever, anorexia, and cyanosis. Congenital mitral valve prolapse is a vāta-type heart disease as well as rheumatic valvular heart diseases.

### Samprāpti (Pathogenesis)

If there are causes that provoke vāta, then vāta from the colon undergoes sanchaya (accumulation), prakopa (aggravation) and prasara (spread), thereby entering into general circulation. If the heart has been weakened by the factors mentioned above, the circulating dosha finally lodges in the heart and produces vāta-type heart conditions indicated by one or more of the following symptoms: churning, pricking, or stabbing pain in the heart area, breathlessness, fear and cold sweat. On the other hand, if the causes are pitta-provoking, then pitta from the intestines undergoes the same changes of sanchaya, prakopa and prasara and lodges in the heart, producing typical pitta symptoms such as sharp, burning pains in the heart, nausea, vomiting ,and syncope. Kapha dosha, owing to its causative factors, also moves away from the stomach and enters the heart producing a sense of heaviness, tightness in the heart, anorexia, edema, or congestive heart failure. On entering the heart, these doshas affect ojas, tejas, and prāna within the heart. Initially the presence of the aggravated doshas in the heart creates functional changes and subsequently more serious structural changes.

The cardinal signs of heart disease are:

* *vaivarnya* – discoloration, cyanosis, due to poor circulation
* *mūrchā* – syncope, transient loss of consciousness, owing to sādhaka pitta disorder
* jvara – fever, due to the entry of pitta into the rasa dhātu

- *kāsa* – cough, congestion of prāna vaha srotas
- *hikkā* – hiccough, owing to ischemia of diaphragm
- *shvāsa* – breathlessness, prāna vata dysfunction
- *āsya vairasya* – perverted taste in the mouth, due to *bodhaka kapha* dysfunction
- *trushnā* – excess thirst owing to congestion of palate
- *pramoha* – mental confusion due to lack of prana to the brain
- *chhardi* – vomiting, pāchaka pitta disorder
- rujā – cardiac pain, congestion of heart muscles

## General Management

Even though heart disease is a serious condition, with the help of your cardiologist you can monitor your heart condition while using the Ayurvedic remedies that follow in a preventative manner.

Arjuna powder enhances the tone of the heart muscle.

Katukā powder improves coronary circulation.

Ashvagandhā helps to protects the ojas in the māmsa dhātu.

Punarnavā a mild diuretic that helps to regulate blood pressure.

Gudūchī is anti-inflammatory and anti-pyritic.

Shatāvarī is a general rejuvenative tonic for the heart muscle.

Triphalā is a colon cleanser and detoxifier.

Pippalī is a broncho dilator and relieves pulmonary congestion.

Shringa Bhasma is a specific cardiac tonic that improves the tone of the heart muscle, increases oxygenation of the heart and relieves cardiac ischemia.

Dashamūla is a general tonic for all bodily dhātus, but is specifically effective for calming vāta and reduces palpitations.

Lasuna (garlic) is used as a seasoning in the food, reduces cholesterol and has pain-killing properties.

Onion (cooked) is also used as a seasoning in the food and reduces heart rate, acting in a manner similar to digitalis.

Gold Water improves coronary vaso-dilation, coronary circulation, and protects the heart muscle from dying. It is made by boiling 24 carat gold (coin or your own jewelry) in 2 cups of water. Boil this down to one cup of liquid. Take 1 teaspoon every 15 minutes.

Yashthi Madhu is a decongestant, expectorant and helps ease breathing.

Yoga Postures: Sun Salutations (10 postures done in a specific order) is an ancient Vedic cardio-vascular exercise. One should gradually work up to repeating the cycle 12 times per day. Yoga postures increase the movement of prāna and help the processing of ojas by tejas into the protection of prāna. Every yoga posture has therapeutic value as it enhances tone, coordination and power of the muscles. Some that are helpful in cardiac conditions are: camel, cobra, cow, boat, bow, bridge, tree, triangle, and corpse poses.

*Mantra* meditation: Sound is energy and every cell has an affinity toward certain sounds. When one repeats a particular sound, the cell recognizes it and becomes harmonious. Cellular function becomes rhythmic, bringing a balance in the rhythm of the cell. To balance vāta, the mantra is *hrim,* pronounced "hreem." For pitta, *aim*—"I'm." For kapha, *klim*—"kleem." And for the heart chakra, *yam*—"yum."

Walking for ½ an hour is good cardio-vascular exercise. It helps to improve circulation, kindles fire and reduces cholesterol. It is an exercise that is mild enough for anyone to perform.

Rudrāksha beads have a spiritual energy to protect the heart chakra. They improve coronary circulation and give spiritual support to the patient of heart disease.

Rose Quartz bead necklaces improve warmth in the heart and are recommended for vāta- and kapha-type conditions.

Limited sexual activity decreases the wasting of vital fluid which is eliminated during the secretion of orgasmic fluid. This will indirectly protect one's ojas and prāna.

Herbal wines, like *drākshā,* kindle agni, performs vaso-dilation, improves circulation and is good for the heart. Take 4 teaspoons with an equal amount of warm water before meals.

Regular checkups with your doctor.

Chapter 15

# An Ayurvedic Perspective on Fevers
## Jvara Roga

Fall 1997, Volume 10, Number 2

THE CONCEPT OF FEVER in Ayurvedic literature is interesting. The Sanskrit quote, *"Jvara deha indriya manasa santapa"* means that fever is heat in the mind and senses as well as the physical rise of body temperature. *Deha* is the physical body; *indriya,* the senses; *manas,* the mind; and *santapa* means heat.

There is a wonderful Vedic story about fever. Lord Shiva was in deep meditation on Mount Kailas. There was a demon known as Tripurasura. *Tri* means three and *pura* means city, so his name refers to the 'three cities' of body, mind, and consciousness. This demon was destroying these cities and only Shiva could stop Tripurasura. But Shiva was in deep *samādhi,* a transcendental state of meditation. Who would disturb his samādhi? All the gods were worried. When Shiva is in samādhi, no one should disturb him. So the God of Love, Madana, said, "I will disturb the samādhi of Lord Shiva." By his magnetic power, Madana created a wonderful garden with birds, swans, a lake, lotus, peacocks, and beautiful fragrant flowers.

Then Madana started throwing arrows of flowers toward Lord Shiva. Symbolically, an arrow is an object of perception. Arrows of flowers are symbolically arrows of senses—sight, smell, sound, taste and touch. In other words, the God of Love was stimulating Shiva's senses while he was in a deep state of meditation. Shiva opened his third eye, the eye of wisdom, and fire came through it and burned Madana. Madana's wife, Rati, whose name means romance, came to Shiva and prayed, "Lord Shiva, you have killed my husband and I am now a widow." Lord Shiva, being full of mercy and compassion, looked at the ashes with intense love and Madana came back to life. The Fire God, who had been burning Madana, came out of his body and said to Shiva, "Where can I go now? You have created me through your third eye and my job is to burn. Where can I go?" Lord Shiva said, "Go to the earth and afflict those people who do not follow the laws of nature, the laws of health." Those laws of nature refer to following a daily and seasonal routine, eating a proper diet, and avoiding abuse of the senses. Those who do not follow these rules become ill.

Since then, fever has been on this planet. This is a mystic story, but it tells us the truth that fever happens to those who eat the wrong food, indulge in excessive physical activity, and otherwise burn their ojas. Fever also happens to those who are consumed by excessive sensual temptation, which burns the body's intelligence and immunity.

## The Stages of Fever

Anger, hate, envy, jealousy, and criticism provoke a kind of fire in the consciousness. This is a type of feverishness that affects the mind. According to Ayurveda, fever begins with judgment and criticism. For example, when you feel that your husband or wife is supportive of you, fever is absent. However, the moment you feel that your partner is confused or critical or that the relationship is not working in your favor, you become furious. That furiousness may become a physical fever. There is even a fever of love. When you fall in love and sing, "I'm crazy for you, I'm dying for you," it is a sort of fever. A newly married couple can get honeymoon urethritis or cervicitis and may even develop a fever called *kāma jvara*.

Before the rise of body temperature, the senses become agitated and then the mind gets confused. This confusion leads to improper food choices. For example, in the summer you may work all day in the hot sun and your body may become hot. Then if you come home and drink chilled water, it is a shock to the system. Ayurveda says to drink warm or room temperature water, even in summer. When you are hot from working outside, wait a bit before rushing to the refrigerator. Give your body time to cool down and then take a sip of room temperature water. People tend to drink cold fluids when the body is hot. This shock to the system affects agni and displaces ojas.

Consuming fluids in this way is similar in its effects to incompatible food combining, such as eating bananas with milk, yogurt with fruit, melon with grains, fruits with cheese or milk, and eating dairy products with meat. Such combinations affect agni and create āma (toxins). Then samāna vāyu pushes āma and pāchaka pitta (the gastric fire) out of the stomach into rasa dhātu and produces fever.

### Explanations of Fever: Modern and Ancient

Fever is a disease in itself, but it can also be the symptom of another disease. According to ancient Vedic science, the entry of dosha and āma into rasa dhātu creates fever. Whichever dosha goes into the rasa tissue will create a specific type of doshic fever.

According to Ayurveda, there are many kinds of fever, including continuous and interrupted fevers, such as when a person runs a fever every second or third day. Fever is classified as mono, dual or triple doshic—vāta, pitta or kapha type, or vāta-pitta, pitta-kapha, or kapha-vāta, or even vāta-pitta-kapha type of fever. Triple doshic fever can be compared with septicemia in modern medicine.

When fever is itself the disease, modern science calls it a fever of non-specific origin. In such cases, there is no septic infection in the body, urine and blood cultures are normal, and there is no strep throat. This fever of non-specific origin is called *jvara roga* in Ayurveda. It is caused simply by the entry of āma into rasa dhātu, the plasma-protein pathway. There is an origin, but it is different from that understood by the modern definition, which has a septic focus. According to modern medicine, fever is a sign of infection such

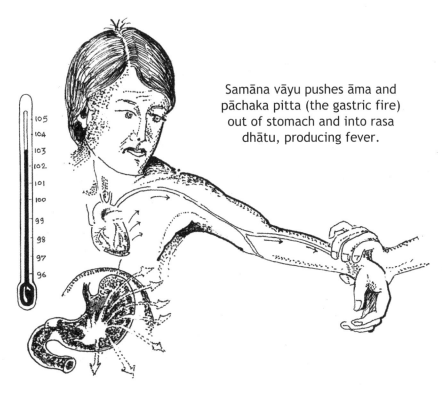

Samāna vāyu pushes āma and pāchaka pitta (the gastric fire) out of stomach and into rasa dhātu, producing fever.

as acute conditions of tonsillitis, pharyngitis, bronchitis, pneumonitis, hepatitis, cystitis, or meningitis.

Some people feel feverish but the thermometer doesn't show a rise of temperature. They are running an internal fever. This is called internal jvara. Such a person has the cardinal signs of fever—headache, bodyache, and malaise, but the skin is cool to the touch. According to the thermometer, there is no fever, but Ayurveda says the person has an internal fever.

How can there be internal fever without a rise of temperature? This condition causes a subjective feeling of feverishness, whereby the person may feel heat going out of the eyes or ears and even the breath becomes hot. The person *feels* on fire, but the external temperature is cool. In these cases, āma and pitta are moving in the sthāyi rasa dhātu, the fully processed rasa tissue. Some people have a burning sensation while passing urine without a clinical diagnosis of urethritis. That is also a symptom of internal fever. Internal fever creates canker sores, fever blisters, or aches and pain in the lymphatic system. When the samprāpti of fever affects mano vaha srotas, the mind becomes irritable, judgmental, critical, and even furious. This is a fever in the mind. There are people who have an internal fever but they do not know it. They continue to take fever suppressants, such as acetaminophen and aspirin, and the cause is never treated.

## Signs and Symptoms of Fever

Ayurveda says that kapha fever begins in the stomach, pitta fever starts in the small intestine, and vāta type in the colon. In a fever, the dosha undergoes sanchaya (accumulation), prakopa (provocation) and prasara (spread).[26] When the dosha goes into the second stage, prakopa, it will disturb agni, creating toxins. In the third stage, prasara, the dosha will push that āma into rasa dhātu and create fever.

During a fever there is no appetite, because jāthara agni is pushed into rasa dhātu and is no longer present in the stomach. This lack of fire in the stomach creates āma. However there is too much fire in rasa dhātu, which enters into mano vaha srotas, the mental channels, and causes fever in the mind. Mental fever can be due to incompatible food combining, wrong lifestyle and diet, and the application of extremes of hot and cold, such as a hot shower followed by cold shower. If it is vāta fever, the person experiences fear and anger together. Anger has the qualities of fire, while fear is vāta. If a person has a kapha fever, he or she experiences greed or attachment along with anger. Pure pitta fever is mainly anger and irritation.

In fever there is no sweating—except in pitta type of fever—because āma clogs *sveda vaha srotas,* the channels of perspiration. This āma also creates generalized bodyache. A function of rasa dhātu is nutrition. Because rasa dhātu is not functioning properly during a fever, there is poor cellular nutrition and the tissues suffer from lack of nourishment. When nutrition of the dhātus is affected, the body and the internal organs start aching. Even the hair aches, because āma in rasa affects the skin at the roots of the hair. These three signs must happen together: internal heat, lack of perspiration, and generalized bodyache. Then you can say that it is jvara. These cardinal signs of fever indicate that the dosha and āma are moving in rasa and looking for a place to stay.

## Prodromal Symptoms

Two of the symptoms of fever are low appetite and feverishness. What are the prodromal symptoms before a fever begins? The person feels exhausted and fatigued. He or she doesn't feel OK with his or her life or with anything. There is no charm in life. A smoker doesn't feel like smoking. A drinker doesn't feel like drinking. There is an aversion toward external sensory stimuli. If it is a vāta type of fever that is coming, the person's skin looks dark. If it is pitta type, the skin appears flushed. If kapha type, the skin is pale. This discoloration is because of āma moving in rasa dhātu. There is no sense of taste in the mouth, because taste comes from agni. The taste of food lies not only in the food but also in the quality of agni.

Frequent yawning and goosebumps also presage a vāta fever. Hot flashes, burning, and dizziness as well as a burning sensation in the eyes indicate a potential pitta fever. Chills, runny nose, and loss of appetite are present before kapha fever manifests. Apathy can lead to fever, as can too much sympathy. Intense crying and grief can also create a fever.

Another indication of fever is constant lacrimation or tears in the eyes. Those tears are hot at one moment and cold the next. At one moment the person wants food, while the next moment all desire to eat has gone. Or the person feels like watching TV and then loses that desire. At one moment the person feels chilled and sits by the fire, then the next moment he becomes hot and throws off the blankets. Or craves cold things, but the

---

26. See Table 1, "Gunas (Qualities) Relating to Each Stage of Samprāpti," on page 7.

moment he touches cold, he craves heat. In the prasara stage of āma, when toxins are circulating, these opposite symptoms occur. Some people can experience these prodromal symptoms of pūrva rūpa for a considerable period of time.

*Vāta Fever.* In vāta fever there is constipation, shivering, and a craving to be bundled in many blankets. There is also generalized bodyache, headache, ringing in the ears and muscle stiffness. The symptoms are similar to malaria. Vāta fever creates insomnia, anxiety, headache, muscle pain, and joint ache. Many times vāta fever is diagnosed as rheumatic fever. The pulse is fast and temperature is not that high, just 99.5 to 99.7 degrees Fahrenheit.

*Pitta Fever.* In a pitta type of fever, there is a high temperature of 102 to 103 degrees, bloodshot eyes, and temporal headache. The person is irritable and throws off the blankets. There is nausea, vomiting, nosebleed, and dark yellow urine. The body is hot. Some pitta prakruti children get convulsions when they have fever. There is photophobia and sometimes diarrhea or dysentery. In pitta fever there is sweating, but that sweat doesn't bring down the temperature.

*Kapha Fever.* Kapha fever is accompanied by a cold, congestion, and cough. The temperature is not that high and sleep is not a problem, because a person can sleep with a low-grade kapha fever. There is a runny nose, excess salivation and no appetite.

*Other Fevers.* Continuous fever is present in acute rheumatic fever, typhoid, septicemia, and tuberculosis. In typhoid, fluctuations of temperature are also present. In the morning there is a rise of temperature and in the evening the temperature comes down. Sometimes the high temperature appears twice, in the morning and evening, and the temperature comes down only during midday. This is typical of a vāta type of fever. The interruption is due to fluctuations of the dosha. Some people will have a fever on every second or third day.

## Fever in the Dhātus

Fever can go into each of the biological tissues, or dhātus: rasa (plasma), rakta (blood), māmsa (muscle), meda (fat and adipose), asthi (bone), majjā (bone marrow and nerve), and shukra/ārtava (male/ female reproductive). By studying the fifth level radial pulse you can find exactly where the fever is lodged.

*Rasa Dhātu.* When fever is in rasa dhātu, the person has kapha symptoms—heaviness in the heart, congestion in the lungs, generalized bodyache, and excess salivation. The by-product of rasa dhātu is stanya (lactation) and *rajah* (menstruation) and the waste product of rasa is kapha—hence, the kapha symptoms. When āma goes into rasa dhātu and creates fever, these symptoms appear. Even if the predominant dosha is vāta, the symptoms will be mainly kapha, although in that case, the rasa dhātu pulse will show a vāta spike. Rasa dhātu has kapha characteristics, so any dosha that goes into rasa dhātu during a fever creates kapha symptoms. However, in a vāta type fever there will be less congestion, in a pitta type more inflammation, and in kapha more congestion.

Palpitations and swelling in the heart or lungs are also common when fever goes into rasa dhātu. If it is vāta fever, there will be more palpitations. Pitta fever will create inflammation of the heart. If it is kapha fever, there will be pericardial effusion.

**Rakta Dhātu.** When rasa is strong, it will not allow āma or a dosha to enter. Then the āma and dosha will go to rakta, the next dhātu. If rakta dhātu agni is low, the āma will enter rakta and create the following symptoms: bleeding of the nose, mouth, stomach or lungs, vomiting with blood, dizziness, delirium, or hemorrhage under the skin. When fever goes into rakta vaha srotas, it creates bleeding. But in vāta, the bleeding is scanty and will be accompanied by clots and more palpitations, in pitta there is more bleeding and in kapha there is bleeding with mucus.

**Māmsa Dhātu.** If rakta dhātu agni is strong, then āma will go to māmsa dhātu. If māmsa dhātu agni is low, āma will lodge in māmsa and create *māmsa gata jvara,* which means fever in māmsa dhātu. This fever produces symptoms of bursitis, tendonitis, or fibromyocitis. Many people today have a form of fibromyocitis called fibromyalgia, inflammation of the muscle sheath. Individuals who take synthetic estrogen disturb their māmsa dhātu agni and may develop māmsa gata jvara or fibromyalgia. These people can also have acne, hives, rash, and boils.

**Meda Dhātu.** In *meda gata jvara* there is profuse, foul smelling sweat, dehydration, and pain in the kidneys or omentum, the fatty protective layer around the abdomen. This condition can create peritonitis, which indicates the fever has gone into meda dhātu.

**Asthi Dhātu.** If fever has gone into asthi dhātu, there will be pain in the joints and bones as well as hair loss. The nails become brittle and the person may lose teeth.

**Majjā Dhātu.** *Majjā gata jvara* leads to rigidity in the neck. Meningitis and encephalitis are serious problems of majjā gata jvara. The person gets headache, meningeal irritation, stiff jaw, and tightness in the neck; he or she may become irritable or even lose consciousness.

**Shukra/Ārtava Dhātu.** When fever goes into shukra dhātu, the person burns ojas and death is sure. Any fever can go into any of the dhātus and create serious complications. Therefore, don't take fever lightly, as it can become serious.

If a patient of fever comes to you, read the pulse and examine the patient. If the person shivers with cold, it is a vāta fever. The subject may subsequently have light bleeding of the nose, but with a little bit of clotting. At that point, the vāta fever has gone into rakta dhātu. If within three days, the subject gets pain in the muscles, the fever has gone into māmsa dhātu. If the person comes to you within the next four days with pain in the joints, the vāta fever has gone into asthi dhātu. This is the logical progression of an untreated vāta fever through the dhātus.

## The Role of Bacteria, Viruses, and Āma

The modern scientific approach says that bacteria or viruses induce disease. Ayurveda says if you eat incompatible foods until your tongue becomes heavily coated, then depending on your level of immunity, you may get a fever. If you really want to have a fever, eat banana milkshakes or fish with yogurt for a couple of weeks. The results depend upon your gastric fire, agni. Ayurveda also thinks along the same lines as Western medicine in this way. Western medicine posits that a bacteria or virus creates an infection, subsequently causing a fever. Ayurveda says that one cause of fever is bacteria and viruses, which create āma on the cellular level. That āma is circulated through rasa dhātu and creates fever.

If tubercular bacteria are introduced into a person's system, that person may not get pulmonary tuberculosis, but rather bone TB or some other type of TB. This is explained by the Ayurvedic concept of khavaigunya, defective space. If there is khavaigunya in the lungs, the person will get tuberculosis in the lungs. If it is in the knee joint, that person will get TB of the knee joint. What Ayurveda wants to convey is that fever is the entry of āma into the dhātu, not the direct result of bacteria or viruses.

# General Management

Whenever an individual has fever, the first treatment is fasting, *langhana*. If the person eats, that food will not be digested but will instead produce more āma and toxins. Whenever there is fever, starve it. The kapha person should take nothing by mouth. This is difficult for vāta and pitta people, who may become dehydrated. There is an herbal tea that induces swedana (sweating) and it can be drunk during langhana. Use equal proportions of ginger, lemongrass, tulsi, and fennel and steep this mixture in hot water for 10 to 15 minutes. The ginger will burn āma and kindle agni; lemongrass is diaphoretic and will promote sweating; tulsi is decongestant and anti-pyretic; and fennel stimulates pāchana, the burning of āma. Just by kindling agni and burning āma, the fever will come back to normal. This is a simple home remedy.

When a person has fever, it takes time to make the body work and regain balance. One should not just take aspirin to bring down the temperature. A person with fever should wait, rest, sleep, and bundle up with blankets. Give the above tea. There should be no reading, watching TV, or talking on the telephone.

Once the person passes an entire day without fever, give softly cooked rice water. Use two cups of water and only a handful of rice. Make a soft gruel, which will be easy to digest. That should be given when the person regains the urge to eat. Generally, a person with a kapha fever has no appetite. Pitta people may become hungry, because pitta is hot, sharp, and penetrating. Because of those qualities, pitta people have strong fever. They may also feel dizziness, nausea, and vomiting, and if these symptoms are present there is no urge to eat. Vāta people with fever have variable appetites.

## Specific Doshic Management

*Vāta Jvara.* For a vāta person you can use this herbal tea:

| | |
|---|---|
| Dashamūla | 500 mg |
| Sudarshan | 400 mg |
| Tagara | 300 mg (for headache) |

Put 1 teaspoon of this mixture in a cup of hot water, let it steep for 10 minutes and then drink it. For headache, put ginger or calamus root paste on the forehead. A nutmeg powder paste on the forehead is also helpful. Never do oleation (snehana) during fever.

A vāta type of fever subsides simply with rest. Cover the patient with two or three blankets and keep the room warm. Give hot herbal tea. For vāta fever, svedana can be more intense. Even under two or three blankets, a vāta person tends to shiver and feel cold.

These treatments are effective, but your diagnosis must be accurate. If you use the wrong tea, it could increase the temperature. Be cautious. Ayurveda is not simplistic; it requires understanding and knowledge of basic principles.

***Pitta Jvara.*** For pitta jvara give:

Gulvel Sattva    400 mg
Mahāsudarshan 400 mg
Kāma Dudhā    200 mg

Take 1 teaspoon, two or three times a day, with warm water, to pacify pitta. In a pitta fever, svedana should be gentle. The pitta subject should be in a closed warm room with dimmed lights, because a bright light will create a headache. Pitta people throw off the blankets because they are hot, but they should cover the body with something light, such as a cotton sheet. If pitta people have too high a fever, they can become delirious or have convulsions. To bring down temperature, sponge them with tepid rose or khus water. Or take white sandalwood powder, add a little cool water, make a paste and apply it to the forehead. Camphor can also be used if the person is not sensitive to it. Mix the camphor with some cool water, dip a cloth into that camphor water and put it on the forehead to bring down the temperature.

***Kapha Jvara.*** In the kapha type of jvara, there is a cold, congestion, cough, runny nose, postnasal drip and bronchial secretions with bronchitis or pneumonitis. For kapha fever, svedana can be more intense. For this condition you can use:

Sitopalādi        500 mg
Mahāsudarshan 300 mg
Abrak Bhasma  200 mg

Take ½ to 1 teaspoon of this mixture two or TID. When a person has bronchial congestion and secretion with a cough, you can use vāsaka, which acts like codeine, to sedate irritation of the cough center. Give ½ teaspoon TID.

Give the above treatments for four or five days. Fever from flu will come down within three days. If it is bronchitis, it must be treated for five to eight days. Pneumonia will take 10 days. It is a potentially serious condition and this formula should be used with the approval of your physician. For a child, use the same treatments, but with a smaller dose.

Influenza is a vāta and kapha disorder. You can use:
Sitopalādi        500 mg
Mahāsudarshan 400 mg
Tagara           300 mg

This combination brings down temperature and soothes body aches. Ideally, a person should not take a bath during a fever or flu. Taking a bath may make the lungs damp and cold, potentially causing pneumonia. Once the fever has been gone for a couple of days, then take a shower. Similarly, when a baby has high fever, sponge the baby with tepid water but don't give him a bath. For high fever in children, grate an onion and divide the pulp into two parts. Put one part of the onion pulp in a cloth soaked in hot water, then fold the cloth and place it on the belly button. Wrap the other half of the onion pulp in another hot, wet cloth and place it on the forehead. Onion pulp on the forehead and the belly button can bring down temperature within 20 minutes. This can be used with children as well as with adults.

When a person has extreme thirst, make an herbal tea out of equal parts of cumin, coriander, and fennel. This tea relieves thirst, stimulates agni and digestion, burns āma, and improves the taste in the mouth. Another combination for extreme thirst during fever is tea made of mustā, khus, sandalwood, and ginger in equal parts. This tea will relieve dehydration, especially in a pitta type of fever. The same mixture is good in a kapha type of fever, if there is nausea and vomiting. Kapha nausea and vomiting is mucous type, whereas in pitta it is bilious.

There are certain fruits that bring down temperature. For pitta and vāta, use pomegranate, cranberry, or purple grape juice, or sugarcane juice. Give a light diet with no cheese, yogurt, ice cream, or heavy meat. Never eat animal flesh during a fever. It will not be digested and will produce āma.

A cup of lemongrass and cilantro tea with a teaspoon of honey is anti-pyretic and also tridoshic. The lemongrass is good for vāta, the cilantro acts on pitta and kapha, and honey is a good anupāna.

If a person with pitta fever has diarrhea, use ½ teaspoon of kutaja. If you don't have kutaja, then cook an apple and mash it. Add a pinch of nutmeg and cardamom and a teaspoon of ghee. Cooked apple is a good source of pectin, which will help to control diarrhea.

In fever, don't use lemon, lime, or any sour juice. They increase pitta and kapha and will create congestion, cold, and cough.

Chronic fever continues because of the debility of the body and dhātus. Hence, one should maintain a diet that will promote the strength of the dhātus. If the tissues are weak, give:

| | |
|---|---|
| Shatāvarī | 500 mg |
| Balā | 400 mg |
| Ashvagandhā | 300 mg |

This is used as a rasāyana (rejuvenative) to strengthen the dhātus. If the weakness is still there, the person may get *dhātu jvara* related to tissue deficiency. In all types of chronic fever, it is beneficial to give a teaspoon of tikta ghrita (bitter ghee) TID, followed by ½ cup of warm water. This will protect ojas and promote the strength of the dhātus.

*Please Note:* Although fever results from the entry of tridosha into rasa dhātu, there may be a serious viral or bacterial infection. One should always consult with one's physician to rule out these possibilities.

# Chapter 16

# An Ayurvedic Perspective on Hypertension
## Sirābhinodhana and Dhamanī Pratichaya

Summer 1993, Volume 6, Number 1

HYPERTENSION IS A MODERN TERM, but in ancient Vedic literature there is a description of something similar. That condition is called *sirābhinodhana*. Sirā means the blood vessels and *abhinodhana* means tension, which corresponds to the modern concept of hypertension. Sirābhinodhana is a condition where venous blood stagnates and exerts pressure on the blood vessel wall. When pitta is involved, venous hypertension may lead to varicose veins, hematomas, and a tendency to bruise easily. The literature also describes *dhamanī pratichaya,* which means increased intra-arterial pressure. Dhamanī pratichaya corresponds more closely to arterial hypertension, and sirābhinodhana indicates venous hypertension.

When referring to hypertension, modern medicine does not give much importance to the veins, only the arteries. In Ayurveda, venous circulation is related to rasa dhātu and all nutrients enter into the veins. The chyle duct, which carries the end products of digested material from the gastro-intestinal tract, opens into the subclavian vein. The venous system is connected to the arterial system via the heart, which is the junction between venous and arterial circulation. The heart is a most vital organ, not only pumping the oxygenated blood, but also receiving venous blood.

Venous blood that comes into the heart has received food nutrients through the subclavian vein. The blood is then carried through the pulmonary artery from the heart to the lungs, where it is oxygenated, and then through the pulmonary vein back to the heart. The Ayurvedic concept of hypertension includes both venous and arterial circulations. Ayurvedic literature states that dhamanī pratichaya (arterial hypertension), the type most commonly referred to, is a tridoshic disorder.

## Doshic Types of Hypertension

The main site of vāta in the human body is the colon. When there are toxins in the colon, they can be absorbed into the blood and may cause constriction of the blood vessels, especially the arteries. Detoxifying the colon can treat this kind of hypertension. Psychologically, it is often associated with fear, anxiety, stress, and insecurity, which may lead to constriction of the blood vessel walls and produce hypertension.

In Ayurveda, the small intestine is the seat of pitta. Toxins from undigested foodstuff in the intestines produce āma, which moves into the general circulation. Hypertension of this type is due to increased viscosity of the blood. Bile is pitta in nature and this fatty, oily substance makes the blood viscous. Because of its increased viscosity, the blood exerts pressure on the blood vessels. In this pitta type of hypertension, the person may exhibit psychological symptoms of judgment, criticism, anger, hate, envy, and jealousy. These emotions themselves can also trigger an increase in blood pressure.

Kapha type of hypertension originates in the stomach, which is the main site of kapha. Kapha-like gastric mucosal secretions are involved in the digestion of carbohydrates, starch, and glucose. The end products of this phase of digestion are triglycerides. When kledaka kapha from the stomach is disturbed, there is an increase in triglycerides and cholesterol (also kapha molecules). The result is that the blood becomes more viscous. This kapha type of hypertension causes fatty molecules to deposit on the blood vessel walls, which leads to narrowing of the arteries (arterial sclerosis) and possible heart attack.

Another important factor in hypertension is the functioning of the kidneys, which regulate the entire water system in the body. In Ayurveda, the kidneys belong to mūtra vaha srotas, the urinary system. Urine (*mūtra*) has the important function of carrying excess kledaka kapha out of the body. People who do not sweat sufficiently can also accumulate excess kledaka. There is no equivalent word for kledaka kapha in modern medicine, but it may be responsible for secretion of chemicals known as vasopressins. These stimulate the adrenals and in excess can lead to hypertension. Various urinary dysfunctions may also lead to hypertension. Acute glomerulonephritis is due to excess pitta in the kidney; hydronephrosis is caused by excess kapha in the kidney; and renal failure, which leads to total absence of urinary function, is due to the dryness of vāta dosha. All of these conditions may lead to hypertension.

## Ayurvedic Diagnosis

Ayurvedic texts describe three types of hypertension: vāta, which begins in the colon; pitta, which starts in the small intestine; and kapha, which originates in the stomach. Although there are seven classical types of dhamanī pratichaya, these basic three types can be diagnosed through the clinical barometers of inspection, palpation, and auscultation. For example, the vāta type of hypertension, which begins with toxins in the colon, constricts the musculature of the blood vessels. Pitta usually affects rakta dhātu (blood tissue) and the kapha type generally affects rasa dhātu (plasma).

Traditional Ayurvedic pulse diagnosis assesses blood pressure by feeling the velocity of the blood flow. In vāta hypertension, the radial pulse will be feeble, empty, and superficial, with prominent throbbing felt under the palpating index finger. The person might also have anxiety, nervousness,, and tachycardia. The diastolic blood pressure will be relatively higher than the systolic pressure, which indicates vāta type of hypertension. In addition, the tongue may become dry and the person might have insomnia. The lower eyelids may also be swollen and there will be constipation. If you give dashamūla basti, all of these symptoms will likely subside. This vāta type of hypertension is often temporary.

In pitta type of hypertension, the radial pulse will be felt most predominantly under the middle palpating finger, and it has a collapsing nature, with high volume and low tension, along with full, bounding, hot qualities. Both the systolic and diastolic blood pressures are high. As a general rule, a person's age plus 100 is the optimal systolic blood pressure. Hence, if a person's age is 30, the systolic pressure should be approximately 130 and if a person is 50, the pressure should be around 150. The diastolic pressure should normally be around 90. In this pitta type of hypertension, the person might get hot flashes, a red nose, and prominent blood vessels. Sometimes the person bruises easily and has headaches, dizziness, nausea, vomiting, or nosebleeds. These people are also prone to bloodshot eyes, retinal hemorrhage or cerebral hemorrhage. Pitta hypertension can be a dangerous acute situation needing prompt medical treatment, or it may cause serious cerebral vascular accidents (CVA).

In kapha type of hypertension, the person is often overweight or obese and may have an underactive thyroid gland. In this kapha condition the pulse is best felt under the ring finger, and it is slow, deep, full and wavy or watery in quality. In kapha type of hypertension, both the diastolic and systolic blood pressures increase somewhat, but the diastolic pressure remains steadier. It may be between 85 to 90. The person may also be diabetic, because hypertension with diabetes is a kapha condition. People with this condition tend to get edema and frequency of urination and there may also be diabetic retinopathy, cardiopathy, renopathy, or cerebropathy. Kapha type of hypertension is as serious as vāta type and this condition may even become what is called malignant hypertension.

Vāta-kapha type of hypertension is another form. It causes blood clots (thrombosis). This can be very serious, as it may cause a sudden cerebral or pulmonary embolism or heart attack.

Ayurveda has also explained some of the complications of dhamanī pratichaya and sirābhinodhana. These disorders may lead to cardiac complications (*hridrogam*) or, if they affect the higher cerebral blood vessels, can lead to paralysis, Bell's palsy, stroke paralysis or, in pitta conditions, cerebral hemorrhage. The Ayurvedic concept of hypertension understands the condition as a whole. Not every hypertensive case should be treated with diuretics, which are effective only in some kapha types of hypertension.

## Ayurvedic Recommendations

Ayurvedic literature has specific recommendations for each type of hypertension and its corresponding samprāpti (etiology). In general, a person with hypertension should follow a lifestyle and diet that reduces the primary dosha. In addition to this there should be no consumption of caffeine, salt, sugar, or fatty, fried foods. Deep breathing, daily walks of three miles, and meditation are all beneficial as well.

*Vāta Remedies.* The samprāpti of vāta hypertension begins in the colon and the second chakra due to repressed fear, anxiety and insecurity. Ayurvedic literature says that one should treat the colon, the main seat of vāta, using dashamūla basti, which is an enema made of dashamūla tea. Herbs like kaishore guggulu, yogarāja guggulu, or sarpagandha may help to reduce hypertension and regulate blood pressure, while panchakarma is also useful, followed by a vāta pacifying diet and lifestyle. In addition, the following herbal program is suggested.

1. An herbal mixture of:

Dashamūla　　500 mg
Ashvagandhā　500 mg
Shatāvarī　　　200 mg
Tagara　　　　200 mg

¼ teaspoon of this mixture taken after lunch and dinner, with warm water.

2. Triphalā, ½ teaspoon at night. Or one to three teaspoons of castor oil, mixed with one cup of ginger tea, taken at night. This helps to clean the colon.
3. In certain toxic colon conditions one should take dashamūla tea basti three times a week.
4. Rub warm sesame oil on the feet and scalp at bedtime to help relieve stress and normalize blood pressure.
5. Practice the following yogāsanas: camel, cobra, cow, cat, spinal twist, palm tree, and corpse pose, with deep, quiet breathing into the belly button. This will help to relax the blood vessels and therefore lower the blood pressure.

***Pitta Remedies.*** The samprāpti of pitta type of hypertension begins in the small intestine and liver, and may be accompanied by gallbladder toxicity and unresolved anger in the solar plexus. Job responsibilities, stressful relationships, and the combined action of hot, spicy, and salty foods act as precipitating causes. Here one should detoxify the small intestine, liver, gall bladder, and solar plexus with panchakarma. The person should follow a pitta-soothing diet and take pitta-soothing herbs like shatāvarī, gulvel sattva, and jatamāmsi, which help to regulate pitta in the blood, thereby decreasing its viscosity and the arterial tension.

Generally, the following program would be suggested.

1. An herbal mixture of

Shatāvarī　　　500 mg
Shankha pushpī 300 mg
Brahmī　　　　200 mg
Sarasvatī　　　100 mg

¼ teaspoon of this mixture taken after lunch and dinner, with warm water.

2. Virechana (administration of intestinal purgatives) with āmalakī, nishottara, or sat isabgol at night with warm water.
3. Brahmī ghee nasya: three to five drops in each nostril on an empty stomach, morning and afternoon.
4. Practice these yogāsanas: hidden lotus, boat, bow, fish, and the cooling shītalī prānāyāma.
5. No one with high blood pressure should do headstands, the breath of fire (bhastrikā prānāyāma), heavy weight lifting or vigorous exercise. One should sleep on the right side and rub brahmī oil on the soles of the feet and scalp at bedtime.

***Kapha Remedies.*** The samprāpti of kapha hypertension begins in the stomach and spleen, with associated lymphatic congestion and sometimes an underactive thyroid. Since kapha's main sites are the stomach, lungs, and lymphatic tissue, one should cleanse these organs to eliminate the root cause of kapha hypertension. Undigested and unutilized kapha molecules from the plasma cause an increase in cholesterol or triglycerides, which leads to increased viscosity of the blood, causing hypertension, diabetes, obesity, and renal dysfunction. According to Ayurvedic literature, these can be managed by panchakarma, herbs, and the correct diet and lifestyle.

1. One can take the following herbal formula:

| Shilājit | 200 mg |
|----------|--------|
| Punarnavā | 500 mg |
| Mūtrala | 200 mg |
| Kutki | 200 mg |
| Sarasvatī | 100 mg |

¼ teaspoon after lunch and dinner, with warm water.

2. Bibhītakī, ½ teaspoon in a glass of hot water, taken before bedtime.
3. Cumin, coriander, and fennel tea (equal parts of each) drunk throughout the day.
4. The yogāsanas: palm tree, turtle, spinal twist, lion, half bridge, and modified peacock pose. Alternate nostril breathing with outer retention is also beneficial.

## Summary

In Ayurvedic literature, hypertension is not a disease, but rather a symptom of doshic changes, and/or toxicity within the gastro-intestinal tract, and/or emotional or stressful conditions. One should understand the doshas involved and whether it is a sirābhinodhana or dhamanī pratichaya condition. Each type of doshic hypertension should be treated individually, by understanding the particular samprāpti (pathological process) as well as the person's prakruti and vikruti. Then and then only can perfect healing of these particular conditions be achieved.

Please note that hypertension is a serious condition, possibly involving or leading to complications. One should not try to treat oneself using this article as a substitute for consultation with a qualified medical doctor.

# Chapter 17

# Cholesterol and Excess Kapha
## An Integrated Approach

Winter 1989, Volume 2, Number 3

AYURVEDA SAYS THAT cellular metabolism is governed by agni, the fire principle, which is present in pitta dosha. Through metabolic, biochemical reactions that occur within the cells, we utilize carbohydrates, proteins, and fats to release energy and produce new structural cellular material. Agni also maintains and regulates the life span of cells. Organic catalytic agents called the three doshas also control these metabolic reactions. The production of these doshas (vāta, pitta and kapha) is controlled by the genetic code, called prakruti (constitution) in Sanskrit, which is held within the molecules of the cells. This genetic code instructs the cells to behave in a certain way to synthesize specific kinds of food molecules.

Metabolic processes can be divided into two major types: The first is anabolic, which stores energy and involves the build-up of larger molecules from smaller ones. This type of change is governed by kapha dosha. The other type, catabolic, involves energy loss and the breakdown of larger molecules into smaller ones. That type of change is governed by vāta dosha.

## Samprāpti (Pathogenesis)

Kapha, which contains earth and water elements, is heavy, thick, oily, cool, and cloudy, and it moves slowly in the plasma. It has a tendency to deposit on the vessel walls, causing thickening and narrowing of arteries, and increasing the viscosity of the blood. This results in hypertension and ischemic or congestive heart disease. Kapha molecules comprise a group of organic compounds that include fats, lipids, triglycerides, lipoproteins, and other fat-like substances that are used to supply energy and lubricate the cell membranes. Triglycerides are present in foods of both plant and animal origin. They are found in meats, eggs, milk, and lard as well as in various nuts and plant oils such as corn, peanut, and olive. Cholesterol is present in relatively high concentrations in shrimp, liver, egg yolks, and fatty meat. It is present in lower concentrations in whole milk, butter, cheese, and dark meats. These animal and plant food products also increase kapha, so a kapha-increasing diet also increases cholesterol.

During digestion, triglycerides are broken down into fatty acids and glycerol. The metabolism of these substances is mainly controlled by the bhūta agni (digestive fire of the five elements) in the liver and indirectly by the jāthara agni in the stomach. The liver, with the help of bhūta agni, breaks down triglycerides and lipoproteins, which may then be released into the blood.

The liver is the root of rakta vaha srotas (the blood-carrying channel) and is largely responsible for controlling the circulation of lipids. The liver regulates the total amount of cholesterol in the body, either by synthesizing cholesterol and releasing it into the blood, or by removing excess cholesterol from the blood and converting it into bile and bile salts. Bhūta agni in the liver further uses cholesterol to lubricate cell membranes, provide structural material for the nerve cells (majjā dhātu) and synthesize various hormones.

Due to low agni in the liver, triglycerides and fatty molecules may not be utilized properly. They then begin to accumulate in the adipose tissue, resulting in obesity. Low agni is also responsible for an under-active thyroid gland, slow metabolism, and the release of excess kapha molecules into the bloodstream, which increases the cholesterol level in the blood. As a rule, an individual below the age of 50 years whose cholesterol concentration exceeds 240 mg per 100 ml, or whose triglycerides exceed 200 mg per 1 ml, is considered to have high cholesterol.

Primary hyperlipidemia, or high cholesterol, is classified in Ayurveda as a kapha disorder. This condition is uncommonly common in those individuals with a kapha-predominant constitution, liver or kidney dysfunction, low agni (low metabolism) and/or a diet high in saturated fat and kapha-producing foods. These individuals may also be at risk for ischemic heart disease.

Among the signs of high cholesterol are multiple hairs in the ear passage, a crease on the ear lobule, white rings around the irises of the eyes, and hypertension. Another indication is a broad, deep, slow, wavy and thickened pulse that shows low liver, kidney, and stomach energy. The serum looks cloudy due to excessive kapha molecules in the rasa dhātu (plasma tissue) and there is an accumulation of water in the adipose tissue, resulting in excess weight or obesity and hypertension. There is also clogging of the arteries (atherosclerosis).

## Causes of High Cholesterol
- Low agni
- Low metabolism
- Hypothyroidism
- Lack of regular exercise
- Sedentary job
- Kapha producing diet: fatty meat, dairy, fried food
- Kapha prakruti
- Heredity

## Possible Results of High Cholesterol
- Liver dysfunction
- Pancreatitis

- Gallstones
- Diabetes mellitus
- Low kidney energy

## Management of a Case of High Cholesterol

Those whose cholesterol count exceeds 200 mg should:

- Avoid fatty fried foods.
- Follow a cholesterol free diet. See the kapha-soothing diet in *Ayurveda, the Science of Self-Healing,* page 82.
- Walk three miles daily at a brisk pace.
- Use garlic and onion in cooking.
- Drink "copper water." (*Ayurveda, the Science of Self Healing,* pages 142-143).
- Use the herbs and compounds chitrak, chandraprabhā, ārogya vardhini, and lasunadi vati.
- Drink a cup of madhudaka, which is hot water with a teaspoon of honey, every morning before breakfast.
- Yoga poses: sun salute, shoulder stand, peacock, cobra, spinal twist, locust, and lotus as well as breath of fire (bhastrikā) prānāyāma. (see yoga poses page 450)
- Meditation.

Chapter 18

# Chronic Lyme Disease

Fall 2008, Volume 21, Number 2

LYME DISEASE IS a multi-systemic disorder caused by a spirochete, called borrelia burgdorferi, which enters the skin through a tick bite. It is a common disorder in spring and summer seasons, when the deer tick vectors are most active. This is the time when more people go camping and hiking in the mountains.

Lyme disease is epidemic in certain parts of the United States, such as the New England states (especially Connecticut, Rhode Island Massachusetts), New York, New Jersey, Pennsylvania, Delaware and Maryland as well as Wisconsin, Minnesota and the Pacific Northwest.

When the tick bite occurs, if the tick is promptly removed and the area is washed, the toxin will not gain access to the blood stream. This will prevent the occurrence of long-term symptoms. It is still important to see your health care professional at this time, especially if symptoms occur at this early stage.

If the tick is not quickly removed, a characteristic rash develops at the site of the bite, within 12 to 24 hours. It begins as a red ring and then gradually expands to leave a typical "bull's eye" pattern. Not all bites have this bull's eye pattern, but most produce a large rash that is circular in shape. This is caused by the localized reaction of bhrājaka pitta under the skin, which produces a rash called erythema chronicum migrans.

There are three stages to Lyme disease:

1.  Localized infection at the site of the tick bite. The incubation period is 7 to 14 days. Erythema (redness of the skin) develops during this period as well as headache, stiff neck, muscle spasms and joint pain. It is easy to forget the tick bite occurred if it is only a small injury. Some or all these signs and symptoms can develop within a couple of weeks of being bitten. Many times, stage one of Lyme disease is misdiagnosed as arthritis, muscular pain, migraine or (because of the stiff neck) meningitis. It is not any of these diseases. It is the entry of pitta into rasa, rakta, and māmsa dhātus.

2. This second stage occurs after the initial one to two weeks of stage one. The spirochete produces non-protective antibodies, which spread throughout rakta vaha srotas (the blood system). This further disturbs rañjaka pitta, moving into the muscles and joints and producing muscular pain and arthritis. It can also result in cardiac arrhythmia or pericarditis due to *avalambaka dushti*.

   Entry of the spirochete into the lymphatic system produces lymphadenopathy. The lymph nodes become enlarged, tender and painful. If majjā dhātu is involved, meningoencephalitis symptoms can be produced. These antibodies are pitta-genic āma (toxins), which produce inflammatory changes in the muscles, pericardium and the joints.

3. The long-lingering pitta āma stays in the deep connective tissue, where it can produce chronic infections over a period of several years. In this third stage of Lyme disease, the patient may develop severe arthritis or encephalitis. However, these diseases are rarely fatal. Examination of the blood serum typically shows the presence of antibodies. Many times, chronic Lyme disease is misdiagnosed a rheumatoid arthritis, fibromyalgia or fibromyositis. Hence, it is important for the patient to remember the incident of the tick bite.

In addition to seeing their health care professional, the person can be given the following herbal remedies to promote healing and a full recovery from this debilitating disease.

## Herbal Treatment

In general, one needs to use Ayurvedic herbal antibiotics, such as:

Neem          200 mg.
Turmeric      200 mg.
Echinacea     200 mg.
Goldenseal    200 mg.
Vidanga       200 mg.

These herbs help to control the development of the illness, preventing it from moving from stage one to stages two and three. They can be used separately, or can be mixed together to create a broad-spectrum antibacterial formula.

The pratyanika (specific to) herbal remedy for pitta dosha:

Shatāvarī        500 mg.
Gudūchī          300 mg.
Mahāsudarshan 200 mg.
Kāma Dudhā       10 mg.

This mixture can be given ½ teaspoon TID. These herbs are all anti-inflammatory and help to balance pitta dosha.

## Topical Treatments for Erythema

1. Make a paste from a teaspoon of sandalwood powder,[27] a pinch of edible camphor, and a pinch of moti bhasma (pearl powder). An alternative to this combination is red sandalwood and turmeric. Apply this to the site of the erythema.

---

27. Sandalwood is considered an endangered species by CITES. The Ayurvedic Institute does sell some sandalwood but only in limited quantities.

2. Drink 2 tablespoons of cilantro juice TID. Also, apply the cilantro pulp topically to the erythema.
3. Apply equal parts of coconut oil and neem oil topically to the site of the erythema.
4. Eat ½ cantaloupe and rub the inner white portion (found near the skin of the fruit) onto the erythema.

# Treatment of Specific Complications

## For Pericardisis or Cardiac Symptoms

| | |
|---|---|
| Punarnavā | 500 mg. |
| Pushkaramūla | 300 mg. |
| Arjuna | 300 mg. |
| Shringa Bhasma 10 mg. (or Shanka Bhasma) | |

Give ½ teaspoon of this herbal mixture TID.

> T.I.D. = from the Latin means *ter in diem,* three times a day

Topically, apply shringa shunti lepa, which is a paste made from equals of ginger powder and shringa bhasma (deer horn ash).

## For Muscle Pain or Spasms

| | |
|---|---|
| Ashvagandhā | 500 mg. |
| Balā | 300 mg. (or Ātmaguptā) |
| Vidārī | 200 mg. |

Give ½ teaspoon of this herbal mixture TID.

Topically, apply mahānārāyana oil onto the site of the pain.

## For Arthritis

Lyme arthritis is an intermittent particular inflammatory arthritis that is due to tick-borne viral disease. It can appear to be rheumatoid arthritis, as it is found in only a few joints. To treat it, one can use:

| | |
|---|---|
| Amrita Guggulu 300 mg. (or Kaishore Guggulu 200 mg.) | |
| Gulvel Sattva | 200 mg. |
| Mahāsudarshan 200 mg. | |
| Kāma Dudhā | 10 mg. |

Take ½ teaspoon of this mix TID with aloe vera gel. The person should also take half to one teaspoon of bhumi āmalakī nightly.

Topically, apply mahānārāyana oil at the site of the pain. Also, apply sandalwood and edible camphor paste, made from 1 teaspoon of sandalwood powder mixed with a pinch of camphor and some water.

# Treatment of Chronic Lyme Disease

This line of treatment will help to control the Lyme disease. However, in reality, chronic Lyme disease is a long-lingering multi-systemic disorder that needs periodic panchakarma (detoxification) treatments and a rasāyana (rejuvenation) program.

## Panchakarma

First, do snehana with sunflower oil and svedana (steam therapy) using sandalwood essential oil or nirgundī essential oil added to the steam box or bath. You can also use ginger or eucalyptus oil instead of the nirgundī. Then the patient undergoes gentle virechana (purgation) with nishottara or bhumi āmalakī. Rakta moksha is also done whenever possible, to cleanse the blood.

## Rasāyana

The following remedies are used to rejuvenate the tissues affected by Lyme disease:

- Mahārasnādi kvath, as a rasāyana for the joints, or kumārī āsava.
- Mahā sudarshan kvath, as a rasāyana for erythema and pyrexia, or kumārī āsava.
- Ashvagandhā arishta, as a rasāyana for māmsa dhātu, or drākshā.
- Arjuna arishta, as a rasāyana for the heart, or drākshā.

In general, the person should eat a pitta pacifying diet and avoid foods that are vāta aggravating. He or she should also follow a pitta pacifying lifestyle and avoid aggravating vāta dosha.

Chapter 19

# Chronic Fatigue Syndrome

Spring 2000, Volume 12, Number 4 and Summer 2000, Volume 13, Number 1

CHRONIC FATIGUE SYNDROME is a complex illness now commonly found in this society. The condition called chronic fatigue syndrome (CFS) is not a new disease. In modern medicine, this illness is associated with an acute viral infection and is often called myalgic encephalomyelitis (ME). Chronic fatigue syndrome is similar to the Gulf War syndrome and it is closely associated with fibromyalgia, myasthenia, neurasthenia, or atypical encephalitis. Its latest name is "Chronic Fatigue Immune Dysfunction Syndrome" or CFIDS. It has been given many names, but I will refer to the condition as chronic fatigue syndrome or CFS.

## The Role of Digestion and Cellular Metabolism

We will begin by studying the important role that digestion plays in health. This is a key to understanding the reasons someone develops CFS. Ayurvedic concepts of digestion, nutrition, and metabolic functions are quite different from western understanding and we will review some of those basic tenets here.

The end product of digested food, called āhāra rasa, is carried to the various tissues. Bodily tissues are called dhātus in Sanskrit. For instance, rasa dhātu is the blood plasma and the lymphatic system. Rakta dhātu is the red blood cells. Māmsa dhātu is the muscles, meda the fatty tissue, asthi the skeletal system, majjā the nervous system and bone marrow. Finally, shukra is the male reproductive system and ārtava the female reproductive system. We will consider these different tissues as we discuss the various manifestations of chronic fatigue syndrome (CFS).

The digestive fire is called agni in Sanskrit. The functions of agni include transformation of food, thoughts, and emotions into the substance of the body and mind. Its strength and capacity determine how well nutrients are utilized by the body. Each stage of digestion has its own agni and the various organs important to the digestive process all have their own digestive capability. The central digestive fire is called jāthara agni. It manifests as hydrochloric acid (HCl) and the various enzymes that are present in the stomach and small intestine. Bhūta agni can be defined as the digestive enzymes and hormones in the liver. Each tissue has dhātu agni, which further transforms the raw materials from food and water into the tissues and their by-products. Bhūta agni in the liver is a bridge between jāthara agni and the dhātu agni and utilizes the end products of digested food to nourish every tissue, organ, and system. Bhūta agni is often affected in CFS.

The smallest unit of the human body is a single cell. Cellular metabolism is related to the fire component of all cells, called pīlu agni and pithara agni. Pīlu agni is the digestive fire in the cell membrane, which converts the āhāra rasa into cellular plasma. Then pithara agni transforms this subtle essence of the food into consciousness. The pure essence of pīlu agni and pithara agni is tejas. Tejas maintains the cellular metabolic activity and is responsible for cellular intelligence. Every cell has this intelligence, which manifests in pīlu agni as selectivity.

There is a constant flow of communication between cells. That flow of communication is prāna. The mitochondria, genes, RNA and DNA molecules, and even the movement of cytoplasm are all governed by prāna. Prāna is responsible for the flow of cellular intelligence and cellular respiration (oxygen exchange). Because of prāna, every cell is a conscious living being. Ojas is the end product of cellular digestion and the pure essence of all bodily tissues, and it is responsible for maintaining the immune response. It governs cellular and systemic immunity. Ojas corresponds to the pure essence of kapha dosha; tejas to the essence of pitta dosha; and prāna to the essence of vāta.

The Ayurvedic concept of CFS is that it is primarily a disorder of imbalanced agni and depletion of ojas. CFS is called *bala kshaya* in Sanskrit, which means depleted strength. One's biological strength is the integration and functional synchronization of jāthara agni, bhūta agni and dhātu agni. Jāthara agni is responsible for digestive strength and capacity in the gastrointestinal tract. The strength of each dhātu is maintained by dhātu agni. Dhātu strength is defined as the tone of the tissue, the resistance of the tissue and its capacity for self-repair. If there is wear and tear of the tissue, it heals itself because of dhātu agni.

Any imbalance in agni causes problems with digestion and disturbance of ojas, tejas, and prāna. In CFS, ojas becomes depleted, but there is also disturbance of tejas and prāna.

## Causes of Chronic Fatigue Syndrome

If we look at the etiological factors of CFS, an important one is incompatible food combining. An example is eating dairy products and fruit together, such as banana milk shakes, banana splits, yogurt with fruit, and so on. Because of incompatible food combining, we develop cellular toxins (āma). These undigested food particles then float through the system, unable to be further digested. Āma is one of the factors involved in the onset of parasites, bacteria, viruses, or repeated allergies.

Incompatible food combining or eating foods that are unsuitable for one's constitution put an undue strain on agni and cause it to become imbalanced. When the agni system (jāthara, dhātu, and bhūta agni) is adversely affected, production of toxins (āma) results. Āma is a toxic, morbid substance that circulates throughout the body and invades the dhātus. Undue production of āma—systemic āma, dhātu āma, or cellular āma—can be a primary cause of CFS. There are some cardinal signs and symptoms of āma:

- *Sroto rodha* – clogging of the channels
- *Bala bhramsha* – profuse fatigue
- *Gaurava* – physical and mental heaviness, or depression, or mental dullness
- *Anila mūdhatā* – mental confusion
- *Ālasya* – malaise
- *Apakti* – indecision
- *Sangha* – stagnation of tissue, of toxins
- *Klama* – extreme fatigue

These toxins, along with aggravated doshas (vāta, pitta, or kapha), can create disease by invading any cell or dhātu that has a weakness in its cellular (pīlu) agni or dhātu agni. These weaknesses are called khavaigunya. They can be caused by genetic factors, accident or trauma, or chronic factors that imbalance the agni. If there is a khavaigunya in the dhātu agni, something like a short exposure to chemicals can aggravate a dosha and then fatigue can set in. Hence, environmental and food allergies are often present with CFS.

Endocrine imbalance or emotional stress can affect cellular metabolism and produce a profusion of microcytes (abnormally small red blood cells), resulting in anemia. This is common in CFS. Impaired metabolism can also be a factor, including thyroid dysfunctions such as hypothyroidism, which is a kapha disorder; or hyperthyroidism, which is a pitta or vāta disorder. Hepatitis, which is high pitta in the liver, is another disease that can lead to CFS. Other causative factors include acute stress or psychological causes. Feeling unloved, childhood abuse, or rejection can all affect dhātu agni, pīlu agni and pithara agni, causing us to carry these unprocessed cellular memories in our connective tissue. How we are brought up and the events of the first seven years of life stay with us.

Multiple pregnancies can induce CFS in a woman, because she loses ojas in the gestation of the fetus. Between pregnancies, there is a need to recover. Before planning a future pregnancy, the prospective mother should undergo panchakarma, rejuvenation, and a rasāyana program.

This multi-faceted etiology shows us that CFS is a complex illness. The modern medical system believes that a virus may be the most immediate cause. The Epstein-Barr virus (EBV) creates mononucleosis, which is an undue production of mononuclei or pitta-type of molecules. The latent form of this virus is found in the majority of people with CFS. Another virus involved in CFS may be the herpes virus, which causes a person to get repeated outbreaks of oral or genital herpes.

In Ayurvedic terms, these viruses increase pitta and tejas, which burns ojas. When tejas is burning ojas, the cellular immune mechanism is affected and the person feels exhausted. This increased tejas can create a mild inflammation in the central nervous system and may even create atypical multiple sclerosis (MS).

Before a person develops CFS, they have subtle weaknesses at the cellular level. Something like a virus or cellular toxins can cause further doshic imbalance and create the symptomology of CFS. Some individuals show pitta symptoms, some show kapha symptoms, and others may show vāta symptoms. Let's look at the different signs and symptoms.

## Signs and Symptoms of CFS

Chronic fatigue syndrome is the journey of āma from the GI tract into different dhātus. *Rasa dushti* (disorder of rasa) creates lymphatic node congestion and the lymph nodes become tender. Other common symptoms are mild fever, sore throat, muscle weakness, and generalized fatigue, which means that āma is moving in the rasa dhātu. *Rakta dushti* can result in anemia or hepatitis; the person looks pale and tired. Then the āma can move into māmsa dhātu. This creates symptoms similar to fibromyalgia such as muscle pain, pain around the joints, headache, insomnia, and depression. A person may have CFS and be treated for fibromyalgia, in which case other symptoms will probably remain.

Muscle pains, headaches, and fatigue are pitta symptoms that commonly happen in the māmsa dhātu. This fatigue may remain for a few weeks, months or even years, and it is not relieved by rest, massage, or any external means. The person has restricted activities, mild fever, and a sore throat. Āma and dosha dushti (imbalance) can create these symptoms of CFS. *Meda dushti* makes the person extremely sensitive to fatty food, to the point that even a small amount of ghee creates a headache. *Asthi dushti* creates pain in the joints and migraine headaches. *Majjā dushti* creates MS-type symptoms (it looks like MS but it is not typical MS), while *shukra* or *ārtava dushti* can create sexual debility.

Symptoms can also be examined according to the various subtypes of the doshas. For instance, if āma goes into the eyes it creates photophobia, which is *ālochaka pitta dushti*. If it affects sādhaka pitta, the person has difficulty concentrating, mental confusion, forgetfulness, and irritability for no reason. Tarpaka kapha disorder creates insomnia and depression. So, if you look at the symptomatology, it is a multi-factorial, multi-dhātu manifestation.

## Chronic Fatigue Symptoms

- Malnutrition due to low agni
- Psychogenic emotional factors
- Circulatory disturbances
- Low ojas
- Excess pitta in the liver
- Excessive activity
- Anemia
- Viral infection
- Accumulation of metabolic waste (ama) in the muscle(s)
- Menopausal hormonal changes
- Lack of prana to the tissues

## Assessment of CFS

Whenever you see a patient with CFS, look for the signs and symptoms she or he has. The patient knows all the symptoms, but you know the signs. Symptoms are subjective; signs are objective. In front of every sign and symptom put a V for vāta, P for pitta, or K for kapha. That means you are allocating all the signs and symptoms according to vāta, pitta, kapha. We also have to find out the person's prakruti (constitution), their vikruti (current imbalance), and how CFS manifests in this individual. That is the unique approach of Ayurveda. If you see ten people with CFS, they will each have a different disease process that created the illness.

During the physical examination, the patient will explain and convey to you his or her symptomatology. Then you can touch their skin and find out if the person is running a fever. Look into the throat and find out whether there is a sore throat. Examine the lymph nodes—anterior, posterior, mandibular, sublingual, and supraclavicular—to see whether any are tender, swollen, or enlarged. Then check the liver and spleen. Are they enlarged? Many times a person with CFS has a history of Epstein-Barr virus (mononucleosis) in high school and the liver is often enlarged and tender. Just make a note of each thing.

You can inquire if there is a family history of MS, or of optic or auditory neuritis, which suggests MS. In an MS patient, there is muscle fatigue even from checking the reflexes. Muscle power and coordination may be slightly affected, but neurological motor system examinations (and in some patients' sensory system examinations) will show extreme muscle fatigue. This is the book picture of MS. In CFS, there can be extreme muscle fatigue but not the severe demyelination found in MS.

Then try to find out whether there is any tumor, checking for tremors in the outstretched hands. Check the reflexes; listen to the heart for tachycardia or palpitations; look at each conjunctiva to see if it is pale or anemic. Look at the fingernails and see if they show calcium, magnesium, or zinc deficiency (white spots). If the patient brings a lab report, you will often see low hemoglobin, increase of white blood cell (WBC) count, and / or erythrocyte sedimentation rate (ESR), or there may be lymphocytosis, an excess of lymph cells in the blood. If the patient has had a magnetic resonance imaging (MRI) test, it may show swelling in the brain and even demyelinating changes, but it is still not MS.

We can use the help of a lab report and MRI to confirm what is going on, since we live in a high tech society, but our diagnosis cannot depend on those tools. We must read the patient's pulse, to determine his/her prakruti and vikruti and which dhātus show a vāta, pitta, or kapha spike. You can find the dhātu pulse at the fifth level. Then inquire about past history, present symptoms, and other personal issues, so we can come to the right understanding regarding the patient's problem.

If you view the CFS patient's tongue, it looks coated, white, and indented around the edges, which indicates malabsorption. Ask the person to swallow and see if there is a lump or impulse on swallowing, indicating that the thyroid gland is enlarged. To rule out thyroid dysfunction, you can listen to the thyroid gland. In such cases, the blood vessels of the thyroid become dilated and there is a 'bruit' or murmur. This physical examination will help you to understand if the patient has CFS.

Modern food is missing vitamins, minerals, and amino acids because of the use of additives and preservatives in the processing of foods. People go to the health food store and buy amino acids and vitamins, but they still show a deficiency of these things. That means that their cellular systems are clogged with āma; their pīlu and pithara agnis are suppressed by āma. There is malabsorption and āma is clogging the channels.

Some individuals with CFS show the characteristics of parasites. If you look at the tongue there are shaved patches. This means that these people have giardia, which can release āma. Parasites, bacteria, candidiasis, or amoebiasis can also be factors involved with CFS.

A person with CFS may have a history of hepatitis B, herpes, EBV, or other virus. These viruses can be related to unprotected sex with an infected partner or drug use involving shared needles. The CFS patient's partner may even be a carrier of herpes or the Epstein-Barr virus.

Some people get CFS after a blood transfusion. Mercury fillings can also be one of the factors of CFS. While eating hot food, molecules of mercury vapor enter into the nervous system. Even social isolation can cause CFS. Here, the person's relationships are the main issue. If relationships are stressful, the cause becomes the effect and the effect becomes the cause. Depression can also develop with CFS. Many times psychiatric doctors treat patients for depression, but they really have CFS. Every neurologist, psychiatrist, and physician should pay more attention to CFS. It may be that the depression is just a symptom, not the disease. The cause is elsewhere.

## Treatment of CFS

The important issue behind any kind of CFS is the long-standing, lingering systemic āma. The root cause of āma is impaired agni. The aim of Ayurvedic treatment is to balance the doshas, balance agni, and eliminate āma. Depending upon the strength of the person and the strength of the disease, there are various options to cleanse the body and mind. The two main approaches are called shodana and shamana.

If the person with CFS has some underlying strength, shodana is recommended. This is commonly called panchakarma, which means "the five cleansing actions." panchakarma is a wonderful detoxifying program that eliminates toxins through one or more of the five methods. Shodana also includes oil massages, steam treatments, eating a mono-diet of easily digested food, and other treatments that help the toxins to loosen their grip, so they can be eliminated by the panchakarma. For a person with CFS, five to seven days of panchakarma may not be enough. They often have to do 2 to 3 weeks.

However, panchakarma is not recommended for an extremely tired and weak person; only if the person has the strength to bear the strain of panchakarma. For many people with CFS, the best treatment is shamana. Shamana means seven palliative measures that help a person to regain balance. They are:

- Kindling agni (digestive fire)
- Detoxifying āma (toxins)
- Fasting, mono-diet, or eating easily digested food
- Limiting fluid intake
- Exposure to the sun or moonlight
- Appropriate exercise
- Prānāyāma

The important point is that these need to be undertaken according to an individual's needs. For example, one person with CFS may need to increase agni, eat a mono-diet and lie in the sun, but should not limit their fluids or do exercise. Another may need to do exercise and prāṇāyāma, but keep out of the sunlight. Shamana is useful for anyone, but particularly for someone with CFS who is too weak to undergo strenuous cleansing.

After panchakarma or shamana, the person needs to do rasāyana (rejuvenation). For CFS patients, this would include an immune system booster. Generally an herbal mixture is given to balance the doshas and treat the CFS. Then we have to suggest a proper ongoing diet and lifestyle. If it is vāta type of CFS, we have to give a vāta pacifying diet and lifestyle; and the same is true for pitta and kapha.

Whenever we are dealing with CFS, we will try to create a balance between prakruti and vikruti, based upon the history of the patient and his or her prakruti and vikruti. Our treatment will be directed to agni and the doshas involved, the particular kind of āma, and which dhātus are affected. With knowledge of the prakruti and vikruti, we will understand which dosha is out of balance. It is the skill of the clinician that will find out where this disease is heading and the treatment will vary according to that.

In Ayurveda, we always treat according to vyādhi pratyanika (specific to disease), dosha pratyanika (specific to dosha), dhātu pratyanika (specific to dhātu) and *ubhaya pratyanika* (specific to agni as well as dosha and disease). This is the basis of Ayurvedic herbology. We will use balā as the vyādhi pratyanika for CFS. CFS is called bala kshaya, or depletion of strength, and the very name of this herb means strength, so it is a great herb to build strength and energy. I am just giving you a direction on how to think. You must have a deep understanding of gunas, doshas, and dhātus; then you'll know what you're doing. We cannot treat every syndrome with one medicine; that is not scientific at all.

Ayurveda treats every case of CFS based upon the individual's prakruti/vikruti paradigm. So, forget the label CFS. It is not going to help us understand exactly what that person's problem is. I can use the words CFS just as a broad window through which I am looking, but there are many different shades of the disease process. Any dhātu depletion can manifest as CFS, so it depends upon each person's prakruti, vikruti, lifestyle, and level of stress.

## Vāta Type of CFS

We know the main site of vāta is the colon and that vāta has an affinity to the asthi dhātu, thighs, pelvic girdle, ears, and skin. If the person has more vāta aggravation, we'll definitely find symptoms that are related to vāta, such as dry, rough, or scaly skin, ringing in the ears, constipation, or bloating. Which symptoms manifest depends upon whether this vāta type of CFS is moving in the colon or going into any of the other dhātus. That is why it is so complex.

When vāta dosha creates manda (slow) agni or vishama (imbalanced) agni, the person's digestion is affected. Manda agni means that appetite and digestion are low. Vishama agni means sometimes the appetite is good and sometimes not; sometimes the digestion is ok and other times it isn't; sometimes there is constipation, bloating and distension, while other times there is not.

If vāta goes into the rasa dhātu, the person will have a rise of temperature in the evening, lymphatic congestion, cold (shivering), and fatigue. Fatigue here is due to a defficiency in the functioning of rasa dhātu, which has the function of nutrition. If rasa (and hence, nutrition) is lacking, the person will have progressive fatigue and weakness. This is a vāta type of CFS samprāpti associated with the rasa dhātu.

If vāta goes into the rakta dhātu, the person will feel anemic. This means that the disease process is creeping from one dhātu to another dhātu. If it goes into the māmsa dhātu there will be muscle tics, spasms, twitching, tremors, and fatigue. If it goes into the meda dhātu, the person will have a severe loss of meda (adipose tissue). The person loses fat, the muscles lose their bulk, his/her cholesterol goes extremely low, and the joints crack. When vāta type of CFS goes into the asthi dhātu, the person will get osteoporosis or osteoarthritis. When it goes into the majjā dhātu, there will be neurological symptoms such as neuralgia, tingling and numbness, or loss of sensation. And when vāta goes into the shukra dhātu, the person will have sexual debility and premature ejaculation.

I am just sharing with you a mono-doshic vāta type CFS. We give balā as the vyādhi pratyanika. If we are dealing with vāta dosha, we need one herb that is vāta pratyanika, another that is specific for agni (*agni pratyanika*) and one specific for the dhātu involved (dhātu pratyanika). For vāta pratyanika, we often use purified guggulu. But for vāta type of CFS, since āma is moving into the deep tissue, I'd use yogarāja guggulu. An alternative in cases where there is less āma is ashvagandhā.

But now I have to kindle the agni, otherwise the yogarāja guggulu is not going to work. Here I can use chitrak, which kindles and balances agni. Next, I have to pay attention to the dhātu. If it is rasa dhātu, I'll use tulsi or fresh ginger, or sudarshan if there is fever. So, the first herb deals with the fatigue and weakness, the second with the dosha, the third herb deals with the agni and the fourth deals with the dhātu. This formula of balā, yogarāja guggulu, chitrak, and tulsi will work for a vāta type of CFS only if it is in the rasa dhātu.

If CFS goes into the rakta dhātu, we would use something to pacify vāta in the rakta dhātu, such as loha bhasma or abhrak bhasma. Either one will be good for CFS associated with rakta dhātu. If it goes into the māmsa dhātu, we can use ashvagandhā. Yasthi madhu and vidārī are good for meda. Kāma dudhā (a great source of calcium) is good for asthi. Jatamāmsi, brahmī, shankha pushpī, and sarasvatī are good for majjā dhātu; ashvagandhā, vidārī, or ātmaguptā (kapikacchū) for shukra dhātu.

## Pitta Type of CFS

When systemic pitta is increased, it becomes like hot water. Pitta is liquid, hot, sharp, light, and oily. When it increases, it disturbs agni and that agni creates āma with a pitta quality. Agni becomes tīkshna—strong appetite, but poor digestion. That āma moves and creates diarrhea, then malabsorption, and slowly it will create fatigue. So in pitta type CFS, if pitta goes into the liver, the person will often get a viral infection of the liver. If it goes into the rasa dhātu, the person will have a sore throat and pyrexia, and the lymph nodes will be tender. Since we are dealing with CFS, the first herb to think of is again balā, to give energy. We will use shatāvarī because it is a dosha pratyanika for pitta. Agni is tīkshna (sharp but weak), so we need gulvel sattva or gudūchī to balance it. If pitta is in the rasa dhātu, we use neem or mahāsudarshan, which will take care of fever without aggravating pitta. If the pitta goes into the rakta dhātu, we still give balā (vyādhi pratyanika), shatāvarī (dosha pratyanika), and gudūchī (agni pratyanika), and we can add manjishthā or āmalakī to work specifically on the rakta dhātu (dhātu pratyanika).

If pitta enters māmsa dhātu, there will be fibromyalgia or fibromyositis, so we need an anti-inflammatory herb for māmsa, such as kaishore guggulu. When pitta moves into the meda dhātu, there is profuse sweating and the person cannot digest fat. A good herb for pitta in meda is shankha pushpī. If it goes into the asthi dhātu, the person gets periostitis or osteoarthritis. For this we can use pravāl pañchāmrit. If pitta goes into majjā, it can create irritability and pitta type of depression. We use jatamāmsi or brahmī, which is a great formula for pitta in the majjā dhātu. Finally, for pitta in shukra/ārtava dhātu, one can use shankha pushpī.

## Kapha Type of CFS

Now we will switch our attention to kapha dosha. We will keep balā, since it is vyādhi pratyanika. A great herb for kapha dosha is punarnavā, so we can use this as the dosha pratyanika. We can again use chitrak or trikatu for agni. CFS of kapha type will create dullness. When the kapha goes into the rasa dhātu there will be a generalized swelling of the lymph nodes. To remove kapha from rasa dhātu, we can use kāñcanāra. If it goes into the rakta dhātu, it will slow down the erythrogenesis process and create megaloblastic anemia. For this we can use manjishthā, which will reduce leukopenia. If kapha enters the māmsa dhātu, we have to protect māmsa with karaskara or vidārī. These herbs will increase and maintain the muscle tone.

If kapha CFS goes into meda dhātu, we can use kutki or shilājit. Kapha in the meda dhātu will create lipoma and fatty degenerative changes in the liver, and then the person can get CFS. For kapha in the asthi dhātu, we can use punarnavā guggulu if there is swelling of the joints, or even triphalā guggulu if there is systemic āma. If kapha CFS enters majjā dhātu, the person gets depression. We can use brahmī, jatamāmsi, or sarasvatī. For shukra and ārtava dhātus, use shilājit or ātma guptā. Kapha in the shukra/ārtava dhātu will create premature ejaculation, sexual debility, or benign prostatic hyperplasia.

## Summary

We have the discussed the causes, signs, and symptoms of chronic fatigue syndrome as well as the assessment of this condition in Ayurvedic terms. We have also covered the treatment of CFS according to the doshas, dhātus, and the condition of the patient's agni. In Part Two, we will talk about the use of supplements, treating the causes of CFS, and working with balancing the mental and emotional states of the client to fully recover one's strength and health. We will also consider the subtle aspects of healing this multi-faceted condition.

## Table 5: Herbs for Specific Dhātu Dushti

| Dhātu | Vāta | Pitta | Kapha |
|---|---|---|---|
| Rasa | Adrak (fresh ginger)<br>Tulsi<br>Sudarshan | Mahāsudarshan<br>Neem | Kāñchanār<br>Ginger<br>Mahāsudarshan |
| Rakta | Loha (iron) Bhasma<br>Abhrak Bhasma | Manjisthā<br>Gudūchī<br>Āmalakī | Manjisthā<br>Katukā |
| Māmsa | Ashvagandhā<br>Balā<br>Vidārī | Kaishore Guggulu<br>Gulvel Sattva | Karaskara<br>Shringa Bhasma<br>Vidārī |
| Meda | Yashthi Madhu (licorice)<br>Vidārī | Shankha pushpī<br>Neem | Kutki<br>Chitrak<br>Shilājit |
| Asthi | Yogarāja Guggulu, etc.<br>Kāma Dudhā | Kaishore Guggulu<br>Pravāl Pañchāmrit | Punarnavā Guggulu<br>Gokshurādi Guggulu |
| Majjā | Jatamāmsi<br>Sarasvatī | Brahmī<br>Jatamāmsi | Brahmī<br>Vacha<br>Sarasvatī |
| Ārtava | Ashoka<br>Vidārī | Shatāvarī<br>Ashoka<br>Aloe Vera Gel | Shilājit<br>Ātmaguptā |
| Rasa | Adraka (fresh ginger)<br>Tulsi<br>Sudarshan | Mahāsudarshan<br>Neem | Kāñchanār<br>Ginger<br>Mahāsudarshan |

## Part Two: The Ayurvedic Concept of Chronic Fatigue Syndrome

In the first part of this article, we saw that chronic fatigue syndrome (CFS) is primarily a disorder of imbalanced agni and depletion of ojas. CFS is called bala kshaya in Ayurveda, which means depleted strength. Strength depends upon balanced agni (digestive fire). Any imbalance in agni causes problems with digestion and disturbance of ojas, tejas, and prāna. In CFS, ojas becomes depleted but there is also disturbance of tejas and prāna. The typical patient of CFS has low prāna and high tejas of poor quality.

The most common manifestation of CFS is in pitta-predominant people with high pitta in the liver. Epstein-Barr Virus, hepatitis, and other viruses directly affect the liver, and these viruses and other pitta-aggravating causes can disturb the five bhūta agnis in the liver. When the bhūta agnis are increased, the digested food does not retain enough nutrients to optimally nourish the tissues. Rasa, rakta, and māmsa dhātus are most commonly affected, but pitta can move into any of the tissues. This can lead to extreme fatigue and all the other symptoms we discussed as being typical of CFS.

Pitta-type of CFS is most common but, as noted earlier, any of the doshas can disturb any of the dhātus and create a condition of chronic fatigue. We will consider some treatments for specific causes, such as the viruses mentioned above, but first we will consider the use of supplements from an Ayurvedic perspective.

*The Use of Supplements.* CFS is a complex condition. We have discussed the different types of formulas for CFS according to the specific dhātu. Modern medicine does not have a drug for CFS. They often use antiviral, anti-bacterial, and anti-parasitic drugs. In some therapies, they give certain amino acids that may enkindle the agni, such as tyrosine, phenylalanine, tryptophan, or glutamine. You can buy these at the health food store. Melatonin is now a popular supplement. Although it has been said that melatonin boosts the immune system, excessive amounts can create depression.

Some practitioners prescribe chelation and multi-vitamin and mineral therapies, but when agni is low and the dhātus are clogged with āma those vitamins and minerals will just create more āma. There is also a condition called hypervitaminosis, which is the result of taking high quantities of vitamins. Some people take 3000 mg of vitamin C at a time. That is too intense; more than 1000 mg at one time can become toxic to the liver. If the person shows a deficiency of vitamins, Ayurveda says that before putting any vitamins into the body we must cleanse the body through panchakarma or one of the cleansing methods mentioned in the first part of this article.

The aim of Ayurvedic treatment is to address the underlying cause and balance the doshas. By kindling agni, the person with CFS can better absorb the nutrients from food and eliminate unwanted toxins. However there are sometimes additional factors that contribute to CFS and these too need to be treated.

## Treating a Specific Cause

CFS is called bala kshaya, or depletion of strength. When we talked about herbal formulas, we used balā as a common herb to promote strength. Other herbs were chosen according to the specific dosha and dhātu involved, because the disease can take different paths. However in some cases, there is a specific cause of CFS that also needs to be addressed. Then we need to add one further herb to our original formula that is *hetu pratyanika* (specific to the cause), because to treat the cause is to treat the effect.

For instance, if we have detected that the cause is parasites (krumi), we need to know what type of krumi (pinworm, tapeworm, roundworm, amoebae, giardia, etc.). We have different herbs for the different parasites. Vidanga is good for pinworm, roundworm, and threadworm. For giardia, we can use neem, while for candidiasis, use shardunikā or hingvastak chūrna.

Herpes virus is a long lingering virus in the neuromuscular cleft that tends to flare up when the person becomes stressed or engages in sexual activity. If the cause of CFS is herpes, we can use kāma dudhā, moti bhasma, or indra and also tikta ghrita topically. In India we also use raupya bhasma or chandrakalaras. Other viruses may also need specific treatment.

If hepatitis is a complication of CFS, we have to treat the hepatitis. If CFS is associated with diabetes, treat the diabetes according to dosha. There is a sūtra that states that one disease can become the cause of another disease. Diabetes itself is a multi-syndrome disorder that can affect the immune system, and therefore we need to treat it first. Our treatment is against the cause: if the cause is a virus, we treat the virus; if the cause is parasites, we treat the parasites; if it is hepatitis, we treat the hepatitis.

If the cause is sensitivity to chemical exposure, the best treatment is to do pancha-karma and then use a rejuvenative tonic such as chyavānaprāsh, Shakti Prāna®, or tikta ghrita. So although the general cause of CFS is cellular weakness (khavaigunya) in one or more tissues, the specific cause or causes also need to be addressed.

Effect can also become cause. For instance, CFS can create a number of psychological symptoms that can in turn exacerbate the CFS. When a person has severe depression, we have to use anti-depressive herbs. If anxiety and tachycardia are present, we have to take care of them along with the main line of treatment. If muscle pain and muscle fatigue are the main symptoms, then we have to use a painkiller for the māmsa dhātu. If there are arthritic changes, we have to take care of the asthi dhātu. If fever is a persistent problem, we have to use antipyretic herbs. People develop drug dependencies, using narcotics, tran-quilizers, or painkillers, because of CFS, so we have to deal with that, too. The treatment plan is multi-factorial.

## Treating According to Physical and Mental Constitutional Imbalances

According to the Ayurvedic system of medicine, every individual has a unique consti-tution, called prakruti. Constitution is of two types: dosha prakruti and *manas prakruti,* respectively meaning the physical and psychological constitutions. Dosha prakruti is also called *deha prakruti* and is governed by vāta, pitta, and kapha with their unique permuta-tions and combinations. For example, in one person a ratio of the doshas may be $vāta_3$, $pitta_2$, and $kapha_1$, while in another it might be $vāta_1$, $pitta_3$ and $kapha_2$. Manas prakruti, or the psychological constitution, is governed by *sattva, rajas,* and *tamas*

Our constitution is the unique genetic code that we are born with. This genetic code of the individual is present in every cell; in every RNA and DNA molecule; in every system and organ. That genetic code can be studied clinically through the ancient Ayurvedic art of darshana, sparshana, and prashna, which are inspection, palpation, and questioning and auscultation, respectively. Through clinical observation, you can determine the individ-ual's genetic code, or prakruti.

Dosha prakruti is always subject to change, and the altered state of the doshas is called vikruti. The doshas are like protective barriers that are constantly acting and reacting to diet, lifestyle, and environmental changes. When the doshas become overwhelmed and can no longer adapt to these changes, they go out of balance. The dosha that is predomi-nant almost always goes out of balance first. A vāta prakruti has an inclination to vāta vikruti (imbalance) and to vāta disorders. However, if the cause is extremely pitta aggra-vating, even a vāta person can get a pitta type of disorder, but it can be easily controlled because pitta does not have favorable conditions to stay in that particular body. In other words, prakruti is disease proneness. This applies to both physical and mental prakruti.

Manas prakruti can be, for example, $sattva_3$, $rajas_2$, and $tamas_1$. Sattva is clarity, purity, the capacity to understand, comprehend, and realize; it is love, compassion, and care. These are the expressions of sattva. Rajas is activity, movement, planning, aggres-siveness, and competitiveness. Success-oriented individuals are rajasic. They want to be famous, political, and influential people in society. That can also be due to high pitta. Unfortunately, sattvic people typically do not want to become leaders and are not inter-ested in politics. Tamas is darkness, inertia, ignorance, and confusion. Diet, lifestyle, and environmental changes will also affect these psychological qualities. An enlightened person will have sattva$_3$, rajas$_3$, and tamas$_3$ because they counterbalance each other. Such a person is free from the gunas.

CFS can begin with changes to the psychological qualities (gunas) of sattva, rajas, and tamas. Because of high sattva quality, a person may do too much fasting or intense meditations. Intense spiritual practices can deplete the person's ojas and strength. Similarly, if the rajas quality increases, the person becomes hyperactive and does not eat properly, this may disturb vāta dosha and bring on CFS. Or high rajas can cause someone to push one's self to the point of exhaustion, which severely deranges pitta and vāta. If tamas is increased, it slows agni (which is sattvic and light) and the metabolism becomes slow. As a result, the person can become depressed, heavy, and possibly anorexic. Whether the anorexia is physiological or psychological in manifestation, imbalanced agni is the cause.

The sattva, rajas and tamas qualities should be balanced. There must be a balance between the material and the spiritual life. Everything must be in its right place. Any quality that becomes overpowering is bound to affect ojas. Ojas can be depleted by the imbalance of these gunas and by *prajnāparādha,* which means not listening to one's natural bodily intelligence.

In cases of CFS, we should pay attention to these qualities. If kapha is increased, it will induce a tamasic quality. If pitta is high, it may enhance rajasic and sattvic qualities. When vāta is increased, it induces more rajasic quality. The problem of qualitative sattva, rajas, and tamas imbalances can be corrected by treating the dosha. If you understand the doshic changes in CFS, i.e., which dosha is involved, and follow that doshic line of management, you will be a successful healer. CFS is an immune dysfunction condition and immunity can be affected by not only dysfunction of ojas, tejas, and prāna, but also by a chronic disorder of vāta, pitta, or kapha, which may lead to a sattva, rajas, or tamas imbalance. The reverse may also be true, whereby an imbalance of the three gunas can lead to disorders of ojas, tejas, and prāna and the three doshas. So, the most important factor in treatment is dosha, although we also treat according to vyādhi pratyanika (specific to disease) and dhātu pratyanika (specific to dhātu) as well as agni pratyanika (specific to agni) and hetu pratyanika (specific to cause).

## Balancing the Chakras

Along these lines, we can now talk about chakra imbalances, which can go together with endocrine disorders or *kundalinī* syndrome. Anatomically speaking, every chakra is surrounded by a nerve plexus. Physiologically, every chakra is connected to the neighboring organs. Psychologically, it is connected to certain emotions. The chakra system is a complex system of neuro-physiology, neuro-psychology, and endocrinology that is related to the immune system. Any chakra that is working under stress is bound to affect the neighboring organs.

Chakra imbalance, kundalinī syndrome, and endocrine disorders may lead to CFS, which has a psychogenic factor. We may take and do everything so seriously that we burn our ojas. As a result, we may become aggressive, competitive, and success-oriented. We may follow a system or method and take it very seriously, but if we take it to an extreme,

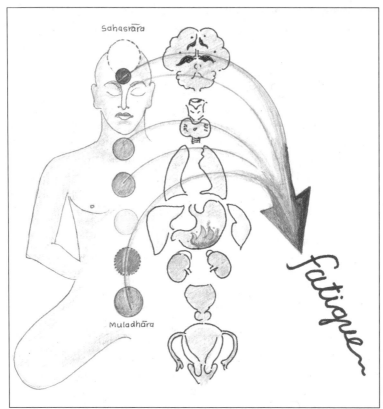

we can deplete our ojas. In life, we have relationships with the world and the chakras are these different relationships with the world.

*Mūlādhāra* is the chakra of survival. We need food, water, and air to survive. Food is energy and the end product of digested food is eliminated through the workings of the root chakra, which is mūlādhāra. Mūlādhāra is the chakra of our basic needs. In this root chakra, there is sex energy. Sex is the highest form of the lowest energy. This is the chakra of material existence.

*Svādhishthāna* is the chakra of procreation. Sva (pronounced swa) means self. The lover meets the beloved on the physical plane. Sex without desire is the highest form of love and sex with desire is the lowest form of love. Sex can transcend into blissful love and become samādhi. In the second chakra is sex in action, that is, procreation. This is also a biological need. When these basic needs are satisfied, then another factor appears in the third chakra, *manipūra,* which is power. In the lowest chakra, matter meets with matter. In the second chakra, man meets with woman. In the third, the leader meets with the follower.

In the fourth chakra, or *anāhata,* devotion meets with the devotee. The lowest three chakras are animal chakras: food, sex, and power. The fourth chakra is the center between the lower three and the higher three. It is the chakra of devotion, love, and trust. If you look into the heart chakra there is a small window and if you enter there, you'll see a staircase that will lead you to the throat chakra, or *vishuddha,* the chakra of communication. In communication, the inner meets with the outer. You communicate with your wife, your husband, your boyfriend, or your girlfriend. This is a very important chakra. Here love becomes song and compassion becomes speech.

Then comes the third eye, or *ājñā* chakra, where *īdā, pingalā,* and *sushumnā* meet. That is why it is called trikūta. Whether kundalinī travels through the right, left, or center channel—īdā, pingalā, sushumnā—she has to come here. Trikūta means three roads meeting together. This is the place to meditate; this is where alpha meets with omega. Alpha is the individual soul, your unique individual atman; omega is the higher self. So, this is the meeting point of alpha with omega, of Shiva with Shakti, Purusha with Prakruti, *jīva* with Shiva. This is the place of the guru, the master.

Chakras are reservoirs of consciousness that contain the neuroelectrical and spiritual energies moving along the ascending and descending tracts of the spinal cord. They also convey the stimuli coming from the higher centers to the lower organs through the sympathetic and parasympathetic systems. The chakra system is connected to the endocrine system. The endocrine system is composed of ductless glands, like the pituitary, pineal, thyroid, parathyroid, thymus, pancreas, adrenals, gonads, and Bartholin's glands in women. This glandular system is under the control of the chakra system and not the other way around. Therefore, endocrine imbalance happens as a result of chakra imbalance.

*Sahasrāra,* the crown chakra, is in the area of the pineal gland. The pineal gland secretes a very superfine essence of tarpaka kapha called *soma.* Inhibition of soma secretion creates extreme fatigue in the crown chakra, leading to indecisiveness, inability to concentrate, depression, migraine type of headache, and insomnia. This kind of CFS also creates forgetfulness, irritability, confusion, and foggy thinking. Before tarpaka kapha, sādhaka pitta and prāna vāta are disturbed, the electrical potential of sahasrāra, the cerebral cortical area, is affected and the energy from the right hemisphere does not flow freely to the left hemisphere. We have seen that these two sides of the brain are bridged together by a primordial brain called the diencephalon. When that bridge becomes blocked, your intuition goes against your intelligence, or your intelligence goes against your intuition. Intelligence and intuition should go hand in hand. Sometimes CFS happens when logic goes against intuition. Logic is beautiful but it has no wisdom. Intuition has great wisdom and wisdom is the application of logic and intuition simultaneously. Even scientists use intuition.

So, if you take a case history of CFS with depression carefully, you'll see that either their logic goes against their own intuition, or vice versa. This is tarpaka kapha encroaching sādhaka pitta and the best herbs for this are brahmī and sarasvatī. Brahmī ghee nasya can be used, or shirodhāra can be done. Cranial-sacral therapy can help, too. Crown chakra disorders of CFS can be managed this way.

Ājñā chakra is connected to the pituitary gland. This gland plays a very important role in the immune system. It is the conductor of the gland orchestra. It secretes and controls thyroid stimulating hormone (TSH), adrenocorticotrophic hormone (ACTH), growth hormone (GH), and the gonadotrophic hormones. So, pituitary dysfunction can be related to CFS and lead to hormonal imbalance. The herbs that act on the third eye are saffron, red sandalwood, jyotishmatī, and sarasvatī to some extent. The third eye is the eye of wisdom, of insight. What the other two eyes cannot see, the third eye sees. Jyotishmatī opens the third eye, so it may help to balance the pituitary functions and maintain the immune response.

The vishuddha chakra is functionally related to the thyroid and parathyroid. If the thyroid gland is overactive, the metabolism becomes fast and in the long term, this can cause the person to feel tired and fatigued. Similarly, the thyroid also plays an important role in metabolic activity and indirectly maintains the immune response. Thyroid dysfunction may be an indirect cause of CFS. The herbs that act on the thyroid are shilājit, gulvel sattva, vacha, and sarasvatī. These herbs are used when CFS is associated with the throat chakra. The cardinal signs of CFS affecting this chakra are repeated sore throats, pharyngitis, and flu symptoms. For flu, we can also use mahāsudarshan and sitopalādi. The herb sarasvatī can be used in a formula for any of the three higher chakras. Sarasvatī is also the name for the goddess of speech, intelligence, and wisdom.

Above the heart is the thymus gland. The thymus produces ojas and T lymphocytes, and plays an important role in the immune mechanism. In children, the thymus is quite large but it shrinks as we mature. In patients with tuberculosis or a chronic illness, the thymus is almost absent, totally consumed by the disease. The thymus gland is under the control of the heart chakra. Generally, when the energy of the heart chakra gets stuck, the person becomes intensely emotional, with a lot of grief and sadness. The chest and lungs are the seat of grief and sadness. For example, when a woman loses her loved one, she may hold intense grief and sadness in her breast tissue, and she is more likely to get breast cancer.

Because of heart chakra imbalances, the thymus does not produce optimal numbers of T lymphocytes, which include the scavenger and killer cells. Naturally, the lymph glands become congested; the axillary and the cervical lymph nodes become tender and swollen, and the person gets a low fever. The lymphatic system, the chyle and the thymus are all linked to rasa dhātu. The job of rasa is to produce white blood cells. In cases of thymus inhibition and CFS, we use yashthi madhu (licorice), neem, golden seal, osha, or echinacea to promote thymus gland activity and produce white blood cells to fight infections.

Manipūra chakra is related to the pancreas. The pancreas can go out of balance because the person is holding anger, judgment, and criticism in the solar plexus. The solar plexus becomes tight, which may build up stress in the pancreas, and slowly inhibit pancreatic secretions. This can lead to diabetes mellitus, or diabetes mellitus may lead to CFS as a secondary complication. The diabetes mellitus patient may get myalgia and sleep disturbance, fluctuation of blood sugar, and extreme fatigue. In this case, we can use chitrak for agni, kutki for lekhana (scraping fat), and/or neem and turmeric to regulate blood sugar.

Svādhishthāna chakra is related to the adrenal glands. The adrenals play quite an important role in CFS. There is a term called professional adrenal burnout. It means people work hard and experience job and emotional stress, and their adrenal secretions become insufficient, causing adrenal fatigue. This could be one of the factors involved with CFS. Herbs that help to normalize adrenal secretions include yashthi madhu, gokshura, punarnavā, ashvagandhā, or ginseng.

Mūlādhāra chakra governs the activities of the gluteal muscles, prostate, testicles, epididymis, ovaries, fallopian tubes, and endometrium. Some women get extreme CFS in their premenstrual period, because there is an endocrine disorder causing fluctuations and imbalance between estrogen and progesterone hormones. Even genital and vaginal herpes can cause CFS. In these cases, we have to give supportive therapy to the mūlādhāra chakra. The herbs that act on this chakra are vidārī, ātmaguptā, shatāvarī, ashoka, and triphalā. In women, the herbs that work on the fallopian tubes are gudūchī, ashoka, and bilva. In men, the herbs that work on the testicles and epididymis are vidārī and ashvagandhā. These herbs will be effective in CFS with special reference to chakra and endocrine disorders.

## Summary of Treatments for CFS

We have seen how to treat CFS using herbal therapy. Take care of the dosha with dosha pratyanika, the dhātu with dhātu pratyanika, the specific disease symptoms with vyādhi pratyanika, and treat the cause with hetu pratyanika. Amino acids, such as tyrosine, phenylalanine, tryptophan, and glutamine as well as various minerals may also be helpful. However you can also recommend natural food sources of these amino acids and minerals. For instance, cow's milk and almond milk are great sources of tryptophan.

In fact, there are a few useful food remedies for CFS. You can soak almonds over-night, then in the morning peel them and blend them with milk, ghee, and date sugar. This is a great drink for CFS. Fresh dates are also good. Wash the dates, dry them, remove the seed, and soak them in ghee for a couple of weeks or more. For a one month supply, you can put about 30 dates in 1 lb. of ghee and eat one every day in the morning. You can also chop a banana, put it in a bowl and add warm ghee, date sugar, and a pinch of cardamom. Eat it between meals and it will give you energy. Since bananas are a good source of potassium, this will help muscle fatigue. At bedtime, you can drink a warm cup of milk with a teaspoon of ghee and a pinch of turmeric. Ghee, milk, and turmeric at bedtime is a general tonic.

The CFS patient should reduce sexual activity, avoid strenuous exercise and work under the hot sun, and minimize anything that causes stress. The person needs a daily regime to avoid burnout. There needs to be a balance of plenty of rest and gentle exercise when energy permits. CFS is a complex syndrome, but Ayurveda can help people with CFS to find balance and health in their life.

# Chapter 20

# Breast Self-Exam

Spring 2006, Volume 18, Number 4

AT THE SAME TIME each month or when your monthly period has ended, check for any change in the normal look or feel of your breasts. If you notice any changes, report them to your doctor or nurse. Have regular breast exams and ask about a mammogram.

- FEEL for any Changes, Standing or Lying Down
- Lie down on your back with a pillow under your left shoulder
- Use the pads of the three middle fingers on your right hand to check the left breast
- Press—using light, medium, and firm pressure—in a circle without lifting your fingers off the skin
- Then press, using an up and down pattern, laterally across the breast
- Feel for changes in your breast, in your armpit, and above and below your collarbone. Gently squeeze the nipple to check for discharge. Discharge during lactation is normal.
- Repeat on the right breast using your left hand
- You can also follow these steps while bathing or showering, using soapy hands.
- Stand and LOOK for Any Changes
- Visually inspect your breasts in four steps:
- Hold your arms at your side
- Bend forward with your hands on your hips
- Hold your arms over your head
- Press your hands on your hips and tighten your chest muscles
- TELL a Doctor or Nurse about Any Changes from Normal
- See your doctor or nurse if you notice any of the following in your breasts:
- A lump, hard knot, or thickening
- Any swelling, warmth, redness, or darkening
- A change in the size or shape
- Dimpling or puckering of the skin
- An itchy, scaly sore or rash on the nipple
- A pulling in of your nipple or other parts

- ◆ Any nipple discharge that starts suddenly
- ◆ New pain in one spot that does not go away

## Breast Self-Exam Methods

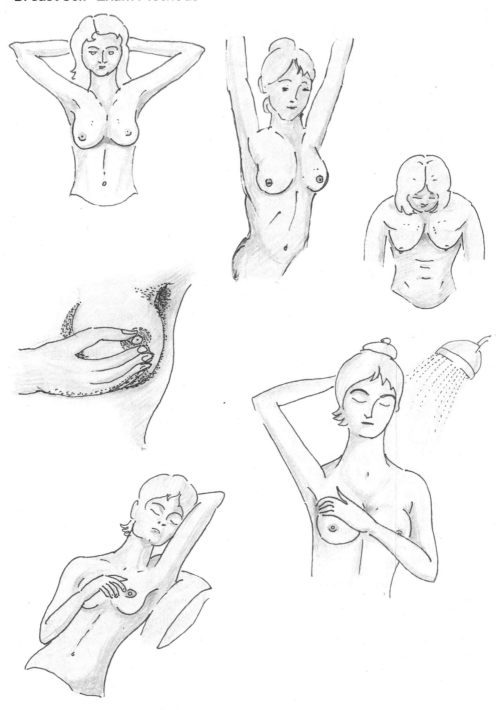

# Chapter 21

# Liver Disorders

Fall 2012, Volume 25, Number 2

ACCORDING TO AYURVEDA, the three doshas, seven dhātus (tissues), and three mala (excreta) govern an individual's unique psycho-physiology. Each dhātu has its own srotas (channel), and generally, each srotas is made up of its related dhātu. For example, rasa vaha srotas governs the functioning of rasa dhātu.

The srotas governs the nutrition of its respective dhātu and the creation of its upadhātu (superior by-product/s) and mala (other by-product/s). For example, the upadhātus of rasa dhātu are stanya (lactation) and rajah (menstruation). The mala is poshaka kapha, and that poshaka kapha nourishes all bodily kapha. Likewise, each srotas has its own unique *sroto mūla* (root), *sroto mārga* (passage), and *srota mukha* (opening). In the root of a srotas, there is the *dhātu dhārā kalā*. This *kalā* is a membranous structure that separates two dhātus from one another. For instance, *rasa dhārā kalā* is a membranous structure that governs the functional aspects of the root of rasa vaha srotas. Each sroto mūla also contains the *asthāyi* (immature) *dhātu* and the dhātu's ojas, tejas, and prāna. To take another example, *rakta vaha srotas* has its *mūla, mārga* and *mukha*. According to Shush-ruta, the mūla of rakta vaha srotas is the liver and spleen. This mūla governs the function-ing of *rakta dhārā kalā,* and rakta mūla contains *asthāyi rakta* and *rakta prāna,* tejas, and *ojas*.

The liver is called *yakruta* in Sanskrit, while the gallbladder is called *pittāshaya* (the vessel of pitta). *Ya* means to circulate and *kruta* means to create. Hence, yakruta can be defined as that which helps to create and distribute āhāra rasa (microchyle). The liver also governs protein, carbohydrate, and fat metabolism. In embryonic life, it is the liver that produces red blood cells. Any red blood cell born into the body of an adult will live for about 120 days. After that time, it will be destroyed in the liver—hence, in this regard, the liver has both creative and destructive functions. Additionally, the liver is both a secretory and excretory organ. It secretes liver enzymes and excretes bile and heavy metals.

## Bile

Bile is a complex fluid created from the disintegration of the old red blood cells. It is excreted by the liver and stored in the gallbladder. Bile is essential for life. In the gallbladder, the bile is concentrated ten times more than in the liver, so it is oily and extremely alkaline in nature. The quantity of bile that is produced daily varies from person to person. In people with *vāta prakruti,* it is generally around 500 ml a day, while in pitta types it may be as much as 1000 ml, and in kapha people is around 700 ml per day. The color of the bile is due to rañjaka pitta. In the liver, it is pale green, whereas in the gallbladder it is dark green, because it is more concentrated. However, when that bile comes into the duodenum and mixes with the digestive juices and pancreatic enzymes, it becomes less concentrated and turns yellow.

The taste of bile is bitter. It is oily, liquid, viscous, and slimy. Bile plays an important role in the digestion of fats. Bile salts are present within the bile and these salts act as a buffer to reduce surface tension, so that fat is converted into an emulsion. The surface area of fat is increased, which improves digestion of the fatty substance.

Bile is also a good solvent for splitting enzymes. It improves the absorption of minerals, such as calcium and magnesium, and fat-soluble vitamins A, D, E, and K. Bile also has the important function of excretion. Bile excretes metals such as copper, zinc, mercury, and other toxic heavy metals as well as dead bacteria. Because bile is liquid and oily, it acts like a laxative. Bile in the colon gives the stools a yellowish-brown color and helps mass peristaltic movement and elimination of feces. Bile maintains an appropriate pH balance in the digestive system.

## Functions of the Liver

The liver is one of the vital organs. One can live without a spleen; one can live without one kidney, or without testes or ovaries. However, no one can live without a liver. Mother Nature hides the liver under the rib cage. You can say we live due to the liver.

According to Ayurveda, a primary function of the liver is the formation of rañjaka pitta. Rañjaka pitta in the red bone marrow gives the reddish color to red blood cells. This is the same rañjaka pitta as in the liver and stomach, so the liver plays an important role in the formation of red blood cells and nourishing rakta dhātu. The erythrogenic formation of red blood cells is an important function of the liver in an embryo, whereas after birth this is done by the red bone marrow. Blood formation in the fetus is called mesoblastic hematopoiesis and hepatoblastic hematopoiesis. After birth, the rounded ends of the long bones, the femur and humerus, contain red bone marrow, which continues to form red blood cells. The ribs, vertebrae, and flat bones also produce red blood cells. When doing kapāla bhāti prānāyāma, there is a peculiar movement in the ribs and vertebrae, so if you do hundreds of this prānāyāma daily, it will improve blood.

In adults, the liver has a destructive function, as it destroys old red blood cells. From these destroyed red blood cells, the hemoglobin is split into heme and globin. The heme becomes the bile pigment, while the globin becomes globulin and promotes immune functions. Globulin contains a high level of ojas, so the liver produces ojas. This is why a doctor can give a gamma globulin shot to prevent hepatitis.

Every dhātu has its own ojas, and globulin is *rakta ojas*. Ayurveda says that rakta ojas is very important for the protection of the hematopoietic system. The reticuloendothelial[28] system of the liver produces this ojas, so the liver helps to govern the important function of immune mechanism.

The liver is also the home of tejas, which is the pure essence of pitta. Additionally, it is the seat of the five bhūta agni, which are related to the five elements: *ākāsha* or *nābhasa* (ether) *agni*, *vāyavya* (air) *agni*, *tejo* (fire) *agni*, *āpo* (water) *agni*, and *pārthiva* (earth) *agni*. These bhūta agni are the fire components of the five great elements of Ayurveda.

The bhūta agni play an important role in manufacturing cells in the body. The size and shape of cells is governed by nābhasa agni. Permeability and cellular respiration are maintained by vāyavya agni. Cellular metabolic activity is governed by tejo agni. The extracellular fluid becomes intracellular cytoplasm due to āpo agni. Finally, mineral metabolism is regulated by pārthiva agni. The liver ultimately governs all these functions.

The liver is a storehouse of blood and it helps to regulate the blood volume. Every day, approximately one pint of blood is stored in the liver. The liver also manufactures prothrombin, which along with vitamin K, produces fibrinogen. This fibrinogen is essential for clotting, so the liver has a blood-clotting function. If the liver is damaged, the person can get a bleeding disorder.

Mast cell formation is another role of the liver. Mast cells are essential for inflammatory reactions in the body, mediated by immunoglobulin. If these mast cells are covered by āma (toxins), they produce histamine when they come into contact with foreign proteins, resulting in allergic reactions. Therefore, the liver is related to hypersensitivity reactions such as allergic rhinitis, urticaria, and asthma. That is why a patient with asthma will usually show low liver energy (and often, low lung energy) in the organ pulses. Heparin is similar to hirudin, a naturally occurring peptide that is present in the saliva of leeches. It has blood anticoagulant properties. The mast cells of the liver also form heparin, which prevents intravascular clotting.

The liver transfers blood from the portal hepatic system to the general circulation. The liver manufacturers all plasma protein, which means that the liver nourishes rasa dhātu. It also governs carbohydrate metabolism, and the liver metabolizes even alcohol. Excessive amounts of alcohol can cause chronic inflammation that damages healthy liver tissue, replacing it with scar tissue.

A protective organ, the liver protects the bodily tissues from heavy metals, by temporarily storing them in the liver and then excreting them through the bile. Various toxins, bacteria, and drugs are also excreted through the liver, via the bile. Therefore, the liver has the important function of detoxification.

About 3% of the body's fat is stored in the liver. It helps in the process of oxidation of fat and plays an important role in releasing energy in the body. The liver is affected in chronic fatigue syndrome, resulting in tiredness and fatigue. In fact, whenever there is

---

28. An older term for the mononuclear phagocyte system, a part of both humoral and cell-mediated immunity consisting of the phagocytic cells located in reticular connective tissue.

fatigue, it indicates the liver is not working at par. The synthesis of cholesterol from acetate occurs in the liver, which also synthesizes carbohydrates and proteins as well as fat-soluble vitamins A, D, E, and K, which are all stored in the liver.

The liver uses iron, folic acid, and vitamin $B_{12}$ for the production of red blood cells. The liver is the principle storehouse of vitamin $B_{12}$, which is necessary for red blood cell formation. Chronic liver disease is associated with $B_{12}$ or folic acid deficiency. Therefore, if the liver is affected, the person often gets anemia. If there is $B_{12}$ deficiency anemia (pernicious anemia), the individual gets angular stomatitis: inflammation of the angle of the mouth—a clinical sign of vitamin $B_{12}$ deficiency. If there is folic acid deficiency, the tongue looks pale and there are raised bumps. These raised papillary cause the tongue to look like a strawberry. Hence, we can say that "strawberry tongue" is due to folic acid deficiency. If there is iron deficiency, the fingernails show a spoon-shaped depression. That is called koilonychia. Whether anemia is due to iron deficiency, $B_{12}$ deficiency, or lack of folic acid, the liver is at fault.

The liver plays an important role in the formation of uric acid and urea, and the manufacturing of plasma protein. It also governs the synthesis of testosterone from cholesterol, and estrogen from estradiol. Lastly, the liver produces a large amount of heat in the body and regulates bodily temperature.

## Rakta Dhātu

Rasa (plasma) and rakta (red blood cells) flow together throughout the body. They are liquid and maintain the lubrication of the blood cells. This function is called *prasādana*. Rakta maintains circulation up to the capillaries, a function called *rudhira-abhisarana*. Rakta is also slow (manda), and due to this quality, the blood nourishes the muscles (māmsa dhātu) and brings stability. Rakta is oily (snigdha) due to the presence of cholesterol and triglycerides. Lubrication of the blood cells is maintained by this oily quality, and this attribute also assists in the synthesis of hormones and protection of nerve endings.

Rakta is mrudu (soft). It softens the capillaries, muscles, and *kandara* (muscle-tendons). The blood is picchila (sticky) because of fibrinogen, which is why it coagulates and causes blood clotting. Blood looks like *indra gopa sama varna*—indra gopa is a kind of bloody red-colored insect, so it means blood looks like the red color of an indra gopa. Finally, the blood is said to be slightly *madhura* (sweet), due to blood sugar, and *lavana* (salty). This salty taste of

**DEFINITIONS**

**Bilirubin:** Orange-colored or yellowish pigment in bile. Derived from the hemoglobin of destroyed red blood cells (RBCs) that have completed their life span and are ingested by the macrophage system of the liver, spleen, and red bone marrow.

**Cholestasis:** Arrested bile flow due to obstruction of the bile duct by gallstones, or any other process that blocks the bile duct.

**Hemolysis:** Destruction of RBCs because of disease or exposure to drugs, toxins, antibodies, infections, artificial heart valve, or snake venom.

**Hepatocellular:** Concerning the liver cells.

**Urobilin:** is the chemical primarily responsible for the yellow color of urine.

blood maintains the correct electrolyte balance in the body. Blood also has a metallic taste because it contains iron and other minerals.

## Liver Diseases

The liver can be affected by many viruses and bacteria, making its health imperative. Hepatitis A, B, and C viruses can enter through infection or blood transfusion as well as from contaminated water or food. Pre-pathological lesions (khavaigunya) can occur in the liver due to genetic predisposition, making the person susceptible to various types of liver disease.

The liver is the seat of anger and the gallbladder is the home of hate, so unresolved anger can affect the liver. The hepatic parenchyma becomes constricted because of anger, and the bile in the gallbladder becomes stagnant due to hate. The liver is also badly affected by drinking alcoholic beverages, especially distilled liquor ("hard" liquor).

### Table 6: Urine Testing in Normal and Jaundiced Patients

|              | Bilirubin | Urobilin |
|--------------|-----------|----------|
| Normal       | –         | +        |
| Pre-Hepatic  | –         | +++      |
| Hepatic      | ++        | ++       |
| Post-Hepatic | ++        | –        |

### Kamala (Liver Disorders)

*Kama* means desire, so *kamala* means the ending of desire – the loss of the desire to eat or do things. The liver is the seat of will, so when it is affected, the person's desire slowly starts to slip away. Even an alcoholic or drug addict loses their desire for the addictive substance.

The condition of kamala is the ending of desire or cravings, but this does not mean the person is enlightened. An alcoholic or drug addict has a strong desire to consume these substances, and these desires are rooted in the liver cells (hepatic parenchyma). When the liver is damaged, these cravings disappear. However, by then it is too late; the damage has been done. A patient of jaundice has no desire to eat, drink, or do work. Anyone who has been addicted to a drug to the extent that it damages the liver is likely to suffer from kamala.

**LIVER PATHOLOGIES**

**Pre-hepatic/ hemolytic:** The pathology is occurring prior to the liver.

**Hepatic/ hepatocellular:** The pathology is located within the liver.

**Post-hepatic/ cholestatic:** The pathology is located after the conjugation of bilirubin in the liver.

## Table 7: Types of Jaundice

| | Pre-Hepatic / Hemolytic | Hepatic / Hepatocellular | Post-Hepatic/ Cholestatic / Obstructive |
|---|---|---|---|
| **Location** | Pathology occurs prior to liver | Pathology located within liver | Pathology located after conjugation of bilirubin in liver |
| **Mechanism** | Increased bilirubin formation | Hepatocellular failure | Bile duct obstruction |
| **Skin Color** | Faint lemon-colored | Yellow-colored | Bright yellow-colored |
| **Causes** | Hemolysis | Viral hepatitis, use of drugs, chlorpromazine (Thorazine®), fever, alcohol, cirrhosis | Gall stones, pancreatic cancer |
| **Past History** | Previous attack, family history | Contact with hepatitis virus, drug injections, or use of hepatotoxic drug | Gallstone attack |
| **Development** | Rapid, with anemia, fever, rigor | Gradual onset and recovery, with anorexia and nausea | Rapid, intermittent, progressive, gallstones |
| **Pruritus (severe itching)** | Absent | Occasional | Present |
| **Urine** | Colorless at first; later it is dark (urobilinogen) | Dark (urobilinogen)++ | Very dark (urobilinogen) |
| **Feces** | Normal | Pale-colored | Pale-colored |
| **Gallbladder** | Normal | Normal | Palpable, enlarged, twisted |
| **Splenomegaly** | Usually | Sometimes | No |
| **Bilirubin** | Unconjugated | Mixed | Conjugated |
| **Serum Alkaline Phosphate test** | Normal | Raised + | Raised +++ |

## Jaundice

Jaundice is a yellowish discoloration of the skin, conjunctiva, nails, and mucus membranes due to increased bilirubin concentration in the bodily fluids. This bilirubin is a component of rañjaka pitta. In cases of jaundice, bilirubin concentration increases to more than 3 mg per 100 ml. There are three types of jaundice.

**Pre-Hepatic.** This first type is also called hemolytic jaundice, which is known as *bahu pitta kamala* in Sanskrit. It is also called *koshta ashrita kamala,* because it is located mainly in the *koshta* (GI tract) and rakta vaha srotas (the hematopoietic system). Due to an increased rate of red blood cell destruction, there is excessive production of rañjaka pitta and bilirubin. Red blood cells survive in the body for around 120 days and, in this disorder, the bone marrow can no longer compensate for the extra destruction of blood cells. Hence, there is an increased output of new red blood cells with stressed nuclei. These stress-nucleated red blood cells are immature and rupture readily, which leads to an increase of bilirubin in the blood. The level of bilirubin urea in the urine is not increased, so the jaundice that results is mild.

If rañjaka pitta is slightly increased, it causes mild jaundice. If there is more destruction of red blood cells (called *rakta dushta*), then there is greater production of bilirubin, resulting in rañjaka pitta being further increased. High levels of rañjaka pitta create increased absorption of urobilin (rañjaka pitta in the urine) from the gut into the urine (urobilinuria). This causes dark colored urine and a more severe form of jaundice.

*Pāndurogī tu yo'tyarthe pittalāni nishevate, tasya pittamashrug māmsam, dagdhdvā rogāya kalpate*

Charaka Chikitsa, Sthanam, Ch. 16, Shloka 34

This sūtra says that when a person is anemic and the anemia is a pitta disorder in the hematopoietic system, due to excessive intake of pitta aggravating food, wine, alcohol or cigarettes, or working under the hot sun, then that increased pitta can affect rakta dhātu agni, which burns the red blood cells and causes muscle wasting.

Hemolysis is the breakdown of red blood cells. Extravascular hemolysis is a condition in which extravascular phagocytes occur in the phagocyte cells of the spleen, liver, and bone marrow, which liberate hemoglobin from the red blood cells. Bilirubin is not detected in the urine, so it leads to a mild form of jaundice with anemia. This is often accompanied by enlargement of the spleen. Intravascular hemolysis results from the rupture of red blood cells within circulation, releasing hemoglobin into the plasma. There

---

**SIGNS AND SYMPTOMS OF JAUNDICE**

Yellowish skin, ranging from pale to dark yellow

Pale, clay-colored stools, due to deficiency of bilirubin in the gastrointestinal tract

Yellowish pigmentation in the bile

Steatorrhea, fatty diarrhea

Dark-colored urine

Generalized itching, because of bile salts

Anorexia (poor appetite), due to low bhūta agni

Metallic taste in the mouth, due to excess pitta

Upper abdominal pain, due to inflammation in the liver

Enlarged, irregular liver

Palpable gallbladder

Gallstones

Severe weight loss

Pancreatic cancer (uncommonly common)

Fever with rigor

Hemorrhage

Vitamin K deficiency

Pain due to bone disease and diminished calcium

is reddish-brown colored urine, called hematuria. This can result in a more severe hemolytic jaundice and is a book picture of rakta pitta.

**Hepatic.** The second type of jaundice we will look at is hepatocellular jaundice, which is known as *yakruta janita kamala.* This category includes hepatitis infections. Hepatic jaundice is caused by an inability of the liver to transport bilirubin into bile, due to hepatic cell damage. The hepatic parenchyma (functional part of the liver) is damaged, and there may be inflammation and swelling. Edema can cause an obstruction of the intrahepatic biliary tract tree, resulting in increased bilirubin in the blood. Diseases such as viral hepatitis and fever can result in hepatic jaundice, as can excessive use of alcohol and toxic drugs. Alcohol creates inflammation of the liver cells and that produces intrahepatic jaundice. Finally, metabolic defects in the liver can create this kind of jaundice.

Pre-hepatic and hepatic jaundice are collectively known as bahu pitta kamala and are disorders due to excess pitta.

**Post-Hepatic.** The third disease is cholestatic or obstructive jaundice, which is called *rudha pata kamala* or *shakhashrita kamala.* This is a "blocked pathway" type of kamala, and it is a pitta-kapha disorder. Cholestatic jaundice is due to a failure of the bile to be released into the duodenum. The cause lies between the liver and the duodenum, usually due to an obstruction somewhere. The obstruction can occur in the bile duct, it may be the bile itself, or a blockage in the duodenum. Increased concentration of conjugated bile causes bilirubin to increase, and this concentrated bilirubin is unable to enter into the hepatic canal. Post-hepatic jaundice is also called "surgical jaundice," whereas the hepatic type is known as "medical jaundice." This is because post-hepatic jaundice usually requires surgery.

There are two main subtypes of post-hepatic jaundice.

**Large Bile Duct Obstruction:** The impact of a gallstone can cause an obstruction of the bile duct. This may occur due to a gallbladder disorder, cancer of the head of the pancreas, carcinoma of the hepatopancreatic ampulla[29], a stricture of the bile duct due to previous surgery, a metastatic tumor blocking the bile, or sclerosing cholangitis[30].

**Small Bile Duct Obstruction:** This is caused by drugs (especially alcohol), biliary conditions, viral hepatitis, cirrhosis of the liver, Hodgkin's disease, pregnancy, or pericholangitis (inflammation of tissue around the bile ducts), or ulcerative colitis. This will result in deep jaundice.

## Types and Causes of Hepatitis

All types of hepatitis are due to infectious viruses. Some produce more acute illness, whereas others cases result in chronic illness.

---

29. The union of the pancreatic duct and the common bile duct.
30. A condition characterized by swelling (inflammation), scarring, and destruction of the bile ducts inside and outside of the liver.

**Hepatitis A.** This acute infectious virus spreads person-to-person via contaminated food or water, especially in situations where there is poor sanitation or contact with the stools of an infected person. That's why hepatitis A often occurs as an epidemic in places where water is contaminated. In some cities, the sewage system and drinking water pipes are pretty close together. In effect, the anal canal of one part of the city goes to the oral canal of another area. The incubation period is short: between 14 to 40 days.

**Hepatitis B.** The virus enters through the blood stream. It can come from a contaminated needle used for injecting drugs, an IV blood transfusion, tattooing, or from direct contact with the mucous membranes, such as kissing or sexual fluids. The onset of hepatitis B tends to be more gradual than hepatitis A, with an incubation period of 40 to 180 days.

**Hepatitis C.** Hepatitis C is also known as "Non A, Non B" hepatitis. It is contracted in the same ways as for hepatitis B. The incubation period is also 14 to 180 days.

In pūrva rūpa (the early stages), there is often a sore throat, diffuse adenopathy, atypical lymphocytosis, mononucleosis, a history of drinking, presence of spider naevi (spider veins), extra hepatic obstruction, and red hands as well as the presence of serum antibodies of hepatitis C virus.

These three common forms of hepatitis (A, B, and C) have similar signs and symptoms:

- Fatigue
- Joint pain
- Muscle pain
- Anorexia (loss of appetite)
- Nausea and vomiting
- Diarrhea or constipation
- Weight loss
- Low-grade fever (101° F or less) with chills
- Enlarged, tender liver
- Rashes
- Jaundice (yellowish discoloration)[31]

---

**AYURVEDIC REMEDIES FOR HEPATITIS**

**Hepatitis A**

Shatāvarī 500 mg
Gulvel sattva 400 mg
Neem 200 mg
Kāma dudhā 200 mg
Abhrak bhasma 200 mg

Give this mixture three times daily with sugarcane juice or aloe vera juice

Bhumi āmalakī, 1 teaspoon nightly

Blue light color therapy

With appropriate treatment, hepatitis A can be successfully managed within a few weeks.

**Hepatitis B or C**

**Snehana and Svedana**

1) Ārogya vardhini, 1 tablet three times daily
Sutshekhar, 1 tablet three times daily

or

2) Shatāvarī 500 mg
Gudūchī 400 mg
Neem 200 mg
Kāma dudhā 200 mg
Shankha pushpī 200 mg

Give this mixture three times daily with sugarcane juice or aloe vera juice

Bhumi āmalakī, 1 teaspoon nightly.

As a student of Ayurveda, one should pay complete attention to the patient's prakruti and vikruti, and the dhātus involved. Then create a specific formula to balance the doshas and treat the affected dhātus and organs. By doing this, we can really help the patient of hepatitis. Undergoing a proper panchakarma program with virechana and rasāyana (rejuvenation) will help to reduce the viral load.

◆ **Hepatitis D.** Hepatitis D is a viral infection that only occurs when hepatitis B is present. It is a so-called "defective virus," which means it is atypical, producing illness only in the presence of hepatitis B.

◆ **Hepatitis E.** Hepatitis E is similar to hepatitis A. It is found predominantly in Asia, Africa, and parts of Latin America. The mortality rate for pregnant women is 20%, so it can be very serious. The incubation period is 14 to 180 days.

◆ **Hepatitis G.** This is a new form of liver inflammation that seems to be closely connected to hepatitis C and is most common in people who have hepatitis C, cirrhosis, or liver cancer (hepatocellular carcinoma). It is usually asymptomatic and may cause mild illness in some cases. Like hepatitis C, it is mainly contracted through exposure to contaminated blood.

◆ **Hepatitis H.** This virus can cause significant liver damage and affect the central nervous system, causing hepatic encephalopathy, which means pathological changes in the brain. It can be caused by side effects to hepatotoxic drugs, such as anesthetics, halothane, and tetracycline.

The above list characterizes hepatitis according to modern medicine. The Ayurvedic interpretation is that hepatitis comes under the general heading of kamala, and specifically will fall into one of the two main categories of kamala: 1) bahu pitta kamala (pitta-type) and 2) rudha pata kamala (pitta-kapha type).

## Table 8: Characteristics of Hepatitis Viruses

| Type | A (HAV) | B (HBV) | C (HCV) | D (HDV) | E (HEV) | G (HGV)[a] |
|---|---|---|---|---|---|---|
| Nucleic Acid | RNA | DNA | RNA | Incomplete RNA [b] | RNA [c] | RNA |
| Serologic Diagnosis | IgM anti-HAV | HBsAgF [d] | anti-HCV | anti-HDV [e] | Anti-HEV | No, DNA instead |
| Transmission | Fecal, Oral | Blood | Blood, needle sharing | Blood | Contaminated water supply | Contaminated blood |
| Epidemic | Yes | No | No | No | Yes | No |
| Chronicity | No | Yes | Yes | Yes | No | Yes |
| Liver Cancer | No | Yes | Yes | Yes | No | No |

a  Produces infection only when HBV is present
b  GB Virus C (GBV-C) is known to infect humans but not known to cause human disease
c  Similar to HAV
d  Hepatitis B surface antigen
e  HDV: hepatitis delta virus

---

31. Note that jaundice is a sign of increased bilirubin in the blood. In all forms of hepatitis, apart from hepatitis A, the levels of bilirubin in the blood may not be raised. In those cases, the jaundice will not be visible.

# Diagnosis of Hepatitis

Diagnosis of hepatitis is done by taking liver function tests and checking the liver enzyme levels. The typical case sees the person get a viral infection that causes anorexia, nausea, vomiting, anemia, depression, fever, and malaise. Within a few days, the patient becomes jaundiced, the liver is painful and enlarged, and there is dark-colored urine. The jaundice fades away within about ten days.

## Prognosis for Hepatitis

Someone with Hepatitis A will usually fully recover, whereas hepatitis B can last much longer and hepatitis C may persist for many years, or even the remainder of the person's lifetime. Complete recovery can occur after several weeks in the case of hepatitis A, and after six months or longer for hepatitis B. People with hepatitis C often develop chronic liver disorders. In rare cases of acute hepatitis, necrosis of the liver leads to hepatic coma and death, so don't take hepatitis lightly.

## Treatment Protocol for Jaundice

**Bahu pitta kamala (pitta-type), pre-hepatic or hepatic jaundice.** This category of kamala translates to pre-hepatic or hepatic jaundice. A good protocol for this disorder is:

Soft virechana with triphala ghrita (if constipation or diarrhea), kutki ghrita (for kapha types), or gudūchī ghrita (if itching).

Virechana with āmalakī, bhumi āmalakī, nishottara, or kutki.

200 mg each of ārogya vardhini, sutshekhar, and chandra kala ras, with an *anupāna* of aloe vera juice or gel (kumārī).

Castor plant juice is given at bedtime to detoxify the liver.

**Rudha pata kamala (pitta-kapha type), post-hepatic (obstructive) jaundice.** The obstruction, in the bile duct or elsewhere, is caused by kapha dosha, so treatment needs to remove excess kapha. The best herbs for this purpose are:

200 mg each of ārogya vardhini, sutshekhar, kapha kuthara ras, and trikatu (ginger, black pepper and long pepper).

Also give tikta ghrita as soft virechana to remove obstructions, plus āmalakī or kutki as virechana.

Note that this treatment can cause darkened stools once the obstruction is removed, as bile then enters into the GI tract again.

## Treatment Protocol for Hepatitis

A patient of hepatitis A needs to rest in bed and avoid strenuous activity. There is severe nausea and vomiting, so intravenous feeding is often necessary. The patient should have no alcohol, no fatty fried food, and no spicy food. The herbal protocol for Hepatitis A is given in formula #1 on page 181. Also give one teaspoon of bhumi āmalakī at night, and use color therapy and expose the patient to blue light. With this protocol, hepatitis A can be successfully treated within a few weeks.

Note that a vaccination is available for hepatitis A, and gamma globulin injections can be given on a preventative basis. A vaccine is also available for hepatitis B, but not for hepatitis C.

An antiviral agent, interferon, can cure hepatitis B or C. It is typically given for 16 weeks for hepatitis B, and 48 weeks for hepatitis C. Interferon is a natural cellular product released from infected cells in response to the virus, and is normally detectable two hours after infection. It blocks translation and transcription of viral RNA. However, success rates for interferon therapy vary according to the precise form of hepatitis B or C, and there are significant side effects.

The Ayurvedic treatment protocol for Hepatitis B and C is snehana (oil massage) with pitta tailam and svedana (sweating therapy) with sandalwood. Nasya with brahmī ghee is beneficial, and one 500 mg tablet of ārogya vardhini and one sutshekhar pill three times a day is the best remedy. If those medicines are unavailable, you can use formula #2 on page 181. Give half a teaspoon of this mixture three times daily with aloe vera juice. Also give one teaspoon of bhumi āmalakī at night. This is a good protocol for both hepatitis B and C.

People with hepatitis B or C should avoid sharing cosmetics, toothbrushes, or razors. They should not donate blood. There are support groups for people with chronic hepatitis B and C and this can be a helpful aspect of management.

## Ayurvedic Healing

According to Ayurveda, the liver is the root of rakta vaha srotas, the seat of bhūta agni and a vital organ. It also heals quickly. Nevertheless, when the bhūta agnis are interrupted or disturbed, then the hepatic parenchyma (the functional part of the organ) become a home for viruses, which can stay in the liver for years. I remember one wonderful story about a young boy from California.

I used to do a summer intensive program in California each year. One year a family brought this young boy, about 16 years old. His mother and father brought the boy in on a stretcher. He had swelling of his feet, his abdomen was distended, and he had shortness of breath because of edema. He had been diagnosed with cirrhosis of the liver with ascites (peritoneal cavity fluid). He had been hospitalized and had the fluid aspirated with surgical procedures; about a gallon was removed. Then, he was dehydrated, which was corrected with intravenous fluids, and again the fluid would accumulate. This cycle was ongoing and his parents were exhausted. He was on the waiting list for a liver transplant.

So they brought him; I felt his pulse. His prakruti was pitta predominant and kapha secondary. At that time though, his kapha dosha was very high, leading to retention of water in the peritoneum and interstitial fluid. I recommended to the family that the boy go to India to receive treatment.

They took him to Pune to the Ayurvedic medical hospital there, where they treated him according to Ayurvedic protocols. They used herbs such as ārogya vardhini, sutshekhar, and kutki. They did virechana with triphala and he followed a milk diet only. He was there in the hospital for three months. The hospital kept excellent records of his progress, tracking him. His liver function improved, the edema went away, his appetite came back, and his fatigue diminished. He improved and, after 6 months, he was absolutely normal when he came back to the US.

Then I recommended to his family to have him examined again by his liver specialist. The doctor was amazed; he said, "We thought you'd be dead by this time!" They examined him thoroughly and his liver function was normal as was his biopsy report. The doctor asked what he had done and they told him Ayurvedic medicine in India. The doctor said, "If Ayurveda has cured you, then it was not cirrhosis of liver. Our diagnosis was wrong." I think that doctor was very honest. They removed him from the waiting list for liver transplant and sent him home. This story shows that Ayurveda has some radical answers for liver problems.

~ Vasant Lad, MASc

# Chapter 22

# Skin Disorders
## Kushtha

Winter 2014, Volume 27, Number 3 and Winter 2016, Volume 29, Number 3

ACCORDING TO AYURVEDA, the top layer of the skin is a by-product of rasa dhātu (plasma). When milk is heated and then cools down, the top layer of the milk forms a cream. In the same way, the top layer of the skin is formed in an embryo because of the heat of the mother's womb.

The upadhātus or superior by-products of māmsa dhātu (muscle tissue) are subcutaneous fat and the six layers of the skin. Hence, the top layer of the skin is related to rasa dhātu, while the remaining six layers are connected to māmsa dhātu. Skin disease is mostly rooted in these deep layers of the skin.

The skin is the largest organ, covering the entire body and weighing about seven pounds. It is a waterproof barrier that protects the body from invasion by dirt, dust, bacteria, viruses, and other harmful substances.

The three major types of skin are the epidermis, dermis, and subcutaneous layer. The epidermis has pigmentation cells that contain specialized rañjaka pitta, which governs body temperature and color complexion. It also manufactures keratin, a substance that is found in the hair and nails.

The dermis contains blood vessels, capillaries and nerve endings; and there are hair follicles, sweat glands, and subcutaneous oil glands. Any damage at this level can send an infection into the bloodstream.

The subcutaneous layer of the skin prevents excessive evaporation by coating the surface of the skin with an oily substance called sebum. This sebum is kleda, a type of kapha.

The nerve endings in the skin, which relate to majjā dhātu, create tactile sensations of touch, pain, and temperature. Amazingly, there are no nerve endings within the nails and hair, so we can cut our hair and clip our nails without pain. However, wherever there is skin, there are sensations of touch, pain, and temperature.

The skin has different textures on the forehead, face, arms, legs, soles of the feet, palms of the hand and other parts of the body. Each area can have a slightly different texture, color, and thickness. For instance, the skin of the feet is thick, because it has to carry the load of the body.

The skin is a membranous structure and there is specialized internal skin, such as the mucous membrane. In between two *dhātus,* there is a *dhātu dhara kalā,* which is a skin-like membranous structure that separates the two dhātus. For instance, a kalā separates rasa from rakta, rakta from māmsa, māmsa from meda, and so on.

The skin is related to all seven dhātus. For instance:

- the special membranous structure of the lips is related to rasa dhātu
- skin of the conjunctiva and eyeball is related to rakta dhātu
- skin of the biceps, triceps, and brachialis muscles is related to māmsa dhātu
- skin under the breasts and on the belly is related to meda dhātu
- skin over the forehead, scalp, clavicle, sternum, patella and shin is related to asthi dhātu
- skin around the joints is related to asthi and majjā dhātu
- skin on the lips, areola, nipples, clitoris and glans penis is related to shukra or ārtava dhātu

It is interesting to note that some outer skin is a continuation of the specialized skin called the muco-cutaneous junction. The skin of the lips, areolar tissue of the nipples, the clitoris and glans penis are all connected to *shukra* or *ārtava dhara kalā.* Kissing on the lips and touching the nipples, clitoris or penis will stimulate sexual energy. Therefore, one should kiss most people on the forehead or cheeks. Kissing on the lips is best reserved for an intimate friend, life partner, wife, or husband.

In the nerve endings of the skin, there are special energy points where there is a complex network of capillaries, muscles, tendons, and joints. Those energy points are called marmāni or marma points. A marma is the gateway of inner pharmacy.

The subcutaneous layers contain sweat glands, which is a mala of meda dhātu (the fatty tissue). Subcutaneous fat acts as an insulating material, by which, the skin regulates body temperature. If body temperature gets too high, the sweat glands are stimulated and the person perspires, cooling down the body. On the other hand, if the weather is cold and body is too cool, the pores of the skin are closed and there is no perspiration. This helps the body to retain heat.

The tactile sensation of touch, temperature perception, and stereognosis (the three-dimensional perception of an object) are key functions of the skin.

Any lingering dosha in any layer of the skin can create a skin disease. In *vāta* skin disorders, the skin becomes dry, rough, and scaly. In pitta conditions, the skin is red and inflamed, with burning sensations and rashes, urticaria, pimples, acne, or boils. In *kapha* skin disorders, the skin becomes cold, clammy, shiny, and silvery, with crusting or flakes, and swelling. Skin diseases can be caused by any aggravated dosha or even be a tridoshic disorder.

## General Etiological Factors of Skin Disorders

Wrong diet for the person's prakruti (constitution)

For vāta: dry foods, beans, and excessive raw food

For pitta: hot, spicy, fatty, or acidic foods

For kapha: eating excessive amounts of sweets, yogurt, ice cream, salty food

- Daily application of chemical soap to the skin
- Prolonged exposure to the sun
- Drinking alcohol or smoking cigarettes
- Dry weather
- Allergies or hypersensitivity
- Exposure to bacteria, virus, parasites, fungus, or yeasts

Psychological factors, such as:

For vāta: fear, anxiety, insecurity, and nervousness can make the skin dry, cold and wrinkled

For pitta: anger, hate, and irritability can cause the skin to become red and flushed

For kapha: attachment, greed, possessiveness, and depression can make the skin thick, flaky, and itchy

Many skin conditions have genetic predisposition, and I see this in my clinical practice.

We will now look at some specific skin disorders, with their specific signs and symptoms, and Ayurvedic management techniques.

### Autoimmune Skin Disorders

In some skin disorders, the immune system creates auto-antibodies that attack the skin. The development of auto immune responses results in hidden antigens in intracellular substances being recognized as cells. It releases these into the circulation and they then induce an immune response.

In autoimmune disease, the normal self-tolerance of the immune system breaks down, and the immune system attacks the rest of the body, causing inflammation, irritation and infection. Autoimmune diseases include Type 1 diabetes, erythematosus (lupus), Hashimoto's thyroiditis, rheumatoid arthritis, spondyloarthritis, psoriatic arthritis, irritable bowel syndrome, gout, optic neuritis, and multiple sclerosis. Also in this category are some forms of eczema and psoriasis.

In Ayurveda, these antibodies are seen as cellular āma. They enter into the general circulation and may lodge into the organs and tissues. The job of the T cells is to destroy the foreign bodies, so the immune system starts attacking the cells. For example, it can attack the normal myocardial cells, which is what happens in myocarditis. Likewise, this type of autoimmune response can happen in other vital organs, such as the lungs, liver, and kidneys.

In autoimmune skin disease, this cytotoxic cellular āma lodges in the rasa and rakta dhātus. It then results in skin disorders such as eczema and psoriasis.

# Acne

The first important skin condition we will examine is acne, which in Ayurveda is called *pītika*. Pītika is a condition where small raised bumps, large cysts, or pimples are formed. About 80% of people get acne sometime in their life, and the condition is especially common amongst teenagers.

Hormones can be the causative factor for getting acne—testosterone in boys and estrogen in girls. Those hormones stimulate the sebaceous glands to secrete more sebum, causing oily skin. Oil clogs the hair follicles and creates acne and black heads.

**CAUSES OF ACNE**

Puberty and up to age 25 years of age

Reactions to medication or cosmetics (most cosmetics use chemical substances that irritate bhrājaka pitta, thereby worsening acne)

Use of chemical soaps and cleansing products

Alcoholic beverages

Unresolved anger and emotional stress can be important precipitating factors

A pitta-provoking diet (especially hot, spicy, fatty foods). An allergic reaction to certain acidic foods can also cause acne, so eliminating chocolate, acidic fruits, and other sour foods may help.

**SIGNS / SYMPTOMS OF ACNE**

Raised swellings on the face, neck, chest, or shoulders. There is pain, itching, and burning.

If a person with acne looks in the mirror and sees pimples all over the face, he or she will feel sad and may then get angry and squeeze the pimples, so they break open, releasing the fluid. This discharges blood and pus, spreading bacteria on the surrounding skin. It can leave a dark stain on the skin. Acne lesions can leave a permanent scar or mark on the person's face or body.

Sebum from the subcutaneous glands and bacteria can plug the follicles, which rupture and create a discharge into the surrounding tissue. There is inflammation, acne formation, bacterial infection, irritation, and secretion of fatty acids.

Acne is a condition with increased production of oil, which leads to the blockage of the hair follicles. This disturbs bhrājaka pitta. It occurs most commonly in young people, which is why it is known as *yauvana pītika* (pimples in young people) in Ayurveda.

According to Ayurveda, whenever rañjaka pitta from the blood enters into the skin it creates inflammation, irritation, and fatty acid secretion. Acne is an inflammatory condition of rakta dushti, due to increased pitta in the blood.

One week before a young woman menstruates, her estrogen levels are high. That stimulates rañjaka pitta and bhrājaka pitta, and due to those hormonal factors, the girl can get acne. After menstruation, which is a natural form of rakta moksha (bloodletting), pitta calms down and the acne usually becomes less of a problem.

## Management of Acne

Pitta is hot and oily. Therefore, it is better to avoid hot, spicy food and not eat fatty, fried food. Also minimize processed food, chocolate, acidic fruits, and other pitta-aggravating foods. Drink plenty of fresh water.

It is also important not to drink too much coffee or alcohol, and not to smoke.

Wash the face or affected area twice a day with warm water and neem soap or sandalwood soap. Clean the face with lemon peel. Use only natural herbal shampoo or Ayurvedic shampoo.

Don't apply oil to the skin. Abhyanga (oil massage) is contraindicated if there is bad acne.

Limited amounts of makeup should be used. The skin may heal with exposure to the sun, but a sunlamp or a blue-light lamp should only be used carefully.

Do not squeeze or pick at the pimples, as this will burst them and pus will come out and touch unaffected areas of skin. This can result in an infection. Instead, just gently wash the face.

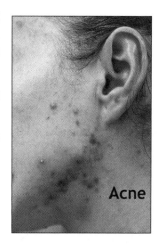

Acne

Benzoyl peroxide often helps. It is used to treat acne and is a useful antiseptic.

Topically, one can apply turmeric and sandalwood paste to the face.

Alternatively, use equal parts of:

Turmeric
Sandalwood
Saffron
Neem
Add milk to make this into a paste and then apply to the skin in the morning and evening.

Orally, take equal portions of:

Coriander seed powder
Fennel seed powder
Turmeric
Āmalakī
Take half a teaspoon of this mixture orally, half an hour before lunch and dinner.

Other treatments include vitamin A and vitamin E. In modern Western medicine, they often prescribe tetracycline antibiotics daily for a couple of months and, in cases of cystic acne, isotretinoin, a retinoid medication derived from Vitamin A. However, there are side effects and a risk of loss of pregnancy as well as severe birth defects, and these drugs are toxic to the liver and hematopoietic system.

The Ayurvedic approach to acne is fascinating. Many times, acne happens because of stagnation of rañjaka pitta in the liver. If tejo (fire element) agni is high, people can get hives, rashes and acne. Ayurvedic treatments aim to pacify pitta in the liver.

A good herbal treatment is one tablet of ārogya vardhini twice daily. Alternatively, the following herbal formula is beneficial for many cases of acne:

Shatāvarī 500 mg
Gudūchī 400 mg
Neem 300 mg
Turmeric 300 mg
Kama dudhā 200 mg
This formula can be taken three times a day.

Do daily virechana (purgation) with one teaspoon of either triphala or nishottara at bedtime, to keep the intestines clean and healthy. Because acne is due to high pitta in rasa and rakta dhātus, virechana removes the excess pitta and relieves the acne.

Yoga and prāṇāyāma can be helpful. Shītalī and shītkāri prāṇāyāma are beneficial for someone with acne. Camel, cobra, cow, boat, bow, bridge, locust, lotus, lion and spinal twist poses, as well as moon salutation, are all calming and soothing *yoga āsana* for acne. (see yoga poses page 450) So'ham meditation is recommended.

Stress management is important. The person should stay cool and calm, and not become irritated about trifling things. Avoid being aggressive or judgmental. Stay out of the hot sun and avoid highly stressful situations.

Just by following this treatment protocol, one can have grand success in treating pītika.

# Dermatitis

Dermatitis (*tvak rāga pāka*) is inflammation of the skin. Tvak rāga pāka means angry, red, and inflamed skin.

## Causes of Dermatitis

The causative factors of dermatitis are similar to acne, with high pitta being the main provoking factor. Pitta from the small intestine undergoes sanchaya (accumulation) and prakopa (aggravation), and can then spread during the prasara (spreading) stage of disease and deposit under the skin, causing dermatitis. Those first three stages are silent. The moment the fourth stage happens, the symptoms of this skin disease flare.

## Signs and Symptoms of Chronic Dermatitis

**Chronic Dermatitis** commonly occurs on the hands or feet and creates constant irritation. There is itching, inflamed skin, and scaling. The person has long-lingering high systemic pitta, which lodges under the skin. Certain factors can trigger the dermatitis, including extensive hand washing with chemical soap or detergent and fungal infection.

**Contact Dermatitis** can be caused by skin contact with chemicals in detergents, powders, salves, cosmetics, lotions, and soaps. In a person with sensitive skin, these can produce an allergic reaction within a few days, weeks, or years of repetitive usage. Poison ivy, as well as chemicals in clothing or even shoes, can also be a cause, as can contact with metal watchbands, rings, or jewelry. Some people are sensitive to ultra violet rays, in which case exposure to the sun can lead to dermatitis. Antibiotic creams are another possible cause. These are all classical characteristics of contact dermatitis due to skin allergy. The cause of this allergy is tejas burning ojas. It is a localized reaction of pitta dosha, and systemic pitta may not be increased.

Under the Chronic Dermatitis category, there are several clinical subcategories.

### 1. Eczema

Is a type of chronic dermatitis. It is inflammation of the skin with small blisters, redness, scales, crusts, and scab formation. There is burning, itching, and dryness or oozing. Most eczema cases are tridoshic, with vāta pushing pitta, which is pushing kapha in rasa and rakta dhātus. Burning is due to pitta, itching is due to kapha, and dryness is due to vāta.

Dry eczema is vāta type; it is more common in elderly people. Angry red eczema rash is pitta type; it is more common in adults. Weeping, oozing type of eczema is kapha type, and it is more common in children.

Individuals with a family history of asthma, hay fever, and other allergies are prone to get eczema. The eczema often subsides by the age of three, but may reappear by age 12 to 15 (teenage), which is the start of pitta age.

Wheat or gluten sensitivity, milk allergy, allergy to eggs, and other food allergies, the main causative factors of eczema, along with exposure to pollen. Areas of skin at the back of the knees and the elbows are commonly affected.

## 2. Exfoliative Dermatitis

After shaving of the skin, those parts of the body can get itching and burning. The skin surface of body becomes red, scaly and thickened. It looks like a drug reaction and can result in a severe skin reaction. In severe cases it may need hospitalization, as it can be life threatening.

## 3. Neurodermatitis

In this chronic inflammatory condition, itching is due to long-lingering pitta in majjā dhātu. There is localized thick, sharp, borderline scaly, breaking of the skin, resulting in leathery skin with little blisters. This localized neurodermatitis may be triggered by habitual scratching at the site of an insect bite or other irritation.

## 4. Nummular Dermatitis

A coin-shaped patch can blister and ooze, creating dry, crusty skin and itching on the legs, buttocks and the trunk. It can look like ring worm and is often misdiagnosed.

## 5. Seborrheic Dermatitis

Seborrhea has scaling and inflammation of the scalp, with dandruff and cradle cap in infants.

## 6. Stasis Dermatitis

This produces stubborn inflammation of the lower legs. There can be mild scaling or brownish discoloration, with red, oozing, scaling, itching patches and the person feels like scratching. This is another chronic dermatitis condition.

## Management of Dermatitis

The treatment of these various types of dermatitis is to clean the affected area without soap. Regular use of any chemical soap is contraindicated, although you can use natural Ayurvedic soaps such as sandalwood or neem soap.

When the skin is sensitive and irritated, oatmeal and other natural cleansers are most effective. An oatmeal, chickpea, neem, or baking soda bath can help the itching and relieve inflammation. In the bathtub, add one-third cup each of oatmeal, chickpea flour, neem powder, and baking soda powder.

In order to relieve itching, you can apply ice, in the form of ice packs or frozen plastic bags, directly onto the itching area. Ice does not feel nice, but it has good medicinal value. Its anti-inflammatory action helps to pacify the itching.

Milk is an effective topical remedy for weeping eczema. Apply a compress of cold milk on to the site of the eczema.

Use no antiperspirants or drying agents, because they can contain aluminum chloride, aluminum sulfate, and zirconium chloral hydrate. These are irritating substances. Baking soda is a good antiperspirant, and it does not have bad side effects.

Stay dry and odor free. Keep fingernails short and the fingers clean. Instead of scratching the itchy areas, press firmly on the surface of the skin for one minute to help relieve the itching. As it displaces the blood, it displaces pitta dosha.

## Some Other Tips

- Hot spicy food, fatty fried food, sour citrus fruit, fermented foods such as pickles, as well as red wine and hard liquor can all provoke pitta and aggravate the symptoms, so avoid these foods and drinks.
- In dry skin conditions, using a humidifier can be helpful.
- Keep showers extra short, or take a warm (not hot) bath for five minutes, to keep the skin moist in dry conditions.
- Use urea or lactic acid to help relieve the itching. Micturition on the site of the itching may help.
- Don't swim in chlorinated pools.
- Rest, read, and relax.
- Check if there is any heavy metal sensitivity. If so, panchakarma is indicated.
- Avoid strong fragrances, colored or scented toilet paper, and stuffed animals and toys – these can all contain chemical irritants that should be avoided.
- Leave Christmas "tree free", as pine needles can irritate the skin. Instead, buy a metal or plastic Christmas tree.

A good herbal remedy to relieve dermatitis is:

Shatāvarī 500 mg
Gudūchī 400 mg
Neem 300 mg
Shankha pushpī 200 mg
Kama dudhā 200 mg
Moti bhasma 200 mg
Adults should take ½ teaspoon of this mixture three times daily; children ¼ teaspoon three times daily.

Also one teaspoon of triphala or bhumi āmalakī nightly as virechana.

Topically, apply a mixture of neem oil and coconut oil – half and half. It is calming, cooling and soothing.

# Psoriasis

*Kushtha* is the name given to any chronic skin condition. *Padma kushtha* means "red skin" and refers to the condition known as psoriasis.

Psoriasis is a persistent skin disease with thick red eruptions and scaly patches. It can cover small areas of skin or a large area of the body. About 2% of people between the ages of 15 to 30 (early pitta age) will get these problems. However, psoriasis needs lifelong treatment.

## Etiological Factors of Psoriasis

Psoriasis is not contagious and its cause is unknown. It is a malfunctioning of the skin growth and regeneration. With normal skin, the old cells change form and are then replaced by new cells. When rasa dhātu agni is vishama (irregular), the formation of skin becomes irregular and there is malformation of the skin.

A deeper layer of the skin may be formed for one month before the skin dies and flakes off. Then the rate of cell growth accelerates and the removal of the dead cells slows down. So more and more skin cells come to the surface and die in a short period of time—usually within four to five days. This results in increased cell growth. Psoriasis is a rasa dhātu nutritional disorder, due to irregular *rasa agni*.

There is a strong hereditary predisposition, caused by high tejas burning ojas, which is an autoimmune dysfunction. The disease can result in psoriatic arthritis, where the pitta-genic āma from the skin enters the joints and causes arthritis.

An injury, cut, burn, or trauma can create a weakness (khavaigunya) at the site of the lesion. Unresolved past *karma* may be one of the causative factors. Stress can be a trigger and there are often emotional factors.

Symptoms are often worse in the winter months, because agni is pulled back from the skin and periphery into the central GI tract. The upper respiratory mucous membrane is connected intimately to rasa dhātu. Therefore, a cold or upper respiratory tract infection can spread *pitta āma* from the throat into the rasa dhātu and into the skin. Hence, strep throat is also linked to psoriasis.

**CAUSES OF PSORIASIS**

Irregular rasa agni

Hereditary factors

Unresolved past karma

Stress

Injury

Dryness

Drug reactions

Infection, such as strep throat

**SIGNS / SYMPTOMS OF PSORIASIS**

Redness of the skin

Itching

Inflammation

Rapid growth of poorly developed skin cells, which pile up and create red scaly plaque

Red patches with silvery scale (plaque)

Dandruff and peeling of skin

Frail, thickened, discolored skin

Nails separated from the beds

Painful red patches around the joints (exfoliative psoriasis)

The symptoms commonly occur on the elbows, knees, trunk, and scalp, under the arms, and in the genital area

## Management of Psoriasis

Keep the skin moist by using some form of moisturizer. Many people apply petroleum jelly or lactic acid, but the best choice is to use tikta ghrita or shatāvarī ghee topically. Moisturize after bathing, by applying the medicated ghee gently onto the skin.

Ultraviolet light treatment, such as a tanning booth, can help to kindle the agni and stimulates synthesis of vitamin D.

Consumption of alcohol affects bhūta agni in the liver and dhātu agni in the tissues, so it interferes with the healing process. Alcohol pushes pitta from the GI tract into the rasa dhātu. Hence, alcoholics are prone to psoriasis. It is best not to consume alcohol at all when there is psoriasis, because alcohol increases capillary circulation (which is pitta in rasa and rakta dhātus) and can aggravate this condition.

Soaking in warm water helps. You can apply neem oil to the affected skin to stimulate the sebaceous glands and then do *avagraha sveda* (hot tub bath). (However, one should not swim.) Alternatively, add half a cup of baking soda, which is alkaline, to one gallon of water and apply to the itching area with a face cloth. Then cover the affected area with gauze or soft cotton soaked in cow's milk and cream.

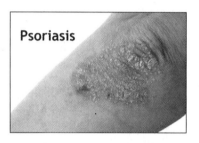

Psoriasis

Watch what you eat. Do not eat sardines, salmon, or tuna fish. Avoid tomatoes, potatoes, pork, fatty meat, caffeine, and sugar. Do not eat extra salt, and avoid fermented food such as yogurt and pickles. Also, try to avoid hydrophilic substances, such as yogurt, cucumber and zucchini.

Use an electric razor to shave, rather than a regular razor that can easily cut the skin and cause a secondary infection. Don't use chemical soap.

## Herbal Protocol for Psoriasis

Ārogya vardhini, 1 tablet three times daily to balance cellular metabolic activity and bring harmony between dhātu agni, bhūta agni, and pīlu agni. It is the best compound for most skin conditions, if you can obtain it.

Kama dudhā 200 mg
Moti bhasma 200 mg

Both are anti-inflammatory and effective in autoimmune dysfunction.

Equal parts of the following herbs:

Manjisthā, rejuvenative for skin
Neem, anti-inflammatory, anti-viral
Turmeric, anti-inflammatory, protects pigmentation cells
Take ½ teaspoon three times daily.

Another useful remedy is equal parts of kumārī āsava and maha manjisthādi kadha. Take 4 teaspoons of each with an equal quantity of water.

Avoid undue stress and take care of the mind by using equal parts of the herbs brahmī, jatamāmsi, shankha pushpī and tagara for tranquility.

Guard against infections by taking equal parts of neem, turmeric, and manjisthā powder. Also, apply neem oil or bhringarāja tailam onto the affected skin areas.

# Athlete's Foot

Fungal infection of the foot (tinea pedis), known as "ringworm of the foot" because it looks like ringworm, though it is not. It is called *dadru*. Many cases are long lasting.

## Management of Athlete's Foot

The following remedies can be applied topically:

- Neem oil with turmeric
- Vacha powder
- Cleansing soaps, such as neem or sandalwood soap
- Remove the dead skin with a brush and rub an antiseptic such as 3% hydrogen peroxide, Lysol, Detol, or neem oil onto the affected area
- Talcum powder
- Baking soda - dust the toes and shoes, and rub in between the toes
- When taking off socks, rub them up and down on the nails of your toes, to keep the toenails dry and clean.
- Blow your hair dryer in between the toes to ensure they are dry
- Place lamb's wool between the toes
- Soak the feet in turmeric water. Take a gallon of water, add a tablespoon of turmeric, and soak your feet in that water
- Nirgundī juice
- Mustard oil
- Bhringarāja oil
- Echinacea
- Gunja tailam
- Jatiadi tailam
- Coconut and olive oil
- Apply a paste made of neem, turmeric, mudgha (gram) and mustard oil

**CAUSES OF ATHLETE'S FOOT**

Tight shoes

Sweaty feet in warm weather

Moisture

Friction

Peeling of the skin

Ingrown toenails

Eczema, psoriasis, and scabies

Exposure to dyes

Builders, whose feet are exposed to cement and sand, and millers exposed to flour dust, are at higher risk.

**SIGNS / SYMPTOMS OF ATHLETE'S FOOT**

Itching, burning, and stinging sensations.

The skin between the toes is reddened, cracked, and crumbly.

The toenails become infected, discolored, and/or malformed.

The fungus can spread to the underside of the foot and beneath the arch.

It causes itching of the arch and the sole of the foot and there may be blisters.

The person's socks stink.

# Scabies

*Pāma* is a highly contagious communicable skin disease, caused by *bāhya krumi* (external parasites, a type of mite that causes itching). In modern medicine, it is called sarcoptes scabiei.

The female mites live in burrows and hatch eggs onto the skin. The larvae spread on the skin surface and mature within two to three weeks.

Scabies most commonly affects the webs of the fingers, the dorsum of the hand, axilla, inside thighs, beneath the breasts and the genitalia. Children are more commonly affected, but adults can also get scabies.

## Management of Scabies

Trim the fingernails and topically apply gandhaka druti, karanja tailam, or chukra tailam.

Only use natural soaps or Ayurvedic soap, such as neem or sandalwood soap.

Daily clean the wounds with an aseptic Ayurvedic medicated oil: ideally either ropanam tailam or shodhanam tailam.

Internally, the person can take 200 mg each of:

| | |
|---|---|
| Ārogya vardhini | Manjisthā |
| Sukshma triphala | Neem |
| Gandhaka rasāyana | Sutshekhar |
| Haridrā (turmeric) | |

Topically, one can apply:

| | |
|---|---|
| Hartal mixture | Brihanmarichadi tailam |
| Shodhan paste | Copper sulfate |

> **CAUSES OF SCABIES**
>
> Scabies can be transmitted by direct skin contact.
>
> **SIGNS / SYMPTOMS OF SCABIES**
>
> Causes itching of the skin; manifesting as papules, vesicles, and pustules.

# Eczema

In Ayurveda, all skin diseases are called kushtha. *Kotha* means local cooking, fermentation and putrefaction. In eczema, which is common disease that falls under the category of kushtha, the skin becomes putrefied. Eczema is a tridoshic disorder.

Eczema is the general term for an itchy red rash with irritation. It can weep or ooze sebum and may become crusty or thickened. The fundamental etiological factor is tejas burning ojas in the skin.

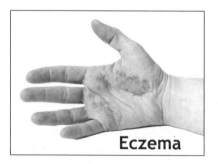

Eczema

## Management of Eczema

Avoiding the cause is the major part of the treatment. So for a rash caused by sun sensitivity, avoid excessive exposure to UV rays. For rashes and irritation due to drugs, poison oak, chemical soaps or perfumes, one should avoid those causative factors. In that way, the skin will not be further aggravated.

The following herbal remedies are recommended in the Ayurvedic literature:

| | |
|---|---|
| Manjisthā | Karanja |
| Neem | Pathola |
| Haridrā (turmeric) | Dāruharidrā |
| Kadhira | Bākuchī |

Usually, these herbs are given in a dose of 200 mg each.

Those herbal remedies are generally pitta pacifying, because skin diseases such as eczema are predominantly due to aggravated pitta. Manjisthā is a blood purifier, while neem is antibacterial, antiviral, and disinfectant. Karanja is good for kapha and pitta, as is turmeric, which is antibacterial, antiviral, and a good blood cleanser. Bākuchī is antiseptic.

The herbs below may also be prescribed according to the specific prakruti-vikruti and the type of eczema:

| | |
|---|---|
| Manahshilā | Swayambhu guggulu |
| Gandhaka rasāyana | Sukshma triphala |
| Vidanga | Tagara |

Certain Ayurvedic herbal wines can help:

Mahamanjisthādi kvatha
Sarasvat arishta
2 to 4 teaspoons of each with equal quantity of water, twice daily after lunch and dinner.

Topically, the following medicated oils may be applied:

| | |
|---|---|
| Maha bhringarāja tailam | Karanja tailam |
| Bākuchī oil | Shatāvarī ghrita |
| Neem oil | |

Use a natural, Ayurvedic soap, such as sandalwood soap or neem soap.

### Dietary Do's and Don'ts

No hot spicy foods, sour fruit, citrus, pickles, yogurt, jaggery, fermented food, idli, dosa, dhokala, fish, yogurt, cheese, wheat, peanuts, mushrooms or yeast containing bread. Reduce salt intake. This is all very important.

Beneficial foods for eczema and most skin disorders include mung dal, masoor dal, bitter melon, drumstick, basmati or jasmine rice, leafy greens, tapioca, millet, amaranth and steamed vegetables.

---

**CAUSES OF ECZEMA**

Chemical exposure, including intolerance (asatmya) of irritating chemical soaps, shampoos or perfumes

A drug reaction

Habitual scratching and rubbing of the skin

Sun exposure

Excessive perspiration, which can cause a fungal infection

Poison ivy

Emotional factors: Psychologically, pitta emotions push pitta from the GI tract into the periphery (rasa-rakta dhātus). When a person is angry, his or her skin becomes flushed, whereas when someone is fearful, his or her skin looks pale. Unresolved anger, irritability, hate, envy, or jealousy can all trigger pitta skin diseases.

**SIGNS / SYMPTOMS OF ECZEMA**

Itching

Rash that initially weeps and oozes and then may become crusty, flakey, thick, and scaly

## Other Recommendations
- Take a daily bath with no chemical soap or shampoo.
- Use no chemical perfume or deodorant.
- Wear cotton or silk.
- Do not wear synthetic clothes, such as polyester or nylon.
- Do rakta moksha, which means bloodletting. This is traditionally done using leeches, but may also be performed by donating a small amount of blood.

### Remedies for Specific Skin Diseases

**Seba (Sidma Kushtha)**

A seborrheic infection that occurs on the neck, cheeks and chest, producing a whitish dry patch. It is a fungal infection.

Apply lime juice topically before showering.

Internally, 200 mg of Vidanga three times daily.

**Tinea Ringworm (Dadru)**

Ringworm infection can happen on the neck, back, or waist. A round reddish patch of rash appears.

Topically, apply leeches for rakta moksha. Also Shodhana paste and Tulsi juice.

Internally, give:

Equal portions of Neem, Turmeric and Sandalwood; 1/2 teaspoon three times daily
Ārogya vardhini; 1 tablet, twice daily
Sukshma Triphala; 200 mg three times daily
Triphala; 1/2 teaspoon daily at night

**Vicharchika, a Type of Eczema**

Application of leeches for rakta moksha (jalauka)
Kampilla (a mineral)          Sandalwood
Yashthi madhu (licorice)    Neem
Ārogya vardhini; 1 tablet, twice daily

**Kitiba, a Type of Psoriasis**

Neem              Kama dudhā
Yashthi madhu    Praval pañchāmrit
Sandalwood
Ārogya vardhini; 1 tablet, twice daily

**Cracked Feet and Hands**

For topical use, combine shankhajira (a mineral), chandan (raw sandalwood paste), and beeswax.

**Dandruff**

For topical use, neem oil, bhringarāja oil, karanja tailam, or shikaki shampoo.

**Herpes Zoster (Chickenpox / Shingles)**

This occurs along the nerve pathways.

Ārogya vardhini; 1 tablet, twice daily

200 mg each of sutshekhar, kama dudhā and moti bhasma; 1/2 teaspoon twice daily

Topically, apply sandalwood paste

# PART TWO: Skin Disorders, Kushtha, Part 2

## Chickenpox

In the ancient Ayurvedic literature, the illness we know as chickenpox is categorized as a form of fever (jvara roga). That fever is called *masūrikā jvara;* masūrikā means blisters.

### Causes of Chickenpox

According to modern medicine, chickenpox is due to a viral infection. The ancient Ayurvedic literature says it is a disorder of extremely high pitta and high tejas.

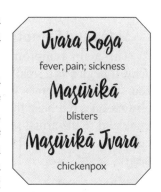

**Jvara Roga**
fever, pain; sickness

**Masūrikā**
blisters

**Masūrikā Jvara**
chickenpox

There is a sūtra that addresses masūrikā jvara. This sūtra says that toxins (āma), especially pitta type of āma from the gastrointestinal (GI) tract, undergo sanchaya (accumulation), prakopa (provocation), and then prasara (spread). During the prasara stage, the āma and pāchaka pitta from the stomach enter into the rasa and rakta dhātus. There, the pāchaka pitta disturbs bhrājaka pitta and rañjaka pitta and creates the typical blisters and rash of chickenpox on the skin.

Chickenpox is an extremely contagious disease that is caused by an infection with the varicella zoster virus, one of the herpes viruses. A rash that forms blisters on the skin characterizes the disease. It occurs mainly in children between the ages of five and eight, although approximately 10% of cases in United States affect people over 15 years of age. Chickenpox is transmitted so easily that everyone in a family can get the disease at the same time.

> A decidedly pitta disorder, people with pitta prakruti and pitta vikruti are most likely to get chickenpox and it occurs mainly in the pitta-predominant season (summer). According to Ayurveda, a pitta-producing diet and lifestyle are two of the primary causative factors.

Chickenpox is a strongly pitta disorder. People with pitta prakruti and pitta vikruti are most likely to get chickenpox, and it occurs mainly in the pitta-predominant season (summer). According to Ayurveda, a pitta-producing diet and lifestyle are two of the causative factors. In previous times, there wasn't the concept of a virus, but Ayurveda talked about *krumi*. The concept of *sūkshma adarshanīya krumi* is a tiny, invisible virus that has an affinity to rasa and rakta dhātus.

Chickenpox is contracted by touching someone infected by the disease, and especially touching a blister or anything that has been contaminated by contact with the patient. The virus is also airborne, so an infected person can transmit it before the rash has even developed.

Another way to get chickenpox is by exposure to shingles (herpes zoster). The same virus causes shingles and chickenpox: varicella zoster. Sometimes the mother gets shingles and, seemingly just by seeing the mother's shingles, the child gets chickenpox.

The incubation period for chickenpox, which is the time between exposure to the virus and appearance of symptoms, is about 10 to 20 days. The illness is highly contagious for about 6 to 8 days after the rash appears, or until the blisters have dried up and formed scabs.

## Signs and Symptoms of Chickenpox

The main symptom is a rash, which can be very itchy. It begins as a small red spot on the trunk. Within an hour, the spot becomes larger and larger with fluid-filled blisters on a red base that begins to spread all over the trunk and to the arms, face, and scalp. The rash is more visible on the trunk and face, and less so on the extremities.

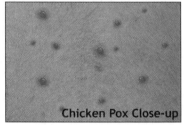
Chicken Pox Close-up

Within a few days, the blisters fill with the pus and then burst. The blisters then form a scab or crust. New spots appear periodically during a two to six day period, possibly spreading to the soles of the feet and palms of the hand. The rash may even affect the eyes, mouth, throat, vagina, and rectum.

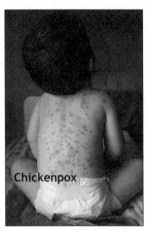
Chickenpox

The rash comes and goes, but in the earliest stage a baby will have a cold, congestion, and cough, be a little feverish and, if you look at the palpable portion of conjunctiva, at the margin of the eyelashes and eyelid, there is a typical fine rash on the conjunctiva. Even a week before the blisters appear, an expert pediatric doctor can see that rash and be able to tell that this child will get chickenpox.

Because of disturbed pitta from the GI tract entering into the hematopoietic system (especially rasa dhātu), there is a mild fever of up to 101 to 103 degrees Fahrenheit (38-39 degrees Celsius). Some children, especially kapha and vāta types, only have a slight fever. They feel slow and sluggish, and then the rash begins. Adults and some pitta prakruti children can get a high fever, with rash, headache and muscle aches. Recovery from all the symptoms occurs within 2 weeks.

Complications seldom develop in otherwise healthy people. However, don't take chickenpox lightly. The most common complication is secondary bacterial infections of the blisters, which can occur if a blister is scratched and the skin is broken. In some instances, the rash spreads to the eyes, causing pain and possibly damage to the eyes.

A rare but serious complication of chickenpox and other viral illnesses in children is Reye's syndrome, which is brain inflammation accompanied by swelling of the liver. Consult a doctor if there are early signs and symptoms of Reye's syndrome. These include extreme drowsiness, confusion, diarrhea, breathing problems, severe headache, nausea, and vomiting. There usually is no fever. This condition will probably last for several weeks before recovery happens. Other complications include pneumonia, encephalitis, and toxic shock syndrome. Although complications are rare, infants whose mothers never had chicken pox, pregnant women who have never had chickenpox, adults, and those whose immune systems are suppressed or compromised can be at risk.

## Management of Chickenpox

The main management protocol is to treat the pitta. Never give aspirin to children or teenagers with chickenpox, because aspirin can trigger high pitta in the GI tract. The best herbal alternative is a combination of mahasudarshan and sutshekhar. Mahasudarshan and sutshekhar are a specific herbal protocol for chickenpox that pacifies pitta. If you also get proper rest and take care of pitta dosha in other ways, the chickenpox will calm down.

> **FOR THE CHICKENPOX RASH**
>
> Apply a sandalwood and turmeric paste to the skin.
>
> One can also use chamomile lotion.
>
> **TO REDUCE ITCHING**
>
> Use fresh-squeezed cilantro (coriander, Coriandrum sativum) juice or cilantro pulp applied to the rash.
>
> **ONCE SCABS ARE FORMED**
>
> Take a warm bath mixed with baking soda, neem powder or oatmeal. This keeps the skin clean and reduces the risk of infection. Gently blot the skin dry with a towel.

> **CHICKENPOX**
>
> If there is fever or respiratory problems, such as cold, congestion, or cough, one can use the following herbal formula:
>
> Sitopalādi 500 mg
> Talisadi 400 mg
> Mahasudarshan 300 mg
> Kanthakārī 200 mg
> Abhrak bhasma 200 mg
> Moti bhasma (pearl ash) 200 mg
>
> Give this mixture ½ teaspoon, three times daily along with tikta ghrita (bitter ghee) or kumārī (aloe vera juice). The person can also take mahasudarshan kadha three times daily.

For the rash, we can apply a sandalwood and turmeric paste to the skin. In modern times, people apply chamomile lotion for itching. This itching is due to aggravated pitta dosha, so if we give 200 mg each of sutshekhar and kāma dudhā, that will also take care of it. Another remedy to reduce the itching is the topical application of cilantro (fresh coriander) juice or cilantro pulp.

The patient should wait until scabs are formed and then take a warm bath mixed with baking soda, neem powder, or oatmeal. This is important, as it will keep the skin clean and reduce the risk of infection. There is a possibility of spreading the infection to other parts of the skin, eyes, nose, and throat.

It is important to gently, yet thoroughly, dry the skin after bathing with a warm soft towel. If the itching is bad, the fingernails should be trimmed and clothes worn at night to minimize any trauma and unconscious scratching in the sleep. Children may need to wear socks and/or gloves during the rash period.

### Prevention of Chickenpox

Because the viral infection can go to the brain, if the child gets bad headaches and rigidity in the neck, it can cause a severe endocrine, neurological, or viral infection in the brain. To prevent that, we can use 200 mg each of brahmī, jatamāmsi, shankha pushpī, and mahasudarshan.

Although almost everyone can contract chickenpox, most people do not get it again because the body manufactures antibodies to fight the virus. This is called acquired immunity. Once a child gets exposure to chickenpox, the immune system knows how to fight off any future infection by producing antibodies.

The chickenpox virus may cause shingles later in life. In modern medicine, vaccination is given against chickenpox and shingles. That way your immune system is trained to fight off the viruses. I'm giving you an integrated approach to masūrikā, with both the Ayurvedic view and the modern concept of chickenpox.

## Shingles

When children get chickenpox, if the illness is not properly treated, the virus remains dormant in the neuromuscular cleft. Then as an adult, especially in middle age, the person can get shingles (herpes zoster).

According to Ayurveda, vāta pushing pitta in the majjā and māmsa dhātus can create disturbed bhrājaka pitta or rañjaka pitta along the tract of the nerves. That is called *nāgina*. Nāgina actually means a red-colored female cobra (*nāga* is a male cobra). The shingles literally look like a cobra creeping under skin.

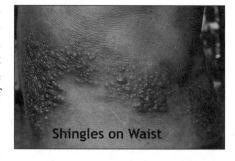
Shingles on Waist

Nāgina or shingles is a painful viral infection of one or more nerves. The infection produces rash, blisters, itching, burning sensation, and severe pain. Even your clothes cannot touch it without aggravating the pain, so some people have to remain without clothes on that area of their body.

In the beginning, the shingles rash looks identical to the chickenpox rash, but whereas chickenpox is scattered on the trunk, face and extremities, the shingles usually appears only in one area.

### Causes of Shingles

Shingles usually occurs only in person who have already had chickenpox as a child. Some authorities believe that after a case of chickenpox has run its course, the varicella zoster virus lies dormant in the neuromuscular cleft and whenever the person gets a fever, suffers emotional stress, physical injury or trauma, or has a pitta-aggravating diet and lifestyle over a period of time, the virus may be reactivated. That triggers a rash along the tract of a nerve or nerves. Ayurveda says that this is due to vāta dosha pushing pitta in the māmsa and majjā dhātus.

Some scientists believe that the number of strains of antibodies that are produced by the body to fight the varicella zoster virus (chickenpox) diminish over time. This makes the person susceptible to another attack. These antibodies linger to ensure that exposure to the varicella virus will prevent recurrence of chickenpox. However, that same person can get shingles.

The incidence of shingles increases with age. It rarely occurs in people under the age of 15. Shingles is uncommonly common in middle age and in the elderly—the later part of the pitta stage of life (especially from 50 years of age) and the vāta phase. The older a person is, the higher the chance they will get shingles if exposed to the virus.

Elderly people get shingles because the chickenpox virus is still lingering in the māmsa and majjā dhātus. This creates a khavaigunya and in old age, when the person's immunity is depleted, any form of stress can activate the virus.

Shingles cannot be passed on to another person. However, because shingles is caused by the chickenpox virus, if an adult who has not had chickenpox is exposed to shingles, he or she will likely get chickenpox. In summary, people can get chickenpox from shingles but cannot get shingles from chickenpox.

## Signs and Symptoms of Shingles

Shingles begins with a prickling tenderness under the skin over the affected nerves. There are burning sensations and shooting pain in the same area. That is pūrva rūpa (early symptoms). Within two to four days, a rash of small red spots appear over the affected area of the body. As the spots enlarge, they become blisters that form in a row, following the tract of a nerve.

Eventually, the blisters fill with pus, then burst and create a crust. The skin around the affected area looks red and there is long-lingering pain. The shingles rash is initially itchy and the pain increases as the rash becomes reddened and more swollen.

Shingles most often attacks the intercostal nerves, with the chest, back, arms, or facial nerves frequently involved. The rash appears in a strip and it is distributed along the pathway of the nerve.

Usually, the shingles blisters persist for two to three weeks before clearing and the pain continues for about four to eight weeks. However, shingles may continue for two or more months, and I have seen patients in pain for six months or longer. In people over age

---

**SHINGLES**

An Ayurvedic herbal protocol for shingles is:
  Ārogya vardhini 200 mg
  Sutshekhar 200 mg
  Kama dudhā with moti 200 mg
  Manjistha 200 mg
  Neem 200 mg
  Turmeric 200 mg

This can be taken ½ teaspoon, three times daily.

Topically, apply sandalwood paste onto the rash.

**PAIN RELIEF FOR SHINGLES**

In modern medicine, there is no cure for shingles. The treatment focuses on reducing pain. A useful Ayurvedic herbal painkiller for shingles is:
  Shatāvarī 500 mg
  Tagara 300 mg
  Gulvel sattva 200 mg
  Kaishore guggulu 200 mg
  Kama dudhā 200 mg

These are all anti-inflammatory herbs that relieve burning sensations and also act as analgesics. The formula can be taken three times daily.

60, the pain can persist for many months or years because of khavaigunya in the nerves. This is called post-herpetic neuralgia.

## Management of Shingles

In cases of post-herpetic neuralgia, antidepressant and anti-seizure medications may be given to the patient, as well as electrical stimulation of the affected area and analgesics to reduce the pain.

Some physicians proscribe a steroid drug to reduce nerve inflammation. To be effective, steroids must be taken soon after the shingles occur. In Ayurveda, a good anti-inflammatory formula is equal parts of licorice, neem, and gudūchi taken three times daily.

Preventing infection is important. A warm bath with baking soda is helpful, as water soothes and cleans the skin. If itching is a problem, apply cilantro pulp topically as needed and also take cilantro juice orally by drinking two tablespoons, two times daily. One can also eat cantaloupe and apply the cantaloupe skin to the rash, as this will help to take care of the rash and itching.

### Prevention of Shingles

There is no guarantee of prevention of this disease because there is no specific vaccination for this disorder.[32] For prevention, Ayurveda suggests the use of maha tikta ghrita, sutshekhar, or mahasudarshan as these herbal remedies have great preventative value.

## Cold Sores

Cold sores (*ostha pitika*) are also known as fever blisters. They are fluid-filled blisters that appear on the border of the lips, around the nose, or at mucocutaneous junctions.

These blisters are due to a highly contagious virus (herpes simplex) that affects much of the population.[33] It enters the body through the nose, mouth, lips or wherever the skin is easy to penetrate – most commonly the mucocutaneous junction at the angle of the mouth.

Between these occurrences of cold sores, the inactivated virus "hides" in the tissue. There is always a possibility of recurrence of this infection, due to diminished ojas or a period of stress. When that happens, the herpes simplex virus becomes active and the person gets another cold sore.

### Causes of Cold Sores

This is a disorder of both bhrājaka pitta and rañjaka pitta. Cold sores can occur due to many reasons:

- skin injury that breaks open the skin
- exposure to heat

---

32. There is a substance called varicella zoster immune globulin that is a human antibody against the virus. It is a purified immune globulin preparation made from human plasma containing high levels of anti-varicella-zoster virus antibodies. It must be used within 4 days after a known exposure to the virus and is recommended only for immunocompromised patients, newborns whose mothers had signs of the virus around birth, and some hospitalized premature infants.
33. The World Health Organization (WHO) estimates that 67% of people under the age of 50 are infected with herpes simplex virus type 1 (HSV-1).

- summer season, sunlight
- working under hot conditions
- emotional stress
- eating hot spicy food, bacon
- excessive consumption of alcoholic beverages
- smoking cigarettes
- fever, common cold, or congestion
- menstruation

dental work

These can all aggravate the virus and cause an outbreak. Whether the person gets cold sores depends upon the individual's immunity.

The virus sheds and is contagious even before the appearance of sores. It is spread through skin-to-skin direct contact, sharing of cups, utensils, and lip balm/lipstick. One can also spread it by touching the sore and then touching an open lesion on the skin.

### Signs and Symptoms of Cold Sores

The virus may be present without any symptoms, which means the virus is inactive. When the virus becomes active, it creates pain, tenderness and sometimes numbness of the affected area, and slowly little fluid-filled blisters appear. These blisters eventually erupt and begin to heal, which can take two to four weeks.

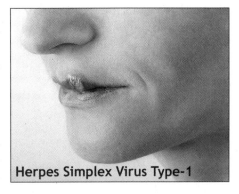

**Herpes Simplex Virus Type-1**

Occasionally there can be excessive pain and swelling. If the herpes simplex virus occurs on the lips, the submandibular and sublingual lymph glands can be swollen. If it occurs on a woman's labia, it can affect the inguinal gland, causing soreness. If any glands are painful or tender, the patient probably has a secondary complication of lymphadenopathy that requires a doctor's attention.

If any labial blisters do not heal within a week, you should consult your doctor, because there is a possibility of secondary bacterial infection. Healing time may be shortened by certain medications, which can help to prevent any secondary infection.

Other complications are herpes simplex keratitis. This is a painful viral infection over the cornea. It creates a white spot and can result in blindness if not treated properly. When inflammation of the eyes is accompanied with fever and blister, a physician should be consulted immediately. Steroid medication should not be applied near the eye during the treatment of this condition.

## Management of Cold Sores

A beneficial Ayurvedic protocol for cold sores is to eat a pitta-pacifying diet, follow a pitta-soothing lifestyle, and to take the following formula, ½ teaspoon, three times daily:

Ārogya vardhini 200 mg
Sutshekhar 200 mg
Kama dudhā 200 mg
Kaishore guggulu 200 mg
Neem 200 mg
Turmeric 200 mg
Manjisthā 200 mg

Topically, apply tikta ghrita or maha tikta ghrita onto the cold sore twice daily.

This is the best protocol for herpes simplex and it can really help this condition.

## Summary

The ancient herbal protocol of turmeric, neem, and manjisthā has antibacterial and antiviral actions. This combination can really take care of these infectious conditions and bacterial invasion. Take a mixture of 200 mg each, ½ teaspoon, three times a day.

These infectious diseases have interacted with humans for thousands of years. Almost all of us have had some exposure to them. Ayurveda has herbal protocols that can support you during an infection and act as preventatives to infection and outbreaks. Maintaining balanced doshas is your best 'defense' in preserving your good health.

# Chapter 23

# Anemia
## Pāndu

Winter 2017, Volume 30, Number 3

*Raktavarahanam srotasam mūlam
Yakrut plīha cha*

. . . . . . . . . . . . . . . . . . . . . . . . . . . . . . . . . . . . . . . . . . . . . . . . . . . .

This famous Ayurvedic sūtra states that the liver and spleen are
the root of rakta vaha srotas and they perform a hematopoietic
function in the body of the fetus. That function is later transferred
to the bone marrow, which in Ayurveda is called rakta majjā.

. . . . . . . . . . . . . . . . . . . . . . . . . . . . . . . . . . . . . . . . . . . . . . . . . . . .

IN AYURVEDIC LITERATURE, anemia is called *pāndu*. The Sanskrit word "pāndu" means
pale white or pallor. In this disease, the skin looks pale, dull and lusterless, due to *rakta
kshaya,* which is depletion of blood. The nails and conjunctiva also look pale. When the
blood volume is low, it may affect the nutrition and oxygenation of all bodily tissues and
diminish ojas, the vital essence.

*Ojas kshaya* means decreased ojas. When ojas is depleted, there is reduced energy, the
complexion has a pale color, and a lack of oiliness of the skin. *Rakta vaha sroto agni,* the
digestive fire in the hematopoietic system, is also impaired.

The seven dhātus (tissues) play an important role in constructing the human body.
These tissues of the body are nourished by digestion of food and its intake into the bloodstream in succession from the first dhātu to the seventh. Each dhātu processes and digests
the nutrients and produces mature dhātu (tissue) and raw tissue that is the precursor nutrient for the next tissue. Each stage takes about five days. The first dhātu is rasa (the plasma
tissue) and the second is rakta (the red blood cells). It takes about ten days for the maturation of rasa dhātu into rakta and it is rakta dhātu that gives color to rasa.

According to Ayurveda, the rasa dhātu is comprised of nine añjali (handfuls) of plasma tissue, while rakta dhātu has eight añjali or approximately 8 pints. In the human body, rasa and rakta move together. The blood contains plasma, red blood cells, white blood cells, and platelets. The plasma and white blood cells are part of rasa, while the red blood cells and platelets are rakta dhātu.

## Functions of Rakta Dhātu

Rakta dhātu is circulated through the heart, arteries, capillaries, and veins. It carries nutrients, hormones, vitamins, minerals, antibodies, electrolytes, heat, and oxygen to the tissues. It takes away nitrogenous waste and toxic gases, such as carbon dioxide, so they can be eliminated from the body. Rakta dhātu also maintains water electrolyte balance and acid-base equilibrium and it maintains body temperature.

Blood contains rasa and rakta dhātus, rañjaka pitta, the 20 *gunas* (which may be related to the amino acids), the five great elements, the six tastes (sweet, sour, salty, pungent, bitter, astringent) and the three divine qualities (sattva, rajas and tamas).

Through a proper blood volume, rakta dhātu maintains blood pressure. When the blood volume is low, it affects the nutrition and oxygenation of all bodily tissues. When it is high, various conditions can result.

Coagulation (*rakta skandana*) is another important function of rakta dhātu. If there is a cut, burn or wound, rakta dhātu coagulates with the help of poshaka kapha and kledaka kapha. Therefore, rakta dhātu and rañjaka pitta maintain an appropriate bleeding time, which is approximately three to four minutes. Within that time, bleeding should stop.

Coagulation happens because of the astringent, dry, rough, and cold of qualities vāta, and the sticky, soft, and stable qualities of kapha dosha. These qualities are connected predominantly to the thrombocytes (platelets), which are a component of kapha dosha. This prevents hemorrhage.

The qualities of rakta dhātu are:

*Drava* – liquid, to maintain lubrication of the red blood cells.
*Sara* – spreading, so it maintains capillary circulation.
*Manda* – slow, which helps to coagulate the blood.
*Snigdha* – oily, to lubricate the tissues.
*Mrudu* – soft, helping to keep the tissues soft and to heal damaged tissues.
*Picchila* - sticky, which creates coagulation and blood clotting.
*Madhura* – sweet, to maintain the blood sugar, acting as a fuel to cellular metabolic activity.
*Lavana* – salty, maintaining water-electrolyte balance.

## ANEMIA

Normal Number of Red Blood Cells          Anemic Number of Red Blood Cells

Red Blood Cell

Platelet

White Blood Cell

NORMAL                              ANEMIC

## Classifications of Anemia

Anemia is a general term referring to the shortage of red blood cells (rakta dhātu) or a reduction of hemoglobin (rañjaka pitta). If hemoglobin is diminished, the blood's oxygen carrying capacity is reduced. Hemoglobin is a pigment that combines with oxygen molecules to carry the oxygen to every tissue in the body. Charaka says prāna runs with the blood in the form of oxygen and it is rañjaka pitta that gives color to the body.

From an Ayurvedic perspective, pāndu happens due to impaired *rakta agni.* Within the root of rakta vaha srotas, the asthāyi (unprocessed) rakta becomes *sthāyi* (processed) due to this digestive fire called rakta agni.

Ayurveda has five major clinical classifications of *pāndu roga:* vāta type, pitta type, kapha type, *sāmnipātika* (tridoshic) and krumi (parasites) type. In modern medicine, anemia is classified as nutritional deficiency anemia, hemolytic anemia, pernicious anemia, aplastic anemia, iron deficiency anemia, and so forth.

### Causes of Anemia

Anemia can be caused by many etiological factors:

- A deficiency of certain vitamins or minerals, or an inability to absorb those substances. Examples are iron deficiency anemia, or anemia due to a deficiency of vitamin $B_{12}$ or folic acid.
- Any long lingering disease, such as tuberculosis.
- An inherited genetic predisposition in the blood (*bīja doshaja pāndu*).
- Depletion of bone marrow, resulting in decreased production of red blood cells (*majjā kshaya*).
- Bleeding disorders such as blood in the stools, upper GI tract bleeding, bleeding ulcer, ulcerative colitis, hemorrhage, hemorrhoids, severe blood loss through menorrhagia, or blood loss due to accident or surgery.
- Drug allergies.
- Cancer, including blood cancer (leukemia), which can be a direct cause of anemia.
- Prolonged exposure to radioactive substances is another factor that can lead to anemia.

## APLASTIC ANEMIA

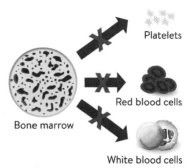

Platelets

Red blood cells

Bone marrow

White blood cells

## HEMOLYTIC ANEMIA

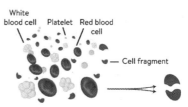

White blood cell    Platelet    Red blood cell

— Cell fragment

*Red blood cells are defective and break down more quickly*

## SICKLE CELL ANEMIA

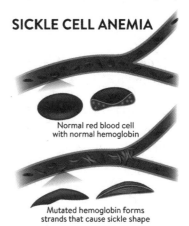

Normal red blood cell with normal hemoglobin

Mutated hemoglobin forms strands that cause sickle shape

## PERNICIOUS ANEMIA

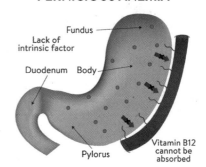

Fundus

Lack of intrinsic factor

Duodenum    Body

Pylorus

Vitamin B12 cannot be absorbed

- Poor diet, which is common for poor people around the world without access to nutritious food.
- Chronic alcoholism; alcohol can disturb pitta dosha and cause pitta type of anemia.
- Insufficient exposure to sunlight.
- A tendency for malformation of red blood cells, which is what happens in sickle cell anemia.
- An autoimmune disorder of tejas burning ojas, causing excessive destruction of red blood cells.

According to Ayurvedic literature, a long lingering doshic imbalance is the underlying cause of pāndu. Protein deficiency can cause *vāta pāndu*. Rañjaka pitta disorder affecting gastric intrinsic factor[34] can lead to *pitta pāndu*. Chronic *sroto rodha* (blocked channels) leading to nutritional deficiency is the cause of *kapha pāndu*.

## Pathophysiological Changes in Pāndu

When we look at different types of anemia categorized by modern medicine, we see that each has certain etiological factors that we can observe clinically.

- Total absence of red blood cells is called aplastic anemia. This is *rakta dhātu kshaya,* the depletion of the dhātu (tissue).
- Destruction of red blood cells can be an autoimmune disease called hemolytic anemia. This is also rakta dhātu kshaya.
- Sickle cell anemia, red blood cells with a distorted form, is tejas burning ojas.

Diagnosis is based upon the findings from a thorough physical examination of the patient and blood tests to detect red blood cells, hemoglobin, iron, and vitamin $B_{12}$ levels.

### Signs and Symptoms of Anemia

Anemia is called pāndu because the skin, conjunctiva, nail beds, creases of the palms, tongue, lips, and genitalia look pale. It is a disorder of rakta dhātu agni and also rañjaka agni. When rakta agni is low, there is undue formation of unprocessed rakta dhātu, which can lead to defective formation of red blood cells.

If we look at the symptoms of pāndu roga, one of the main ones is fatigue, due to lack of *prīnanam* (nourishment) and *jīvana* (oxygenation and life-giving energy). There is often shortness of breath, because of a lack of oxygen-carrying capacity in the blood. There is also often an increased heart rate, because the body demands more oxygen, and the heart compensating by trying to pump more blood. Therefore, there is a pounding, rapid heartbeat, resulting in headaches. This is a sādhaka pitta disorder, due to disturbed rañjaka pitta.

In vāta type of anemia (microcytic anemia, in which the red blood cells are smaller than normal, or aplastic anemia), the skin is dry, rough, scaly and pale. In pitta type

---

34. A glycoprotein produced by the parietal cells of the stomach. It is necessary for the absorption of vitamin $B_{12}$ (cobalamin) later on in the ileum of the small intestine. Retrieved November 14, 2017: https://en.wikipedia.org/wiki/Intrinsic_factor.

(hemolytic, hemorrhagic, aplastic, or pernicious anemia), the skin will have a yellowish tinge. In kapha anemia (megaloblastic anemia, in which the red blood cells are larger in size and smaller in number), the skin will be pale, cold, clammy and swollen.

When there is anemia, disturbed rañjaka pitta affects pāchaka pitta in the stomach and causes gastrointestinal (GI) tract ischemia[35], loss of appetite, and poor digestion.

Due to diminished blood volume, there is dizziness, ringing in the ears, weakness and sometimes fainting. The person can get burning sensations on the tongue or a change in the appearance of the tongue. If there is iron deficiency, there is often a history of menorrhagia, hemorrhage, hemorrhoids, or fissures.

In many serious cases, there are swollen ankles because of hypoproteinemia (lack of protein) edema. The pulse becomes rapid and weak and there is pain in the neck or abdominal muscles.

## Types of Anemia

### Iron Deficiency Anemia (*Vilohita Pāndu*)

Iron deficiency anemia is caused by a shortage of the important mineral iron. This pāchaka pitta disorder results in the individual not processing or absorbing iron, which is necessary for the production of hemoglobin. Rañjaka pitta in the stomach (gastric intrinsic factor) normally utilizes iron, vitamin $B_{12}$, and folic acid to produce red blood cells, so in this type of anemia, a rañjaka pitta disorder can produce iron deficiency anemia.

Pāchaka agni and rañjaka agni can be affected by a variety of conditions leading to blood loss. The person may be losing blood from hemorrhoids, fissures, fistulae, a bleeding peptic ulcer, upper GI tract bleeding, an accident, chronic blood loss, krŭmi (hookworms), or menorrhagia (profuse bleeding during menstruation). These can all create iron deficiency anemia, as can a diet that is lacking in iron.

### Folic Acid Deficiency Anemia (*Pāchaka Pitta Dushti Pāndu*; Pitta-kapha Type)

Folic acid is a B vitamin ($B_9$) that aids in the production of red blood cells. Folic acid deficiency anemia is due to insufficient dietary folate, which is necessary for hemoglobin production. It is one of the most common causes of megaloblastic anemia. Insufficient absorption of folate can be caused by malnutrition, alcoholism, small intestinal disorders, inflammatory bowel, irritable bowel syndrome, Crohn's disease, and regional ileitis. These are due to vāta pushing pitta in the gut. These conditions inflame the villi resulting in malabsorption. The tongue looks like a pale strawberry and the person gets repeated glossitis.

Even though folic acid deficiency anemia looks like pitta type, this rañjaka pitta disorder can inhibit the DNA synthesis during the production of red blood cells, resulting in increased kledaka kapha. This slows down red blood cell formation, which makes the cells larger in size and lower in number.

---

35. An inadequate blood supply to an organ or part of the body.

### Pernicious Anemia (*Agni Dushti Janita Pāndu; Pitta Type*)

Pernicious anemia arises if the body is unable to absorb vitamin $B_{12}$ (cyanocobalamin), which is necessary for the production of red blood cells in the bone marrow. It is the other common cause of megaloblastic anemia. Gastric intrinsic factor, which is a manifestation of rañjaka pitta in the stomach, is affected and the stomach is unable to absorb the $B_{12}$, a form of *rañjaka pitta dushti*.

An individual may suffer from vitamin $B_{12}$ deficiency and this can lead to anemia. It is common in cases of parasitic infection, as well as inflammatory bowel diseases such as ulcerative colitis and irritable bowel syndrome. Vitamin $B_{12}$ deficiency anemia can also create angular stomatitis.

It is important to note that during pregnancy, a woman needs to take supplements of folic acid, vitamin $B_{12}$, and iron to prevent anemia in mother and baby.

### Aplastic Anemia (*Rakta Dhātu Kshaya Pāndu;* Vāta-pitta Type)

Aplastic anemia is a serious condition caused by the inability of bone marrow to produce white blood cells, red blood cells, and platelets. The bone marrow function can be inhibited by cancer, exposure to radiation therapy (where bone marrow functioning is depressed), radioactive substances, chemotherapy, antibiotics, or hazardous chemical drugs. Viral infection or autoimmune disease can result in aplastic anemia, and pregnancy can be a contributing factor.

### Hemolytic Anemia (*Rakta Pitta Janita Pāndu; Pitta Type*)

Hemolytic anemia is caused by the excessive destruction of red blood cells. This type of anemia can either be acquired or developed congenitally, right at the time of birth. Acquired hemolytic anemia can be caused by mismatched blood transfusion, drug allergy, cancer, autoimmune disease, or a serious infection.

Congenital hemolytic anemia is caused by an inherited abnormality in the red blood cells, due to rañjaka pitta dushti. The most common type is sickle cell type anemia, a disorder that predominantly affects those of African descent. In this form of anemia, the red blood cells are distorted, so they look like a sickle shape. These cells cannot carry sufficient oxygen. They become fragile and are easily disintegrated or hemolyzed, breaking down easily. This disease is characterized by a crisis period, with severe joint or abdominal pain, that can lead to complications such as kidney failure, gallstones, or heart failure. Sickle cell anemia is treated with painkillers and blood transfusion.

### Hemorrhagic Anemia (*Rakta Srāva Janita Pāndu or Rakta Kshaya Janita Pāndu;* Vāta Type)

This is either an acute condition, due to a large volume of blood loss over a short period, or a chronic illness, caused by a smaller volume of blood loss over a long period. Hemorrhoids are a common cause of hemorrhagic anemia. It can also be caused by an infection, tumor, leukemia, lymphoma, lupus, or autoimmune disease. Certain drugs can also cause hemorrhaging, which may result in anemia.

Through thorough medical examination, we need to discover the precise type of anemia that the person has and then treat it accordingly.

## Ayurvedic Protocol for the Management of Pāndu

The main treatment of pāndu roga is to improve the blood volume and remove the cause that is resulting in destruction of the blood cells. The basic Ayurvedic approach is to use shamana chikitsā therapies, such as dīpana (kindling digestive fire), pāchana (eliminating toxins), and anulomana (maintains the normal direction of the dosha). We have to kindle the jathāra agni, bhūta agni and dhātu agni, and then balance the doshas.

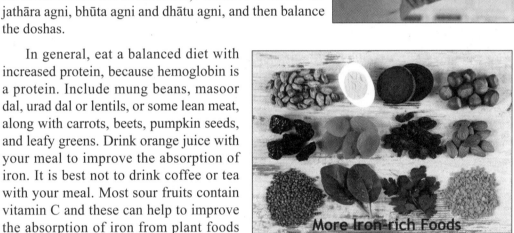

In general, eat a balanced diet with increased protein, because hemoglobin is a protein. Include mung beans, masoor dal, urad dal or lentils, or some lean meat, along with carrots, beets, pumpkin seeds, and leafy greens. Drink orange juice with your meal to improve the absorption of iron. It is best not to drink coffee or tea with your meal. Most sour fruits contain vitamin C and these can help to improve the absorption of iron from plant foods such as vegetables and grains. One can

More Iron-rich Foods

also eat iron-fortified cereals such as bran flakes. Good fruits and vegetables include pomegranates, cranberries, oranges, grapes, broccoli, Brussels sprouts, green peppers, raisins, and currants. Ghee is particularly beneficial in anemia, as ghee kindles agni, promotes ojas and improves digestion.

Most anemic patients have poor circulation and cold extremities, as iron carries heat, so they should keep the body warm. Exposure to the sun is beneficial.

In general, Ayurveda uses remedies such as abhrak bhasma, loha bhasma, raktavard-hak, kumārī āsava number 1, and tamra bhasma. The treatment protocol will vary depending upon the type of anemia and the precise cause. If it is folic acid deficiency anemia, we can add to the diet leafy greens, lettuce, spinach, broccoli, beets, carrots, and juices made from these fresh vegetables. If it is vitamin $B_{12}$ deficiency anemia, one has to take $B_{12}$ supplements.

For snehana therapy, triphala ghee, pancha tikta ghrita, or pancha dravya ghrita are given. Ghee is a standard Ayurvedic treatment protocol for pāndu.

Internally, 200 mg of navayasa churna is administered three times daily along with one teaspoon of tikta ghrita or ghrita madhu yoga (ghee and honey). Navayasa churna combines nine herbal ingredients with loha bhasma. Mandūra bhasma is purified ferric oxide. One can also give 200 mg of mandūra bhasma or punarnavā mandūra with a cup of buttermilk three times daily.

To achieve a proper medical line of treatment, we have to regularize the person's bowel movements. We can use virechana therapy, such as triphala, harītakī, āmalakī, bibhītakī or bhumi āmalakī. These choices of virechana substance will also build up rakta dhātu. Sometimes, because of bleeding, one also has to give piccha basti, which produces a hemostatic action.

This is a bird's eye view of dealing with anemia. If the patient is suffering from severe anemia, we may have to send that patient to the hospital where they might give a blood transfusion.

## Management Recommendations

### Vāta Pāndu (Microcytic Anemia or Aplastic Anemia)

The skin is dry, rough, and scaly. Take this herbal formula three times daily (TID)[a]:
Ashvagandhā 500 mg
Balā 400 mg
Dashamūla 400 mg
Vidārī 300 mg
Abhrak bhasma 200 mg

One teaspoon of chyavanprash each morning. Tikta ghrita to buck up the person's agni. For virechana, one teaspoon of harītakī at bedtime.

### Sāmnipātika Pāndu (Tridoshic Disorder)

Take this herbal formula TID:
Dashamūla 500 mg
Ashvagandhā 400 mg
Gudūchī 300 mg
Kama dudhā 200 mg
Kutki 200 mg
Chitrak 200 mg
Trikatu 200 mg
Navayasa churna 200 mg

This mixture should be taken three times daily with ghrita madhu yoga (a teaspoon of ghee mixed with a teaspoon of honey). The person should also take 2 Tablespoons of triphala ghee at bedtime. Triphala is also good for all three types of pāndu and is often given as an anulomana therapy to buck up the rakta dhātu.

### Kapha Pāndu (Megaloblastic Anemia)

Take the following herbal formula TID:
Punarnavā 400 mg
Mandūra bhasma 300 mg
Kutki 200 mg
Chitrak 200 mg

Also one teaspoon of maha tikta ghrita three times daily before meals.

For virechana, one teaspoon of bibhītakī at bedtime.

### Mrud Bhakshana Pāndu (Pica Disorder[b] Where Child Eats Clay)

Some young children have the urge to eat clay. This can also happen in pregnant women. In both cases, this can be due to a deficiency of calcium, iron or other nutrient. The clay has no nutritional value and eating clay decreases agni. Also the clay may contain parasites that are ingested. This can cause sroto rodha and a type of anemia called mrud bhakshana pāndu. For this condition, one can give the following herbal remedy:
Vidanga 200 mg
Kutki 200 mg
Gairika 200 mg
Indrayava (a form of bitter cumin) 200 mg

Take this mixture TID with meals.

## Pitta Pāndu (Hemolytic, Hemorrhagic, Aplastic, or Pernicious Anemia)

Take this herbal formulation TID:
Shatāvarī 500 mg
Gudūchī 400 mg
Kama dudhā 200 mg
Moti bhasma 200 mg

Take 4 teaspoons of kumārī āsava with equal parts water after lunch and dinner.

One teaspoon of maha tikta ghrita or pancha tikta ghrita three times daily before meals. These are types of medicated ghee that are particularly effective for pitta type of pāndu roga.

For virechana, one teaspoon of bhumi āmalakī or nishottara at bedtime. Āmalakī and bhumi āmalakī are good sources of vitamin C and iron. Give āmalakī with black raisins, honey, sugar and ghee to buck up the blood in people with pitta type of anemia. A decoction of āmalakī and the powdered root of chitrak is given with cow's milk at bedtime in cases of pitta anemia.

## Iron Deficiency Anemia

In iron deficiency anemia, we also have to give iron in the form of loha bhasma. Take the loha bhasma in addition to the remedies specified for the Ayurvedic type of pāndu shown above. One can either use 200 mg of loha bhasma three times daily, or loha āsava, a medicated fermented juice containing loha bhasma. The digestive power of the patient has to be improved so that there will be proper digestion, absorption and assimilation of iron, resulting in improved formation of rakta dhātu.

The best iron supplement used in modern medicine is ferrous gluconate, rather than ferrous sulfate, because the sulfate form can cause constipation. Cooking in a cast iron pan can also provide some iron supplementation, so cook pasta sauce and vegetables in an iron pan.

## Krumi Pāndu (Anemia Due to Hookworm or Other Parasitic Infection)

Vidanga 400 mg
Palash bīj[c] kajjali 300 mg
Krumi kuthar[d] 200 mg
Shigru bīj kajjali 200 mg

This formula should be taken TID.

Take 4 teaspoons of vidanga arishta or palashpushpāsava with equal parts of water after lunch and dinner. Kumārī āsava is also effective.

Additionally, the person should take one teaspoon of chyavanprash twice daily, and 200 mg each of punarnavā mandūra bhasma and loha bhasma taken with 1 teaspoon of panchagavya ghrita three times daily.

One should see an expert Ayurvedic physician to get a proper personalized formula that can treat the specific type of krumi.

## Hemolytic Anemia

Hemolysis is disintegration of red blood cells, which is cellular dhātu kshaya. One has to buck up the rakta dhātu by giving raktavardhak and the person sometimes needs a blood transfusion. A good formula to manage hemolytic anemia is:
Tapyadi loha 200 mg
Swarna makshika bhasma 200 mg
Abhrak bhasma 200 mg
Vanga bhasma 200 mg

Take this mixture TID with one teaspoon of shatāvarī ghee.

In general, to buck up the blood and improve the functioning of rakta vaha srotas, one can use the following formula:

Ārogya vardhini 200 mg

Sutshekhar 200 mg

2 teaspoons of raktavardhak twice daily after meals.

## Ojas Kshaya

If there is ojas kshaya (depleted ojas), one can add the following herbal remedies:

Tapyadi loha 200 mg three times daily with meals.

One teaspoon of chyavanprash each morning.

One teaspoon of ashvagandhā avaleha three times daily with meals.

One teaspoon of shatāvarī kalpa, taken twice daily.

    a.  TID, ter in die, is Latin for three times a day.
    b.  The persistent ingestion of non-nutritive substances.
    c.  Also spelled beej.
    d.  Also spelled krimikuthar ras.

# Chapter 24

# Fibromyalgia

Summer 2017, Volume 30, Number 1

. . . . . . . . . . . . . . . . . . . . . . . . . . . . . . . . . . . . . . . . . . . . . . . . . . . .

Ayurveda says that fibromyalgia could be an autoimmune disorder
caused by tejas burning ojas.

. . . . . . . . . . . . . . . . . . . . . . . . . . . . . . . . . . . . . . . . . . . . . . . . . . . .

FIBROMYALGIA IS MISCELLANEOUS CHRONIC LESIONS of the connective tissue, causing skeletomuscular aches and pain. There is muscle pain, spasm and multiple aches. The neck, shoulder girdles, back, and gluteal region are the most common sites of the aches and pain.

Inflammation of the connective tissue of the muscles is the main symptom. Ayurveda says that fibromyalgia could be an autoimmune disorder caused by tejas burning ojas. It is called *māmsa gata pitta,* which is caused by vāta pushing pitta in the māmsa dhātu.

In old medical texts, fibromyalgia is called muscular rheumatism. One of the diagnostic criteria is an absence of signs and symptoms of other specific systemic illnesses.

## Etiological Factors
  * Prolonged exposure to cold, damp weather, which aggravates vāta
  * Non-articular rheumatic complaints
  * Chronic fatigue
  * Poor posture
  * Proneness to tendon sprain or strain
  * Flabby muscles
  * Obesity

Fibromyalgia is often due to occupational hazards. Some common jobs that can trigger fibromyalgia include miner, dockworker, foundry worker and clerk, as well as any night job under artificial lighting, as that disturbs sleep patterns and can result in muscle pain.

### Signs and Symptoms of Fibromyalgia

The primary symptom is chronic pain in the muscles, especially in the soft tissue surrounding the joints, which is usually difficult to manage. There are typically 11-18 trigger points that are particularly tender, although this test is not used as much today. (See illustration page 20.) This condition often worsens with advanced age. Fatigue and sleep problems are other signs and side effects of fibromyalgia.

### Other Symptoms

- Inflammation
- Lumbago
- Sciatica
- Occipital pain
- Cervical spine pain
- Unilateral pain (on one side of body)
- Hypermobility syndrome
- Shoulder pain
- Supraspinatus pain (tendonitis or pain in the supraspinatus muscle)
- Gout-like attack
- Tendonitis
- Bursitis
- Bicipital tendonitis (frozen shoulder)
- Depression, due to the persistent pain and chronic insomnia

## Management of Fibromyalgia

In modern medicine, a key treatment is local anesthetic injected into the trigger points. It is regarded as a difficult illness to treat.

In Ayurveda, the management protocol is based upon abhyanga (oil massage) or other forms of snehana. If there is āma (toxicity), one can use vishagarbha tailam as the massage oil. For a nirāma condition (no toxicity), use mahānārāyana tailam.

First snehana is done, then svedana (sweating therapy) using a sweat box with nirgundī oil. One can also take a ginger and baking soda bath after abhyanga. This will relieve muscle aches and pains.

The patient should increase gentle physical activity to help cope with his or her illness. Good forms of exercise include walking, cycling and exercising in warm water. Underwater exercise minimizes pressure on the soft tissues and is calming to pitta dosha. Yoga and stretching exercises are also beneficial, as these help to maintain the range of motion without as much pain.

Fibromyalgia patients sleep so poorly that they get depression, so encourage optimal sleep by nightly giving equal parts of tagara and jatamāmsi, or else a teaspoon of Good Night Sleep Tea®[36] in a cup of warm water.

---

36. A formula by Vasant Lad, sold as a tea in the store at The Ayurvedic Institute.

Equal parts of brahmī, jatamāmsi, and shankha pushpī can be used to help with the depression. Give half a teaspoon of this mixture three times daily.

Finally, fibromyalgia patients need cognitive behavioral therapy and spiritual counseling, to allow moment-to-moment awareness of their higher being. Go behind the observer of the pain. Just behind the observer is choiceless, passive awareness. "I am not the body and the pain. I am the watcher of the body and pain." Suddenly, you can use the pain as a springboard to jump into the inner abyss of quantum bliss.

## Herbal Remedy for Fibromyalgia
Take 1/2 teaspoon three times daily

Dashamūla 500 mg – to pacify vāta
Ashvagandhā 400 mg – to relax and build skeleton muscles
Mustā 300 mg – anti-inflammatory and analgesic
Kaishore guggulu 300 mg – anti-inflammatory and analgesic, it specifically pacifies vāta pushing pitta in māmsa dhātu
Tagara 200 mg – tranquilizer

Additionally, take one teaspoon of gandharva harītakī nightly at bedtime, to keep the colon clean.

# Chapter 25

# Obesity
## Staulya

Winter 1988, Volume 1, Number 3

IN AYURVEDA, OBESITY is defined as a metabolic disorder that produces an increase in weight and gradual pendular development of the breasts, abdomen, and hips, later spreading to the extremities. Generally, it occurs in an individual where the caloric intake is more than the physical activity. As a result, there is an accumulation of fat stored as adipose tissue (meda dhātu). The excessive deposition of adipose tissue is commonly in the breast, abdomen, and hip areas. However it may be distributed predominantly in the lower part of the trunk and thighs, which is more common for females, or in the upper part of the trunk and extremities, which is usual for males.

There are certain conditions in which the individual's weight gain is not due to obesity, such as fluid retention in edema, ascites, kidney diseases, and pregnancy. Physiologically, the weight that body builders and weight lifters gain cannot be considered obesity. Similarly, idiopathic (cyclic) edema in females, which is characterized by periodic swelling during the pre-menstrual period, is also not obesity.

According to Ayurveda, obesity is an excess kapha disorder causing low metabolism and low agni. There is a progressive fall in the basal metabolic rate (BMR) due to low agni that accompanies weight gain. There is also lethargy, decreased physical activity, excessive sleep, breathlessness on exertion, and sweating even with minimal physical activity, which results in excessive thirst. Obesity is also associated with serious disorders such as hypertension, diabetes mellitus, cardiovascular disease, and pulmonary insufficiency.

There are seven basic individual constitutions:

+ Three mono types: vāta, pitta, or kapha predominant
+ Three dual types: vāta-pitta, pitta-kapha, or vāta-kapha predominant
+ One triple type: vāta-pitta-kapha, equally distributed, very rare

Through different permutations and combinations of each dosha, there are many variations on these basic seven types of constitution. In all body types, when kapha dosha is increased, the imbalance may become obesity.

Kapha has the following qualities that are present in a person's diet, lifestyle and habits: heavy, slow or dull, cold, oily, slimy, soft, dense, liquid, static, gross, sticky, cloudy, and/or sweet. Heavy, slow, cold, oily and gross qualities are observed in foods such as cheese, meat, and fatty fried foods, while cold, cloudy, and dense qualities are found in ice cream, chocolate, yogurt, and other dairy products. Kapha qualities are also aggravated by constantly snacking, not doing much exercise, sleeping on too soft a bed, prolonged sleeping and napping during the daytime, and drinking alcohol and cold water.

The biological attributes of kapha are similar to those of meda dhātu (adipose tissue). The food products, lifestyle, and habits that have the same attributes as kapha also have the attributes of meda, and are responsible for the pathogenesis of obesity.

A kapha-producing diet, lifestyle and habits that increase the heavy, cold, and slow attributes in the body will in turn reduce the light, hot, sharp attributes of agni, causing slow metabolism, weight gain, and increased deposition of adipose tissue on the breasts, belly, and hips. The same phenomenon occurs in hypothyroidism, anterior pituitary deficiency, Cushing's syndrome, and diabetes mellitus type 2, which are all excess kapha disorders according to Ayurveda.

Obesity may be due to steroid toxicity. Patients who have undergone surgical treatment may have to carry out a prolonged period of steroid therapy. According to Ayurveda, steroids have similar properties to those of kapha, containing the heavy, slow, liquid, and gross properties. The patient retains water, becomes moon-faced, and puts on weight, which results in obesity. Obesity is frequently associated with gonadal deficiency, both in males and females, due to excess kapha dosha and psychological factors. It is also common in females during menopause, when psychological factors can be responsible for increased appetite. Under these circumstances, food is used as a substitute for satisfaction or as an escape from problems. These persons may even become alcoholic.

Depression, anxiety, fear, and insecurity are frequently responsible for increased food intake resulting in obesity. Just controlling the person's diet and food intake under these circumstances is not going to work. The underlying emotional disturbance must also be dealt with. Stopping the use of alcohol and tobacco also results in increased appetite and therefore may produce obesity. Obese subjects do not leave food on their plates. They generally eat a lot and love to drink excessive amounts of chilled water or soda drinks. Over-eating may be a familial and cultural habit. These habits are firmly implanted from generation to generation, beginning at an early age. The mother often compels the child to eat more, out of love. However, watching television and drinking cold drinks can cause obesity even in children under the age of ten.

## Management of Obesity

One must determine the exact cause of obesity in an individual; whether it is due to hypothyroidism, diabetes mellitus, menopause, emotional factors, hormonal imbalances or some other reason. The condition can then be managed accordingly.

According to Ayurveda, obesity is due to excess kapha in the system and low agni. In particular, it occurs when there is a slow fat-dissolving metabolism, which is low meda agni. Hence, we must eliminate kapha-producing foods from the diet and increase the person's meda agni. Herbs that help to increase meda agni and thereby improve the fat metabolism are kutki, chitrak, and shilājit. Herbal compounds include trikatu, ārogya vardhini, chandraprabhā, and triphalā guggulu.

An obese person tends to accumulate fat over the diaphragm and around the heart and lung tissue. There is diminished air entry, pulmonary insufficiency, and breathlessness on exertion. To improve the vital capacity of the lungs, use an herbal compound called trikatu. This contains equal amounts of dried ginger, black pepper, and pippalī (long pepper). Take 300 mg of this twice daily after food with warm water.

Kutki improves liver function, stimulates metabolism, and helps to scrape the adipose tissue. Taking 200 mg of kutki about fifteen minutes before a meal will help to regulate the appetite. An obese person tends to become excessively hungry due to emotional factors and this can be controlled by kutki, thus helping the person lose weight. One teaspoon of honey with one cup of warm to hot water taken early in the morning also does scraping of adipose tissue in an obese person.

Due to an accumulation of fat in the connective tissue, prāna (chi) becomes blocked and this results in palpitations, breathlessness, and low sex drive. This condition can be corrected by using 200 mg of the compound triphalā guggulu, twice daily on an empty stomach. Chandraprabhā is an ancient, authentic herbal formula that is effectively used in obesity due to diabetes mellitus. The dosage is 250 mg twice daily after meals.

Ayurveda recommends that obese people undertake a special cleansing program with oil massage and medicated steam treatments as well as eating a special diet. Fasting also helps to improve the metabolism. Similarly, water intake should be regulated, because excessive consumption of water lowers the person's metabolism by inhibiting agni. Four to six glasses of liquids a day is sufficient for most obese people. These may be taken in the form of herbal teas such as tea made from equal parts of cumin, coriander, and fennel. In order to regulate thirst, one should do shītalī prānāyāma, which involves inhaling through the mouth when making a tube of the tongue and then exhaling through the nose, and the lion pose, which is done by sticking the tongue out as far as possible and roaring like a lion. These exercises strengthen the thyroid and help to regulate metabolic activity, which helps to regulate the deposition of adipose tissue. The sun salutation and other yoga exercises, such as spinal twist, are also of great value in controlling obesity. These should all be practiced on a regular basis.

To deal with the underlying causes of obesity, one must deal with the emotional aspects. However, regular yoga exercise, prānāyāma and medical treatment help the emotional body as well as the physical body. In the old Ayurvedic texts, it says it is easier to manage a thin person than an overweight person.

## Dietary Guidelines for Excess Kapha

*Fruits to Enjoy.* Apples, apricots, berries, cherries, cranberries, dry figs, lemons, mango, peaches, pears, persimmon, pomegranate, prunes, raisins

*Fruits to Avoid.* Most sweet and sour fruits, avocado, bananas, coconut, fresh figs, grapefruit, grapes, oranges, papaya, pineapples, plums

***Vegetables to Enjoy.*** Pungent and bitter vegetables, asparagus, beets, broccoli, Brussels sprouts, cabbage, carrots, cauliflower, celery, eggplant, garlic, leafy greens, lettuce, mushrooms, okra, onions, parsley, peas, peppers, white potatoes, radishes, spinach, sprouts

***Vegetables to Avoid.*** Sweet and juicy vegetables, cucumber, sweet potatoes, tomatoes, zucchini

***Grains to Enjoy.*** Barley, basmati rice, corn, millet, dry oats, rye

***Grains to Avoid.*** Cooked oats, brown or white rice, wheat

***Meats and Eggs that are Permissible.*** Dark meat of chicken or turkey, rabbit, eggs (not fried or scrambled), venison, shrimp

***Meats to Avoid.*** Beef, lamb, pork, seafood (with the exception of shrimp), fried or scrambled eggs

***Legumes.*** All except kidney beans, soy, mung beans, and black lentils

***Nuts.*** There should be no nuts or seeds except small amounts of sunflower seeds and pumpkin seeds

***Sweeteners.*** None except raw honey

***Spices.*** All are good except sea salt.

***Dairy Products.*** None should be consumed except for ghee and goat milk.

***Oils.*** No oils except small amounts of almond, corn, or sunflower oil.

# Chapter 26

# Cholesterol and Management of Fat Metabolism

Winter 2012, Volume 25, Number 3

ACCORDING TO AYURVEDA, there are three doshas (vāta, pitta, kapha), seven dhātus (tissues), and three mala (excreta). The dhātus are the constituents of an individual's constitution and every tissue (dhātu) has a unique function. Rasa dhātu has the function of *prīnanam,* nutrition. Rakta dhātu has the important life function of oxygenation. Māmsa has the functions of *lepana* (plastering), power, locomotion, and strength.

Meda dhātu, the adipose tissue, has the important function of lubrication. Meda is represented by lipids, fats, and cholesterol. Asthi dhātu's function is support; majjā functions are communication and filling the space, while the function of shukra and ārtava (male and female reproductive tissues) is procreation and release of stress and emotions during orgasm.

Cholesterol is connected intimately to meda dhātu, the fatty tissue, which has the functions of storing energy and lubrication. It is also present in the myelin sheath of the brain tissue, spinal cord, liver, kidneys, and adrenal glands. Cholesterol is a precursor for the biosynthesis of bile in the liver, which is then stored in the gallbladder. Cholesterol helps to heal inflammatory lesions anywhere in the body.

### The Five Bhūta Agnis

| Nābhasa Agni | Ether |
|---|---|
| Vāyavya Agni | Air |
| Tejo Agni | Fire |
| Apas Agni | Water |
| Pārthiva Agni | Earth |

Increased cholesterol is a metabolic disorder that is associated with liver dysfunction. When the liver does not fully process fat, it can lead to hyperlipidemia.[37] The liver is the seat of bhūta agni. *Bhūta* means element or that which manifests as matter. Nābhasa agni maintains cellular size and shape, vāyavya agni regulates cellular respiration, tejo agni governs cellular metabolic activity, āpas agni administers nutritional functions, and pārthiva agni governs mineral metabolism.

---

37. Elevated levels of lipids or fats in the blood. Hyperlipidemia includes several conditions but most commonly refers to high cholesterol and high triglyceride levels.

Kapha and cholesterol are almost identical in their attributes, because the Earth and Water elements predominantly make up both kapha dosha and meda dhātu. Kapha, meda (fat), and cholesterol are all heavy, slow, oily, slimy, and sticky. When pārthiva agni and āpas agni (two of the bhūta agni) are low, these attributes are not metabolized, and so the liver doesn't process fat and cholesterol.

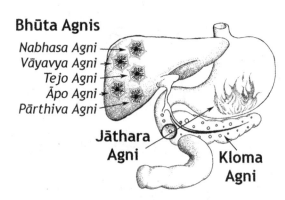

**Bhūta Agnis**

*Nabhasa Agni*
*Vāyavya Agni*
*Tejo Agni*
*Āpo Agni*
*Pārthiva Agni*

**Jāthara Agni**

**Kloma Agni**

When fat metabolism slows, there is often an increase in cholesterol levels. This can lead to deposition of cholesterol and other fats on the walls of the blood vessels, which is a condition called atherosclerosis. In Ayurveda, it is called *sirā kathinya* (hardening of the arteries or blood vessels). If the concentration of lipids is greatly increased, fatty streaks are formed along the arterial walls.

A normal arterial wall is smooth and elastic, but because of this deposition of fat, the lining of the arterial wall becomes rough, thickened, sticky, and inflamed. Fibrous scar tissue grows and attracts fat, calcium, fibrin, and cellular debris onto the wall of the vessel. Accumulation of calcium creates a chalky film called plaque, which makes the blood vessels hard. This lining inside the arterial wall hampers its ability to properly expand and contract, and slowly this vital pathway narrows.

Atherosclerosis generally progresses slowly. The fatty depositions partially clog the affected blood vessels, and then ultimately can totally block the blood flow. That condition is called *sroto rodha* (blocked passage) in Ayurveda, and it reduces the blood flow in that particular part of the body. Such narrowing of the artery or blood vessel can in turn create *sirā granthi,* which means an obstructed artery or vein.

Atherosclerosis is often due to a diet that is high in saturated fat, or one that includes a lot of fatty fried food. Other physiological factors of atherosclerotic changes are hypertension, smoking, increased blood cholesterol, or a family history of high cholesterol, atherosclerosis, or diabetes mellitus.

Hypertension increases the risk of atherosclerosis because it puts constant pressure and therefore increased strain on the arterial walls, which speeds up the hardening process. Smoking is another cause, because the nicotine in tobacco causes narrowing of the arteries. In some families, there is a genetic predisposition to have high cholesterol, so these people need to be more careful.

Generally, individuals with high cholesterol also have high triglycerides. For example, most people with type-two diabetes have high triglycerides as well. However, some individuals have high cholesterol with normal triglyceride levels. Alternatively, others get high triglyceride levels but have normal levels of cholesterol, and these people may suffer a heart attack even though they are within the normal range of cholesterol levels.

It is not the case that only chubby people will have high cholesterol. I have seen many skinny people who have high cholesterol levels. High cholesterol is a metabolic disorder related to the liver not processing fat, so genetic and lifestyle factors, such as insufficient exercise, fatty food, smoking, and diabetes, are the main factors responsible.

Cholesterol has the function to heal trauma and to seal areas of inflammation. This is because inflammation of the arteries attracts cholesterol molecules to seal the area. Nature is a good physician but a bad surgeon. The arterial wall inflammation causes deposition of cholesterol in order to seal the inflamed area, but it sometimes deposits so much choles-  terol that it creates plaque.

## Signs and Symptoms

Diagnosis is carried out by asking about the person's medical history, and using darshana (visual inspection), sparshana (touch), and prashna (questioning). The patient should ideally have a thorough physical examination, blood pressure examination, blood analysis tests, exercise tolerance test, electrocardiogram, and angiography. These normal investigations can be used to assess or rule out high cholesterol.

In the early stages, there are no visible symptoms of high cholesterol. At some point, there may be symptoms related to certain organs. For example if the heart is affected, the person can get angina pain, ischemic pain, or ischemic heart attack.

However, there are some signs of high cholesterol that an Ayurvedic practitioner can assess. If you feel the radial artery and roll it between the palpitating finger and radial bone, it will feel thickened. A second important sign is in the eyes at the sclerocorneal junction, where you may see a whitish ring, which is a sign of high cholesterol and/or atherosclerosis. A crease on the ear lobule, lots of hair in the ears, and xanthoma[38] are other signs of high cholesterol. High cholesterol and hypothyroidism go together. A person with a double chin, which is a sign of low thyroid function, may well have high cholesterol.

The manifestations of high cholesterol will change according to which blood vessels are blocked—the heart, head, kidney, retina, or an extremity. If cholesterol clogs the cerebral artery, the blood supply to the brain will be diminished and it will create dizziness, fainting, cerebral lesion, paralysis, or stroke. A stroke is the death of brain tissue. If sroto rodha happens to the kidneys, it can lead to renal failure. Sroto rodha may occur in the retinal blood vessels, in which case the person can get blurry vision or blindness. If it affects the extremities (*shākhā*), the result may be varicose veins, or thrombophlebitis.

# Management

An Ayurvedic herbal protocol will vary according to the prakruti-vikruti paradigm and the organs affected. It will include a dosha pratyanika (specific to the dosha) and *vyādhi praty-anika* (specific to the disease).

- The basis of any herbal formula is the use of kapha-reducing herbs such as chitrak, kutki, trikatu, neem, and turmeric. Chitrak kindles agni and burns fat. Kutki

---

38. A condition in which certain fats build up under the surface of the skin.

scrapes excess fat and improves the hepatic parenchymal functions. Trikatu (ginger, black pepper and long pepper) kindles agni and improves fat metabolism. Neem is extremely bitter and it helps to reduce fat from the hematopoietic system. Turmeric is a blood cleanser and it activates the secretion of fatty acids.

- A good herbal blood thinner is triphala guggulu, shilājit, chitrak, and trikatu. Arjuna can be added to prevent heart disease. To reduce blood pressure, add passionflower and hawthorn berry or alternatively give sarpagandha.
- For kidney disorders, one can use punarnavā and gokshura, or punarnavādi guggulu and gokshurādi guggulu.
- For dizziness, fainting or blurry vision, use sarasvatī, brahmī, jatamāmsi, and shankha pushpī.
- To reduce angina pain, one can give arjuna, gokshura and pushkaramūla, along with neem, turmeric, and some form of guggulu.
- For symptoms in the shākhā (extremities), give kaishore guggulu, yogarāja guggulu, or rasnadi guggulu.
- For retinal blindness, triphala tea eyewash is a good remedy, or a combination of punarnavā and triphala teas as eyewash. (see instructions page 329)
- Kaishore guggulu is beneficial for thrombophlebitis, while goraksha chincha guggulu will help both varicose veins and thrombotic areas.

The amounts of each herbal remedy vary according to the individual and their specific condition. A typical formula to reduce high cholesterol and minimize the risk of heart conditions is:

Punarnavā 500 mg
Arjuna 300 mg
Shilājit 200 mg
Triphala guggulu 200 mg

This formula would normally be taken three times daily. Anyone with high cholesterol should take triphala each evening, or alternatively take bhumi āmalakī every night to detoxify the liver and reduce cholesterol.

Abhyanga (oil massage) is done with kapha or pitta pacifying oils, and sweating therapy with *nirgundī svedana*. Nasya is applied to the nasal passages, and commonly vacha tailam nasya is given to improve the cerebral circulation.

The person's lifestyle will have to change. If he or she is a smoker, quit smoking. Losing excess weight and increasing exercise will help to regulate the person's circulation. Bhastrikā prānāyāma, kapāla bhāti prānāyāma, and *agni sara kriya* all help to maintain the elasticity of the blood vessels, so they can prevent a future heart attack. The person should also do regular *sūrya namaskāra* and *yogāsanas*.

Ayurvedic dietetics prescribes a kapha-reducing diet with no fatty fried food and minimal butter, cheese, sugar, and saturated fat. One has to regulate blood pressure and reduce cholesterol by use of a low-cholesterol diet. The best oils to use are sunflower oil, safflower oil, flaxseed oil, and olive oil. Steamed vegetables, corn, millet, and buckwheat are all beneficial as well as orange juice, pomegranate juice, or cranberry juice.

Saturated fats are those that usually become solid at cool temperatures. Common sources of saturated fat in the diet include animal fat (meat and lard), dairy products, such as butter, ghee, cream, and cheese, as well as certain vegetable oils like coconut oil, cottonseed oil, and palm kernel oil. Saturated fats consist of triglyceride and saturated fatty acids. If total cholesterol is high, one should even avoid ghee in the diet, because it can also add to the hyperlipidemia.

Modern medicine uses various pharmaceutical products to control cholesterol, in particular statins[39] such as atorvastatin (Lipitor®). However, these drugs are toxic to the liver and increase liver enzymes. Long-term use of these statin medications can also lead to other complications, such as muscle pain and nausea.

It may be necessary to use modern drugs such as nitroglycerin to take care of angina pain, blood pressure-controlling medicine for hypertension, an anticoagulant to prevent clotting, or cholesterol-reducing medicine. However, according to Ayurveda, the best protocol is to control cholesterol by changes in the person's diet, exercise, and lifestyle measures, along with appropriate herbal remedies.

---

39. Statins are a class of drugs used to lower cholesterol levels by inhibiting the enzyme HMG-CoA reductase, which plays a fundamental role in the production of cholesterol in the liver.

Chapter 27

# How to Maintain Healthy Weight

Fall 2015, Volume 28, Number 2

WEIGHT IS A GRAVITATIONAL FORCE exerted on an object. The weight of an individual depends upon a number of factors and, most importantly, on growth, nutrition, and metabolic activity.

All weight-related problems are due to the imbalance between energy intake and energy expenditure. Generally, young children do not have weight problems, although some babies are born overweight or underweight. However, a weight imbalance can occur at any age.

Body weight is inversely proportional to the strength of dhātu agni (the bodily tissues). When dhātu agni is manda (slow), there will be undue production of unprocessed bodily tissue (asthāyi dhātu). That causes excess weight, which can gradually lead to obesity. Whereas if dhātu agni is high, the body burns up more of the unprocessed tissue, resulting in low body weight for the person's height.

From an Ayurvedic point of view, obesity is a disorder where jāthara agni (the gastric fire) is high and dhātu agni is low. In other words, overweight people have strong appetite and slow metabolism. They tend to eat quite a lot, but what they consume is not processed fully. These unburned calories turn into adipose tissue.

Weight problems are uncommonly common these days, and obesity is the most common nutritional disorder in affluent societies. Obesity is associated with increased mortality, a range of diseases, and affects happiness and relationships.

| TYPES OF AGNI |
| --- |
| **Manda Agni** |
| Slow metabolism and poor digestion, related to increased kapha, leads to kapha disorders |
| **Tīkshna Agni** |
| Sharp metabolism and quick digestion, related to increased pitta, leads to pitta disorders |
| **Vishama Agni** |
| Irregular metabolism and fluctuating digestion, related to increased vāta, leads to vāta disorders |
| **Sāma Agni** |
| Balanced metabolism and optimal digestion, brings balanced doshas |

Socioeconomic factors play an important part in weight disorders. In affluent countries, people in lower income groups are most affected. In developing countries, it is the prosperous elite. Nowadays, in places such as China and India, the middle classes can afford a car and the resultant lack of exercise can lead to obesity.

Hereditary factors are also significant. Family background and eating patterns are influenced by the culture and by economic factors. In some societies, overweight men are respected and chubby women are considered to be beautiful, while in other places skinny people are viewed as beautiful.

A person's occupation is another important factor. Barmen and barmaids often have weight related problems, and cooks are almost always overweight. Whereas jockeys have to maintain their weight, or else their poor horse will lag behind. Fashion models are very worried about their weight, and often suffer problems from being underweight.

Twins often become overweight because they are fed more by their parents. Adopted children often become chubby because of overfeeding and emotional eating.

Endocrine factors play a role in weight gain as well. Young women can often become overweight at puberty and women commonly put on weight after pregnancy and during menopause. Hypothyroidism, hypogonadism, Cushing's syndrome, and other endocrine disorders can all result in weight gain and obesity.

When plasma concentration of insulin is raised, cortisol is increased and growth hormone is reduced. If there is a regular, small excess of caloric intake over calories burnt from exercise, the result can be a large accumulation of adipose tissue.

If a person eats two slices of bread (approximately 20 gm) more than is needed each day, and travels by car instead of walking for 20 minutes, there will be an extra 48 calories accumulated daily. This leads to 20 grams of fat deposition every day.

Weight problems may be connected to the use of certain drugs, especially steroids and oral contraceptives. Insulin is an appetite stimulant, so people who are on insulin medication tend to eat more than is ideal.

Business people are busy, with little time to exercise. They often eat emotionally, either because they are unhappy or because of long business lunches that frequently result in overeating. This leads to obesity.

## Weight Gain and Obesity

Obesity is defined as a metabolic disorder that produces an increase in weight and gradual pendular development of the breasts, abdomen, hips, thighs, and extremities. It usually occurs when the caloric intake is greater than the energy consumed by physical activity. As a result, there is an accumulation of fat stored as adipose tissue (meda dhātu).

In females, this excess meda is more commonly distributed in the lower part of the trunk and thighs as well as the breasts. In males, the fat tends to accumulate in the upper part of the trunk and on the extremities as well as the abdomen.

In obesity, there is a progressive fall in the basal metabolic rate (BMR), which is a condition of low dhātu agni. Common signs and symptoms are lethargy, decreased physical activity, excessive sleep, breathlessness on exertion, sweating even with minimal physical activity, and excessive thirst. Associated symptoms are edema, breathlessness, cardiovascular problems, and lymphatic disorders.

Obesity is also associated with serious disorders such as hypertension, diabetes mellitus, hepatic disease, cardiovascular disease, and pulmonary insufficiency. If untreated, weight gain can lead to these and other serious diseases.

According to Ayurveda, obesity is due to excess kapha in the system, along with low agni. In all body types, when kapha dosha is increased, the resulting imbalance may result in weight gain and then obesity. It is most common in people with kapha prakruti and kapha vikruti.

The attributes of kapha are similar to those of meda (adipose tissue). Hence, kapha-promoting foods and habits also have the characteristics of meda dhātu, so these are responsible for the pathogenesis of obesity. A kapha-producing diet and lifestyle will increase the heavy, cold, and slow attributes in the body, which suppresses the light, hot, and sharp attributes of agni. This causes low agni, slow metabolism, weight gain and accumulation of fatty tissue.

The same phenomenon occurs in hypothyroidism (low *jatru*[40] *agni*), anterior pituitary deficiency (which can create diabetes insipidus), Cushing's syndrome, and diabetes mellitus type 2, which are all excess kapha disorders according to Ayurveda.

Heavy, cold, slow, oily, gross, cloudy, and dense qualities are found in fatty fried foods, meat, chocolate, cheese, ice cream, yogurt, and other dairy products. Kapha is also aggravated by constant snacking, lack of exercise, prolonged sleeping, napping during the daytime, and drinking alcohol and chilled drinks.

If an individual with kapha prakruti keeps eating a kapha-provoking diet, kapha will suppress jāthara agni. That suppressed jāthara agni will produce more meda, because the qualities of kapha and meda dhātu are identical—like attracts like. In time, this increased meda will clog the channels and push agni from the periphery to the center (gastrointestinal tract). This will temporarily increase jāthara agni. That is why overweight kapha people are always hungry. Whatever the person eats is not well-processed, because tissue metabolism is slow.

An Ayurvedic sūtra states that in obesity, all srotāmsi are clogged by *asthāyi meda dhātu,* so that whatever the person eats, becomes meda (fat). Hence, overweight people can get sexual debility, osteoporosis, and other conditions because meda is increasing but the other dhātus are not being nourished.

It is important to note that weight gain is not always due to obesity. For example, increased bodily weight can be due to fluid retention in edema, ascites, kidney diseases, and pregnancy. Physiologically, the weight that body builders gain is not considered obesity. Similarly, cyclic edema experienced by some women during the pre-menstrual period, characterized by periodic swelling, is also not obesity.

---

40. Jatru is the Sanskrit word for thyroid.

Obesity may be due to steroid toxicity. Patients who have undergone surgical treatment may have to carry out a prolonged period of steroid therapy. According to Ayurveda, steroids have similar properties to those of kapha dosha, promoting the heavy, slow, liquid, and gross qualities. Therefore, the patient retains water, becomes moon-faced, and puts on weight, which can result in obesity. That is a book picture of steroid toxicity.

Obesity is also associated with gonadal deficiency, in both males and females, due to excess kapha dosha.

People who stop using alcohol and tobacco often find they have increased appetite for food, which leads to weight gain. When the drug is stopped, it creates a vacuum and emptiness. Jāthara agni increases temporarily, as the person seeks comfort from food. A drinking or smoking habit thereby becomes an eating habit.

Psychological factors may create emotional eating. Depression, anxiety, loneliness, fear, and insecurity are frequently responsible for increased food intake, which can result in obesity. If there is lack of love, food becomes a substitute for love. Lonely people often eat more and become chubby.

It is also common for women to put on weight during menopause, when psychological factors can be responsible for increased appetite. Under these circumstances, food is used as a substitute for satisfaction or as an escape from problems. In such cases, controlling the person's food intake is not sufficient. The underlying emotional factors must also be dealt with.

Obese subjects do not generally leave food on their plates. They usually eat more than needed and drink excessive amounts of chilled water or soda drinks. Over-eating may be a familial or cultural habit. These habits are firmly implanted from generation to generation, beginning at an early age. The mother may compel the child to eat more, out of love. In modern times, watching television while eating snacks and drinking cold drinks can lead to obesity, even in children under the age of ten.

## Clinical Features of Excessive Weight

**Appearance:** If the patient looks out of shape, one can assess the body frame and measure the person's height and weight to get the body mass index (BMI). Also, assess the skin fold thickness by measuring over the triceps muscle with spring-loaded calipers. If it measures more than 20 mm in a man, and more than 28 mm in a woman, that indicates an excessive accumulation of subcutaneous fat. That is a sign that the person is overweight.

Metabolic disorders that cause weight gain include hyperlipidemia, high cholesterol, high triglycerides, gallstones, gout and non-insulin dependent diabetes mellitus (type 2 diabetes).

**Psychological factors:** Weight related problems can be psychological. An overweight patient may be disturbed with depression and anxiety, or ashamed of his or her own unattractive appearance. There may be sexual problems, because an overweight person cannot usually enjoy sex. Overweight people can also suffer from mechanical disability, flat feet, backache, osteoarthritis, knee and hip pain, pain in the lumbar spine, abdominal discomfort, diaphragmatic hernia, varicose veins, and sleep apnea.

**Cardiovascular system:** Enlargement of the heart due to increased body weight can cause cardiac output to be diminished. Stroke volume is high, output is increased, blood volume is increased, and blood pressure is increased. That is why obesity and excessive weight can cause cardiovascular disorders.

**Life expectancy:** People with obesity cannot expect to live as long as if they had normal weight. There is a correlation between increased weight and an increased rate of mortality.

# General Management of Obesity and Overweight Conditions

Firstly, one must determine the exact cause of obesity in an individual—whether it is due to hypothyroidism, diabetes, menopause, emotional factors, hormonal imbalance, or some other issue. The condition can then be managed accordingly.

In general, obesity occurs when there is a slow fat-dissolving metabolism, which is low *meda agni*. Hence, we must increase the person's meda agni. Herbs that do so and thereby improve the fat metabolism are kutki, chitrak and shilājit, as well as compounds such as trikatu, ārogya vardhini, chandraprabha and triphala guggulu.

A weekly weight loss program aiming at losing one to two pounds (0.5 kg to 1 kg) per week should be the general aim. It is best to reduce weight slowly but steadily, rather than trying to achieve rapid weight loss.

If you want to reduce your weight, avoid foods that increase kapha dosha. See *Food Guidelines for Basic Constitutional Types* [41] for a complete list of kapha-balancing foods.

Don't eat excessive amounts of meat, sugar, wheat, salt, cheese, yogurt, ice cream, and alcoholic drinks. Instead, have millet, buckwheat, corn, and amaranth. Eat more fiber-rich foods, with lots of vegetables and fruit and some whole-grain cereals. Ensure you get plenty of vitamins by eating lots of green vegetables and fruit. Eat beans several times a week.

Make breakfast your big meal, and then eat a light lunch and dinner. Don't eat too much; don't eat too little. The ideal ratio is to eat about 100 gm of carbohydrates, 50 gm of protein, 30 gm of fat, and 10 gm of miscellaneous things such as minerals.

The amount of food varies according to gender, size, amount of exercise and other factors. For example, a small woman might need only 1,000 calories per day. Whereas a large man doing lots of active physical work might require 3,000 calories per day or more.

Drink a small glass of warm water instead of eating whenever you feel hungry or thirsty. This helps to minimize your food intake. Drinking a glass of hot water with honey and cider vinegar can help with weight loss. Each morning, drink one glass of hot water with one teaspoon of honey and 5-10 drops of apple cider vinegar mixed into it.

Fasting helps to improve the metabolism. Similarly, water intake should be regulated, because excessive consumption of water inhibits agni. Four to six cups of fluids a day is sufficient for most obese people, including tea and coffee. An herbal tea, made from equal

41. Available at https://www.ayurveda.com/pdf/food-guidelines.pdf

parts of cumin, coriander, and fennel, is helpful for overweight people. It is a mild diuretic and regulates agni.

Yoga is beneficial for people trying to increase agni and manage their weight. Sūrya namaskāra (sun salutation) should be done daily, along with camel, cobra, cow, boat, bow, bridge, lotus, locust and lion poses. (see yoga poses page 450) These poses should be learned from a certified yoga teacher. Yogāsanas are of great value in controlling obesity, so these should all be practiced on a regular basis.

Also, do regular prānāyāma. Kapāla bhāti, bhastrikā, anuloma viloma, ujjāyi and utgeet prānāyāma can all help someone trying to control their weight. Do two rounds of 20 bhastrikā prānāyāma, and two rounds of 200 kapāla bhāti, with a rest in between.

In order to regulate thirst and metabolic activity, one should do shītalī prānāyāma, which involves inhaling through the mouth when making a tube of the tongue and then exhaling through the nose. The lion pose also helps to regulate metabolic activity and strengthen the thyroid gland. It is done by sticking the tongue out as far as possible and roaring like a lion.

Being overweight creates gravitational stress, which may cause varicose veins, hiatal hernia, inguinal hernia, lower backache, hypothyroidism, or edema (swelling). An overweight person should not do jumping exercises, because there is the possibility of a slipped disc. Daily walking is a good form of exercise as well as swimming or light weightlifting.

A good herbal protocol for an overweight condition is to take the following formula three times daily with warm water:

Punarnavā 500 mg
Chitrak 200 mg
Kutki 200 mg
Neem 200 mg
Shankha pushpī 200 mg

Regular use of triphala is beneficial. Take one teaspoon nightly at bedtime with warm water. Also, first thing each morning, place 5 drops of vacha oil nasya in each nostril.

Just by following this regimen, one can achieve drastic weight loss.

One teaspoon of honey in a cup of warm water taken early in the morning also helps to regulate appetite and remove excess body fat.

Chandraprabha is an ancient herbal formula that is used in obesity, especially when there is diabetes mellitus. The dosage is 250 mg twice daily after meals.

An obese person tends to accumulate fat over the diaphragm and around the heart and lung tissue. There may be diminished air entry, pulmonary insufficiency, and breathlessness on exertion. To improve the vital capacity of the lungs, use an herbal compound called trikatu. This contains equal amounts of dried ginger, black pepper and pippalī (long pepper). Take 300 mg of this mixture twice daily after food with warm water.

Kutki improves liver function, stimulates metabolism and helps to remove excess adipose tissue. Even taking 200 mg of kutki about fifteen minutes before meals will help to regulate the appetite. An obese person tends to become excessively hungry due to emotional factors and this can be controlled by kutki.

Due to the accumulation of fat in the connective tissue, prāna can be blocked, resulting in palpitations, breathlessness, and low sex drive. This can be corrected by using 200 mg of the compound triphala guggulu. This should be taken twice daily on an empty stomach.

To deal with the underlying causes of obesity, one must treat both the physical and emotional aspects. Regular yoga, prānāyāma, and exercise as outlined above will all help the emotional body as well as the physical body.

## Preventing Weight Loss

Generally, people who have difficultly putting on weight have vāta prakruti and/or vāta vikruti, sharp agni, and fast metabolism. They have a strong appetite and burn up the calories quickly, losing weight and easily becoming fatigued. Their body weight may decline by 10 to 20 pounds below the person's optimal weight.

The ancient Ayurvedic texts state that it is easier to manage a thin person who is underweight, than to treat an overweight person. Weight loss decreases the risk of coronary heart disease, whereas increased weight can result in diabetes, hypertension, depression, and other serious disorders.

However, weight loss is a common symptom in some serious illnesses, such as peptic ulcer, ulcerative colitis, malabsorption syndrome, and cancer. For example, cancer of the stomach can create severe weight loss.

The first thing to do is to find out the cause of weight loss. For example, weight loss can occur in hyperthyroidism or goiter, anxiety, tachycardia, Addison's disease, AIDS, chronic diarrhea, celiac disease, peptic ulcer, ulcerative colitis, chronic infection, type 1 diabetes mellitus, prolonged lactation, and starvation as well as in cases of consumptive diseases, which include tuberculosis, severe anemia, hypoproteinemia, and diabetes insipidus.

The treatment protocol for weight loss can be tricky, because it depends upon the precise etiological factors. For instance, take weight loss due to celiac disease. In that case, we have to treat the celiac disease and not just try to increase the person's weight.

The first category of weight loss is consumption. We can treat tuberculosis and consumptive illnesses with the following formula:

Ashvagandhā 500 mg
Sitopalādi 400 mg
Talisadi 400 mg
Balā 300 mg
Ardrak (Ginger) 200 mg
Laghu malini vasant 200 mg (this is important)

Then we have to give the person goat's milk, cow's milk, yogurt, ghee, cheese, cashews, soaked almonds, pistachio nuts, and a rich protein diet. There should be no strong virechana (purgation) and no drastic basti (enema), because the person will lose too many minerals and nutrients.

You should slowly buck up the patient's energy, giving them saffron, turmeric, and so forth. If they wish, they can have egg omelet, egg curry, chicken broth or other animal protein.

In this anti-tubercular protocol, the patient can have a little Ayurvedic wine: draksha āsava, dashamūla arishta, or ashvagandhā arishta. Ashvagandhā is particularly good for consumption and weight loss.

If the weight loss is due to *grahani roga* (malabsorption syndrome) or sprue syndrome, you can treat that separately with:

Kutaja 300 mg
Balā 300 mg
Pañchāmrit parpati 200 mg
Prevail pañchāmrit 200 mg
Kama Dudhā 200 mg

Follow a healthy, nourishing diet that is easy for the person to digest. This will improve the person's agni and help with absorption.

The third main category is weight loss due to hyperthyroidism. In this case, we have to treat the thyroid gland with the following formula:

Shatāvarī 500 mg
Kaishore Guggulu 300 mg
Gulvel sattva 200 mg
Kama Dudhā 200 mg

This can be followed by a weight-building program, including soaked almonds, cashews and other nuts, rice pudding or tapioca pudding, cream of wheat, and other nourishing foods.

# Chapter 28

# Backache and Sciatica
## Kati Shūla and Grighrasī

Summer 1997, Volume 10, Number 1

*VĀTA VYĀDHI* (VĀTA DISORDERS) include neuromuscular and neuroskeletal problems, such as lumbago and sciatica. *Kati shūla* is the Sanskrit term for lumbago or lower back ache. Kati means lower back and shūla means pain. *Grighrasī* means sciatica.

The entire pelvic cavity, including all of its organs and bones, is under the control of apāna vāyu. If apāna vāyu enters into asthi dhātu (the bone tissue), majjā dhātu (nerve tissue), or māmsa dhātu (the muscles and ligaments) during the spreading stage of pathogenesis, it can, depending upon the site of the khavaigunya (weakness), cause either of these two conditions related to the lower half of the body.

Lumbago (kati shūla) is pain in the lower part of the back, in the lumbosacral joint or sacro-iliac joint, while sciatica (grighrasī) is pain along the pathway of the sciatic nerve. Pain from sciatica is felt in the buttock. From there it radiates down to the posterior aspect of the thigh, then it goes to the calf, following the lateral aspect of the lower leg to the outer border of the toe. The pain starts in the buttock area and it follows the track of the nerve. Lumbago and sciatica are closely associated and can exist together. Aggravation of vāta is responsible for both these conditions.

## Etiological Factors
In the ancient Ayurvedic literature the causes of these two conditions were given in beautiful Sanskrit poetry. The etiological factors include:

***Trauma, such as a car accident, lifting heavy objects, or twisting the spine.*** Exerting oneself beyond capacity will pull the muscle, ligament, or connective tissue and manifest as pain. At times, individuals do yoga without sufficient knowledge and beyond their capacity, twisting the spine. Twisting of the spine can also happen in a car accident, or from lifting a heavy weight with flexion of the spine. While lifting a heavy weight, one should bend the knees and ankles, and then lift, using the support of the muscles of the thighs, gluteus, and calf. If people just bend and then try to lift, at that moment the spine becomes twisted.

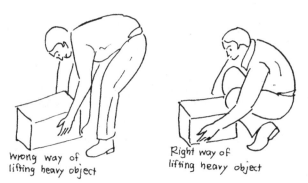

wrong way of
lifting heavy object

Right way of
lifting heavy object

*Constipation with gases in the rectum.* These gases exert pressure on the lumbosacral area and can cause pain. Constipation is a vāta disorder.

*Cystitis.* Any problem in the bladder, such as cystitis, may create referred pain in the lower back.

*Vaginitis, cervicitis, or even colitis.* In these conditions, vāta is pushing pitta in the bladder, vagina, cervix area, or colon, as well as the rectum.

*Congestive dysmenorrhea.* Congestive dysmenorrhea (congestion in the myometrium) will refer pain to the back. That kind of pain is usually associated with the premenstrual period.

*Herniation of an intervertebral disc.* Anterior and posterior ligaments weaken and lose their tone because of aggravation of vāta. This condition can also be the cause of lumbago.

*Gulma.* Spinal tumors, such as neurofibroma or meningioma, are caused by apāna vāyu pushing prāna vāyu pushing tarpaka kapha in the majjā dhātu.

*Ankylosing spondylitis.* Vāta pushing pitta in the majjā dhātu and asthi dhātu can create ankylosing spondylitis, leading to lower back pain.

*Cancer.* Lumbago is also present in malignant diseases of the pelvic cavity. Cancer of the prostate, cervix, or rectum can create pain in the lower back.

*Koch's spine.* In common terms, this condition is called bone tuberculosis (TB). Bone TB is secondary to pulmonary tuberculosis.

People who have open tuberculosis with cavitation, caseation,[42] and infiltration are less likely to develop lumbago. In closed tuberculosis or tubercular lymphadenopathy, where the cervical glands are matted in a chain, the abdomen becomes shaped like a boat. The person has a low-grade fever, nocturnal perspiration, evening rise of temperature, and loses weight. That person is prone to Koch's spine, which is tuberculosis of the intervertebral disc, and can create fusion of the vertebrae L4 and L5, or L5 and S1. When these vertebrae are fused, due to deposition of calcium, there is restricted movement to the lower back that can create kati shūla.

---

42. Transformation of tissue into a soft, cheese-like mass.

*Osteoarthritis.* In osteoarthritis (asthi gata vāta) of the sacroiliac joint, vāta has gone into asthi dhātu. Degenerative changes of the joint, resulting in osteoporosis, are called *asthi saushīrya.* I have even seen a young boy of 20 with degenerative changes. That patient had an underactive parathyroid gland, which governs calcium metabolism, causing the bones to lose calcium.

*Āma.* Metabolic toxins, created by improper digestion, incompatible food combining, or environmental poisons.

*Infection.* Local bacterial infection can produce either lumbago or sciatica.

| OTHER CAUSES OF BACKACHE |
| --- |
| • Strain and stress |
| • Overwork |
| • Under-exercised back muscle |
| • Sudden jerking movements |
| • Reflex actions, e.g., sneezing |
| • Obesity |
| • Pregnancy and childbirth |
| • Dysmenorrhea |
| • Scoliosis |
| • Anxiety, fear, insecurity |
| • Kidney disease |
| • Heart, lung, bone or reproductive organ disease |
| • Malformation due to congenital anomaly |
| • Tilted pelvis — if one leg is shorter than the other |

These are the etiological factors of the lumbago-sciatica syndrome. Sometimes they go together and the patient doesn't know if it is sciatica or lumbago. There can be vāta, pitta, and/or kapha causes. There may be vāta pushing pitta, creating inflammation; or vāta pushing kapha, creating spinal tumor, meningeal tumor, or neurofibroma.

Whenever considering lower back pain, bear in mind all of these etiological factors. Don't jump too quickly to a conclusion. Understand the complete history, including the family history. In some families there is a genetic disposition for lumbago, sciatica, or obesity, which may lead to backache.

## Signs and Symptoms

The onset of lumbago pain or sciatica may be sudden or gradual. There can be attacks of lumbago that precede sciatica by a month or year. It is variable. Just a month ago, someone may have been suffering from lumbago, then today that person has sciatica. Lumbago also may be a complication of sciatica and vice versa. These complications may appear within a short or long period of time. Lumbago may also appear as sudden, severe, low back pain.

*Vāta.* First, you must classify whether the type of pain is vāta, pitta, or kapha. Vāta pain is a shooting, throbbing, and pulsating type of pain. It is increased by movement of the lumbosacral and sacroileac joints. The pain can be so severe that the person is prevented from straightening or can do so only with difficulty. If you ask the person to stand straight, he or she stands slightly bent. The rough quality of vāta creates this stiffness. Vāta type of pain is more severe during vāta times: dawn and dusk, fall season, whenever there is cold or damp weather, a cloudy day, or a storm.

In severe vāta pain, there is parasthesia, loss of sense of touch, with numbness and tingling and sometimes wasting of the calf muscle. Vāta is dry, light, and rough. These qualities create *māmsa dhātu kshaya,* which shows as wasting or weakness of the calf muscle. This may cause foot drop. In *vāta grighrasī,* the quality of pain is shooting, cutting, throbbing, radiating, fluctuating, and migrating. It runs along the track of the nerve. Vāta pain is relieved by support and touch, such as massage.

***Pitta.*** In pitta type of grighrasī, the pain is burning, sharp, sucking, and pulling. There is pain and tenderness on pressure. This pain is exacerabated by coughing or sneezing, which increases pressure in the vein and in the subarachnoid space in the spinal area. Because pitta is sharp and burning, there is a tender spot. If you press the midpoint of the gluteal fold, the patient will jump. Another test is to have the patient lie on his back, with flexion of the leg and extension of the knee, and perform dorsiflexion of the ankle. This action stretches the sciatic nerve and will cause severe pain in the sciatic patient. That indicates pitta type of grighrasī, which is often provoked by vāta.

In grighrasī, if vāta is pushing pitta, there will be inflammatory changes. If vāta is pushing kapha, there will be dull and static pain. Therefore, to bring radical healing, we must clinically distinguish between these three types of grighrasī—vāta, pitta, kapha. There is no pain without vāta, no inflammation without pitta, and no congestion without kapha. It is vāta that causes the pain to move or radiate. When the grighrasī is secondarily pitta, there is inflammation as well as pain. If the secondary dosha is kapha, there is congestion along with pain.

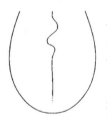

Prolapse of an intervertebral disc may create inflammation. In a prolapsed vertebrae, vāta is involved first and then pitta. Then the person may get lumbar scoliosis and tenderness. If you look at the tongue, there will be a zig-zag line at the back of the midline of the tongue and then a straight line will come forward.

Symptoms may vary in intervertebral disc prolapse, depending upon which root nerve is affected. If the first sacral root nerve (S1) is involved, there will be loss of ankle jerk. Every reflex has a root value. We must know these root values, so that we can know exactly where the lesion is. When the lesion is at S1, there is also weakness of eversion[43] and weakness of the plantar reflex. If L5 is affected, there may be sensory loss, dorsiflexion of the toe, and foot drop. In some patients of prolapsed disc, because of involvement of apāna vāyu, the patient may have incontinence of urine, which is associated with L4, L5, S1 and S2.

Don't treat lumbago lightly. It can create serious problems, such as foot drop, incontinence, parasthesia, numbness, muscle weakness, and wasting.

To understand kati shūla and grighrasī syndrome, first read the person's pulse. Find the prakruti and vikruti. Then go to the fifth level and find asthi dhātu. What kind of spike is present—vāta, pitta, or kapha? Pulse diagnosis is the key to this ancient Vedic wisdom. Then ask the person to stand and observe how he or she stands. Then have the patient lie on the table and observe. Find out if both ankles are equidistant. If the pelvis is twisted, it indicates that one leg is a little longer than the other, which occurs if there are scoliotic changes. Measure the distance on the right and left sides to make this clear. Then touch the dorsum of your hand to the thighs, calves, and foot to determine temperature. If the

---

43. The condition of being turned outward.

temperature is dry and cold on the affected side, it indicates vāta. If the temperature is hot, it is pitta. If the skin is damp and cold, it is kapha.

This differential diagnosis will increase your diagnostic skill. Don't just jump to an herbal solution without developing this knowledge. There are a thousand herbs, but knowing which herb should be used in each condition is a skill we have to develop. When you have knowledge, there is a great deal of security, because you know what you are doing.

## Management

Now we will move to the management of the lumbago and sciatica syndrome. First, find out whether the condition is vāta, pitta, or kapha type, through study, symptoms, and your clinical observation. A thorough examination must be done before you can proceed further.

> T.I.D. = from the Latin means *ter in diem*, three times a day

# Treatment with Āma

If it is vāta type, find out if it is with āma (sāma) or without āma (nirāma). With āma, the person will have coating of the tongue, bad breath, and constipation. In that case, don't do snehana (a specialized Ayurvedic oil massage) or svedana (an herbalized steam bath) because panchakarma is not recommended during a toxic (āma) condition. Instead, use āma pachan with trikatu—ginger, black pepper, and pippalī—¼ teaspoon with honey TID. Also use triphalā guggulu, 200 mg TID. Give gandharva harītakī, one teaspoon at night with warm water. Keep the colon clean and remove āma, but do not suggest oil massage. Doing oil massage during a severe āma condition will actually push the āma into the deep tissues. Even the most expert massage therapist may commit such a mistake in treating a person with an āma condition, if this knowledge of Ayurveda is lacking.

If it is pitta type with āma, use kaishore guggulu, 200 mg TID. Also give trikatu 200 mg with aloe vera juice TID, and bhumi āmalakī, one teaspoon at night with warm water.

For kapha type with āma, use punarnavā guggulu, 200 mg TID, and include trikatu, 200 mg TID, taken with hot water and/or honey. Punarnavā guggulu reduces swelling and congestion. The above program is preliminary therapy to help to move the āma out of the system.

Examine the etiological factors. If constipation is present, triphalā will take care of it. If there is cystitis, cervicitis or colitis, then treat those causes. In these cases, the sciatica or lumbago is a symptom, not the disease. If it is cystitis, cervicitis, or colitis, you have to treat vāta pushing pitta. If it is a spinal tumor, treat vāta pushing kapha and use kāñcanāra guggulu, 200 mg TID. Ayurveda does not treat symptomatically; it deals with the root cause.

If the cause of lumbago and sciatica is ankylosing spondilitis, use anti-inflammatory herbs. The best anti-inflammatory herbs in Ayurveda are kaishore guggulu, gulvel satva, and kāma dudhā. If TB is the root cause, then treat the TB. Laghu mālinī vasanta—a traditional Ayurvedic medicine—is used in India, but not approved in the U.S. One tablet twice a day is the recommended dosage. Trauma, childbirth, and toxic infection also need special treatment.

We have discussed treating the doshas, with attention to vāta, pitta, or kapha with āma. Now we will shift to vyādhi pratyanika, treatment of the disease itself.

### Rest

In vyādhi pratyanika, rest for at least four weeks is essential in severe pain from a slipped disc. Sleeping on a firm mattress supported by boards is helpful for kapha type. Immobilization is important, resting the involved part of the body. A water bed or a soft bed is not good for lumbago. Soft beds are uneven and sleeping on an uneven bed is also a cause of lumbago or sciatica syndrome. Sitting for a long time is also aggravating, because it exerts pressure. Likewise, lifting heavy objects should be avoided. This may seem obvious, but some people continue to do heavy lifting because their job requires it.

### Exercise

Back stretching exercises are quite helpful. Yoga is a good accessory therapy but it is important to guide the patient properly. Beneficial postures include modified camel pose, modified cobra pose, and *mahā mudrā*. Include passive yoga exercises. The person lies on their back and you gently lift their legs, supported with a pillow. The person should learn the squatting pose, which is relaxing. When a woman has recently delivered a child and has a backache, she should sit in a squatting pose. The person should sit with pillow support behind the lower back, which relaxes the lumbosacral joint. Sitting flat on the floor is stressful to the back. When sitting in an armchair, using pillow support is quite effective.

Certain yoga prāṇāyāma (breathing techniques) are effective for lower backache. For example, use alternate nostril breathing with inner retention.

### Additional Management

* Raise your fitness level and increase aerobic capacity
* Wear special shock-absorbing inserts in your shoes
* Find your most restful position to sleep and do so in a horizontal position
* Stop overdoing things
* Try kaishore guggulu, mustā, and mahānārāyana oil massage
* Get a posture check
* Warm up your muscles before exercise
* Try water exercises and yoga
* Marma point, acupressure, or trigger point therapies
* Give up smoking
* Take it easy on sexual activity
* Warm up your lower back by applying external heat

## Treatment without Āma

*Snehana.* When āma is removed, treatment should include snehana and svedana. For a vāta person, use mahānārāyana or sesame oil for abhyanga. For a pitta person, use sunflower oil. For a kapha person, corn oil with vacha oil is effective. But never do snehana when there is āma.

*Svedana.* For svedana, put nirgundī or eucalyptus powder in the sweat box. A ginger and baking soda bath will also help pacify the pain. For a pitta person, give a short svedana, only 5 to 10 minutes in duration, because prolonged svedana is not good for pitta. For a kapha person, give a long svedana, 20 minutes to half an hour. Care should be taken in treating vāta to monitor the person during the svedana.

*Diet.* The person should follow the right kind of diet—vāta-pacifying food in a vāta condition; pitta-pacifying diet in a pitta condition; kapha-reducing food in a kapha disorder.

*Basti (Therapeutic enema).* For vāta, use dashamūla tea basti. Boil 2 tablespoons of dashamūla in one pint of water for 10 minutes. Cool and strain. If there is no āma, add ½ cup of sesame oil. That is called anuvāsana basti. If the person has muscle wasting, numbness, and tingling, use balā tea. Boil 2 tablespoons of balā powder in a pint of water for 10 minutes. Cool it, strain it, and then add ½ cup of sesame oil.

If there is severe tenderness, indicating pitta type pain, use gudūchī basti. Boil 2 tablespoons of gudūchī with a pint of water for 10 minutes. Cool and strain this, then add ½ cup of coconut oil. Coconut oil is anti-inflammatory and this basti will relieve inflammation.

To treat sciatica and lower back pain, you should do a basti every day for the first week, every other day the next week, every third day the third week, then once a week for the next six months.

For slipped disc, use a madhu tailam basti, which is one cup of sesame oil and ½ cup of honey mixed together. First, give a regular water enema and clean the colon. After a good bowel movement, wait for one hour. Then inject one cup of warm sesame oil and ½ cup honey mixed together. Give this once a day during vāta time, either in the early morning or very early evening. Ask the patient to retain it as long as he or she can. In some people it will not be passed, as it will be absorbed into the colon. This basti prevents muscle wasting. It will strengthen the ligament and help the disc to return to normal. It is also effective in treating urinary incontinence, because it enhances the strength of the sphincter muscle. If the nerve is affected in the segment of L4, L5, or S1, it may cause incontinence. Madhu tailam basti improves nerve conduction and is helpful in bringing back sphincter control in a slipped disc condition.

## Herbs

If you do not know the type of sciatica or lumbago, use the following formula:

| | |
|---|---|
| Dashamūla | 500 mg |
| Vidārī | 300 mg |
| Tagara | 300 mg |
| Mustā | 300 mg |
| Kaishore guggulu | 300 mg |

This mixture should be given ½ teaspoon TID with warm water, before food, to work on the lower part of the body.

For specific vyādhi pratyanika use:

| | |
|---|---|
| Yogarāja guggulu | 300 mg for vāta type |
| Kaishore guggulu | 300 mg for vāta pushing pitta type |
| Punarnavā guggulu | 300 mg for vāta pushing kapha type |

There are various guggulus, so choose the guggulu according to prakruti and vikruti.

Sometimes a kidney stone can create lower backache. In that case, use:
Gokshurādi guggulu      300 mg

At the time of pain, give lemon juice and potassium carbonate.
1 cup of lemon juice
pinch of potassium carbonate

The following combination is effective for kapha and vāta type of pain.

| | |
|---|---|
| Deodara | 300 mg |
| Dashamūla | 300 mg |
| Ginger powder | 300 mg |
| Garlic powder | 300 mg |

Give ½ teaspoon TID to relieve pain of sciatica and lumbago.

Ayurveda says that even a fractured vertebra can be healed by mahāyogaraja guggulu, but it contains mercury and so its use is prohibited in the United States.

Rub the lower back with Maha Ganesh® oil and mahānārāyana oil before a bath.

There are also psychological causes for lumbago and sciatica. The sacrum supports the lumbar vertebrae. Whenever there is insecurity and fear, the sacrum moves slightly downward and creates a gap in the lumbosacral area, where vāta is easily aggravated and can cause pain. For a psychological cause, we treat the problem with Tranquility Tea© and support. Psychological counseling is also effective.

## Marma Chikitsā

Trik, Ūrū, Sakthi Ūrvī, Jānu, Gulpha, and Pārshni are marma points that are specific for treatment of this syndrome. Pārshni marma is a point at the central part of the heel that will relieve sciatica pain when it is pressed.[44]

Ayurveda is a fascinating medicine. It gives wonderful information to help the patient of lumbago and sciatica.

---

44. Illustrations are shown in the appendix on page 455.

# Chapter 29

# Diseases of Bones, Joints, and Connective Tissues
## Asthi, Sandhi, and Majjā Roga

Fall 1991, Volume 4, Number 2

AYURVEDA, THE SCIENCE OF LIFE, is an ancient art of healing that deals with all rheumatological diseases, which are called in Sanskrit *asthi, sandhi,* and *majjā roga.* These names indicate disorders of the connective tissue (majjā dhātu) that also involve joints (sandhi) and bones (asthi dhātu). In these rheumatic diseases, the presence of pain, stiffness, and swelling of parts of the musculo-skeletal system are the prominent feature.

According to Ayurveda, vāta dosha and asthi dhātu (bone tissue) are intimately associated, due to the porous nature of the bones. They have a container-content relationship. The large intestine is the main site of vāta, and its mucous membrane nourishes the bones by absorbing minerals. Agni (digestive fire) and apāna vāyu govern this function in the colon. If agni is low, there will be production of āma (toxins) in the colon. Eventually this toxic material will be carried by vāta into the musculo-skeletal system, where it clogs the channels by producing congestion in the connective tissue. Depending upon which of the other doshas are involved, this āma may create various pathological conditions in the connective tissues, bones, and joints. These conditions may be of three types: inflammatory/infective, metabolic, and degenerative.

*Inflammatory/Infective Types.* Inflammatory or infective type of rheumatism is caused by pitta. Systemic pitta dosha and āma can linger in the asthi dhātu and produce acute rheumatic fever and rheumatoid arthritis, or make one vulnerable to infective ailments such as gonococcal or syphilitic arthritis.

*Metabolic Types.* Dhātu agni can undergo metabolic changes when āma is present in the blood. This can cause deposition of crystals in the joints, which, in turn, can manifest as gout and chondrocalcinosis.

*Degenerative Types.* When āma blocks asthi vaha srotas and aggravates vāta dosha, degenerative disorders can result, including osteoarthritis, spondylosis, and other painful syndromes of the connective tissues.

# Rheumatism

Rheumatism is a broad term as used in modern medicine. It embraces a diversity of symptoms and diseases of the connective tissue. Rheumatic diseases affect people of both genders and all ages and ethnic groups. The frequency of rheumatic disorders increases with age. One can observe that about 35% of people over the age of 60 have rheumatic complaints of one sort or the other. These ailments may severely disable a person or even shorten the span of life due to cardiac complications.

## Rheumatic Fever (Acute stage of Āma Vāta)

When an individual has low agni and eats incompatible food combinations, such as milk with fish or banana or meat with dairy), frequent tonsillitis or pharyngitis may result. Eating ice cream and drinking cold liquids may also reduce natural resistance and slow down the digestive fire (agni), which will result in production of āma in the gastrointestinal tract. Āma is then carried by vāta into the general circulation. When āma enters rasa dhātu, it results in further disturbance of agni. This imbalance of the fire principle, together with the invading āma in the rasa and rakta dhātus, causes a systemic inflammatory condition. It is called rheumatic fever, and it comes as a sequel to pharyngitis or tonsilitis. Rheumatic fever principally involves the joints, heart, central nervous system, and subcutaneous tissues. During the acute stage of the condition, vāta dosha carries āma throughout the body; then pain and swelling may migrate from joint to joint, affecting several large joints at once. This can lead to polyarthritis, fever, carditis or rheumatic valvular heart disease with a specific type of murmur. All these symptoms are the manifestations of toxic āma circulating throughout the body. Not everyone who has this kind of infection will develop rheumatic fever, but a subject having low agni, poor resistance, and systemic āma could develop rheumatic fever several days after an acute infection.

## Etiology and Pathogenesis (Nidāna and Samprāpti)

The ancient Ayurvedic literature says a great deal about the wrong kind of diet and lifestyle being important etiological factors in rheumatic fever. Over-active individuals and those who eat incompatible foods and chilled drinks are particularly susceptible. In addition to food-induced āma, other causes include bacteria, chronic constipation, and repressed emotions. Constant exposure to a cold draft, being in a chilly and damp climate, and low natural resistance are among the vāta-aggravating and agni-diminishing components that play a major role in the pathogenesis of this malady. Rheumatic fever can occur at any age, but because kapha and āma are similar in attribute, it is more common in childhood up to the age of 15, which is during the kapha stage of life.

Rheumatic carditis is the result of āma affecting avalambaka kapha and usually manifests first as a heart murmur of either mitral or aortic incompetence. In extreme cases, āma may be responsible for pericarditis and congestive heart failure leading to death. Carditis manifests as increased, irregular heartbeats and enlargement of the heart. This complication needs prompt medical supervision.

Āma can also create painless swellings (subcutaneous nodules) over bony prominences on the muscle tendons of hands and feet, elbow and patella, scalp and scapula.

Vāta pushing āma in the central nervous system can lead to prāna disorders, by creating irregular chorea-form movements. Chorea is a delayed manifestation of rheumatic fever, because it takes time for the āma to enter the nervous system. This vāta condition is associated with emotional instability, ungroundedness, and anxiety. In a pitta individual, rheumatic fever will likely manifest with high fever, abdominal pain, and nosebleeds. A kapha person will exhibit low-grade fever, swelling and loss of appetite.

The duration of rheumatic fever varies according to prakruti. In a vāta person it may last 6 weeks, in a pitta individual about 12 weeks, while in a kapha person it can remain present for 6 months. The chronic nature of the kapha type rheumatic fever may cause dhātu kshaya (degeneration of the tissues), which may lead to vāta disorders and rheumatoid arthritis.

## Chikitsā Sūtra of Āma Vāta (The Management of Āma Vāta)

The ancient Ayurvedic skills used to deal with āma vāta (rheumatic fever) are unique. The following are the basic principles of management of this disorder:

*Langhana.* Langhana is a therapy that involves fasting or eating light foods, which will indirectly bring down the person's temperature by breaking the chain of toxemia. In this case, Ayurveda suggests rice broth, very softly cooked rice, or tapioca as the best foods. All these should be spiced with cumin, mustard and ginger powder. This helps to kindle agni, burn the toxins lodged in the tissues and clear up the clogged channels. After langhana therapy, the tongue will become clean, the pulse will slow and the toxic pyrexia (elevated temperature) will be reduced. Langhana should be continued until positive indications of detoxification appear.

*Svedana.* Svedana means the application of heat. Methods include using a hot sauna, steam bath or shower, or applying a hot sand bag to the inflamed joint or joints. An herbal paste can also be applied directly to the affected joints, followed by application of heat. One such preparation can be made with powders of bachan, dhattūra, and vacha, along with with sufficient water to form a paste. These herbs should not be used internally. After applying the paste to the painful joints, one should sit near a fire or heater. This will dry the paste, pull toxic āma from the synovial membranes, and reduce pain, swelling and inflammation.

In the case of rheumatic fever, svedana should be done using dry heat, not wet heat such as a steam bath or shower. Āma is itself wet, so the dry quality of such heat helps to reduce āma. Dry heat will also help to detoxify the connective tissue and will clear the channels, thereby preventing further pathogenesis.

*Tikta Herbs.* Tikta means bitter taste, and bitter herbs are related to the elements Ether (ākāsha) and Air (vāyu). Thus they spread quickly into the subtle channels of the tissues. While overall the bitter taste is cooling, in this instance we use herbs that are both bitter and heating, such as rāsna, guggulu and parijata. These bitter, heating herbs will do āma pāchana (detoxify āma), clear blocked channels, and have an anti-pyretic and anti-inflammatory action. A few compounds containing these herbs include yogarāja guggulu, kaishore guggulu, mahārasnādi kvath, and parijatak guti.[45]

***Katu Herbs.*** *Katu* means pungent. *Dīpana katu* are pungent herbs that enkindle agni and do āma pāchana (detoxification). Some pungent dīpana herbs include ginger, black pepper, and pippalī. These can also be combined and used as a compound called trikatu. They improve the immune system, circulation and appetite, and clear the tissues. They are also carminative, which means they dispel gas.

## Panchakarma and Rasāyana

Once the fever and toxic manifestation of āma are under control, it is good to do panchakarma therapy for at least seven days. panchakarma should not be done during the toxic, acute stage of pyrexia (fever), as it could then push āma into the vital organs. Once detoxification has progressed through use of the previously mentioned herbs, it will often be helpful to perform vamana (vomiting therapy), which will cleanse the stomach of āma. To induce vomiting one may drink licorice or calamus tea. Three days after vamana therapy, Ayurveda advises taking a dashamūla tea basti (herbal enema). For a total of five days, perform this basti daily, made of one pint of dashamūla tea, to remove residual āma from the colon.

Once the āma is totally removed from the GI tract, one should follow a rasāyana therapy suitable for the individual's prakruti. For vāta prakruti, ashvagandhā rasāyana is effective; for pitta, shatāvarī rasāyana is good; for kapha, punarnavā rasāyana is best. All constitutions may take balā rasāyana.

If there are cardiac complications with a heart murmur, Ayurveda recommends the use of suvarna bhasma (gold ash), arjuna, punarnavā, and deer horn ash at this stage of the treatment. All of these are helpful in cases of carditis.

Two teaspoons of castor oil can be taken along with ginger tea at bedtime when fever is absent, as it is highly effective as an anti-rheumatic. This remedy contains natural steroids and detoxifies the skeleto-muscular system and the connective tissue of the joints.

Garlic, ginger, mustard, and mint chutney can be included in the diet. If vāta dosha is elevated, herbal wines such as mahārasnādi kvath, drākshā, and dashamūla arishta are effective.

Through the use of vamana, basti, and rasāyana as well as proper diet and lifestyle, one can prevent the recurrence of rheumatic fever and rheumatoid arthritis. These disorders are generally complicated cases to manage, so it is advisable to consult an Ayurvedic physician who can offer expert advice on how best to proceed.

---

45. Guti is a round tablet as compared to a vati, which is a flattened tablet.

# Chapter 30

# Arthritis
## Asthi, Sandhi, and Majjā Roga

Spring 2015, Volume 27, Number 4

ARTHRITIS IS A DISEASE of the articular tissue of the joints—either inflammatory or non-inflammatory. It is associated with pain, swelling, stiffness, and sometimes deformity of the joints. There are various conditions of arthritis, such as osteoarthritis and rheumatoid arthritis, which I discuss below.

According to Ayurveda, arthritis is caused by systemic vāta from the colon undergoing sanchaya (accumulation), prakopa (provocation), and then prasara (spread). During the prasara stage, vāta circulates around the body and then in the fourth stage it enters into one or more of the *dhātus*. If there is khavaigunya (defective space) in asthi dhātu, vāta goes into that tissue and creates *asthi gata vāta*. When vāta affects the joints it is known as *sandhi gata vāta* (sandhi means joint).

Where two bony ends come together as part of a joint, it is part of asthi dhātu. The articular tissue of the joint space is part of majjā dhātu. Majjā dhātu includes the joints, articular fluid, synovial fluid, and bursa.

When vāta goes into asthi dhātu, it can cause pain and stiffness in the joints due to excessive dryness. There is cracking and popping of the joints. It is non-inflammatory joint pain.

When vāta goes into majjā dhātu, it can cause pain, stiffness and swelling in the joints, along with possible inflammatory changes. When vāta pushes pitta or āma in majjā dhātu, there is inflammation.

According to Ayurveda, arthritis is usually either:

**A**) vāta type, caused by vāta entering into the joints causing pain and stiffness, or

**B**) vāta pushing pitta type, caused by vāta pushing pitta into the joints, which will also lead to pain and swelling, but it will be a more inflammatory disorder

Additionally, either vāta or pitta can push kapha dosha into the joint space, creating a kapha type of mild congestive arthritis, which is related to obesity and gravitational stress.

When pitta pushes kapha into the joints, it can cause inflammatory exudate, because pitta and kapha are both liquid.

Finally, āma (toxins) can be involved, as in rheumatoid arthritis. This is a bird's eye view of the Ayurvedic understanding about arthritis.

## Types of Arthritis

**Osteoarthritis** is called sandhi gata vāta, which occurs when vāta enters into asthi and majjā dhātus and affects the joints. Osteoarthritis is quite common in old age (after 55), because that is a time of vāta dosha. It is the most common form of arthritis overall, due to wear and tear of the joints. Chronic osteoarthritis may lead to degenerative changes in the joints.

**Bacterial arthritis** (also called septic arthritis) may be due to a staphylococcus or streptococcal infection, which in some cases can produce arthritis. The bacterial toxins can enter into the bloodstream and then into the joints, causing joint pain.

The following are specific forms of bacterial arthritis: 1) **Lyme arthritis** occurs because of a tick bite. Toxins created by the Lyme spirochete (*borrelia burgdorferi*) can lodge into the joints, causing a chronic multi-systemic disorder called Lyme disease. The tick bite season is spring and summer, when deer-tick vectors are most active, particularly in the northeast of the United States. Prompt removal of the tick is necessary before the bacteria spreads into the bloodstream. If not immediately removed, a typical rash begins at the site of a bite, with a red ring and then erythema. The ring expands, so the periphery is red and the central part is clear white. Stage one of Lyme disease is this localized reaction, while in stage two the reaction spreads throughout the bloodstream and can cause arthritis, muscle pain, cardiac arrhythmia, pericarditis, lymphadenopathy and meningoencephalitis. Antibodies are developed during this stage. Stage three sees a chronic infection develop within two to three years. In this phase, the patient develops severe arthritis or encephalitis, which is rarely fatal.

2) **Gonococcal arthritis** (*upa damsha*) results from sexual exposure to a person who has gonorrhea. Generally, in gonorrhea infection, the bacteria infect the glans penis and can create gonorrhea discharge. These bacteria produce toxins that can go into the bloodstream and then enter into the articular tissue of the joints, causing gonococcal arthritis.

3) **Syphilitic arthritis** (*abhyantara phiringa*) is similar to gonococcal arthritis. It is a sexually transmitted disease, in which the syphilitic bacteria transmitted through the blood can lodge in the joints and cause a form of arthritis.

4) **Tubercular arthritis** (*koshtu kshirsha*) can result from tuberculosis (TB), which occurs in the mediastinal lymph nodes. One form of extra-pulmonary tuberculosis is bone TB. When the infection goes into the bones, it can cause tubercular arthritis in the hips, knees, ankles, and intervertebral disks. There is pain, swelling, and inflammatory exudate. Generally, the knee joint is affected, so it is called tuberculosis of the knee joint or Koch's knee.

5) **Suppurative arthritis** is a complication of bacterial arthritis. It occurs due to vāta pushing pitta in the joints, with acute pus formation.

**Allergic arthritis** is caused by serum sickness or exposure to allergenic foods. Someone may be allergic to certain food items such as strawberry, cranberry, potato, eggplant, egg, and so forth, or have celiac disease. This can result in the symptoms of allergic arthritis.

**Enteropathic arthritis** is due to inflammation of the colon. Arthritis can become a complication of ulcerative colitis, irritable bowel syndrome (IBS), Crohn's disease, or regional ileitis. Whenever there is a chronic patch of inflammation within the inner wall of the colon, the person can get enteropathic arthritis. People who have celiac disease, gluten sensitivity, or sprue syndrome are prone to enteropathic arthritis.

**Gouty arthritis** is called *vāta rakta*. It is a metabolic disorder that occurs in certain individuals when bhūta agni and dhātu agni are low. That causes carbohydrate and mineral disorders, leading to increased uric acid within the serum and calcium pyrophosphate crystals within the synovial membrane. The uric acid and calcium pyrophosphate crystals are sharp and lodge into the surface of the small joints—especially the metatarsal phalange joint or interphalangeal joint of the big toe—where they can cause arthritis. Vāta rakta (gouty arthritis) always starts with the big toe.

> **GENERAL ETIOLOGICAL FACTORS FOR ARTHRITIS**
>
> Trauma
>
> Infection
>
> Gravitational stress, such as from obesity
>
> Misuse of the joints – occupational misuse or sports
>
> Food allergies or sensitivities
>
> Incompatible food combinations
>
> Rheumatic fever (leads to rheumatoid arthritis)
>
> Staphylococcal infection
>
> Gonorrhea
>
> Tuberculosis
>
> Metabolic disorders such as gout
>
> Multi-systemic immune diseases, such as Lyme disease
>
> Psoriasis
>
> Endocrine disorders
>
> Systemic Lupus
>
> Neuropathic disorders such as Charcot's neuropathy

**Neuropathic arthritis** is a condition of *majjā gata vāta*. This disease of the nervous system occurs mainly as a result of diabetes, tabes dorsalis (syphilitic myelopathy), neurosyphilis, or Charcot joint (neuropathic arthropathy). *Majjā kshaya* can lead to *asthi kshaya*, causing bone loss.

**Gravitational stress-induced arthritis** generally occurs in people with obesity. It is due to vāta pushing kapha in asthi dhātu.

**Psoriatic arthritis** (*kushtaja*) is another form of arthritis. Psoriasis is an autoimmune skin disease, resulting in skin lesions around the joints—especially the elbows, wrists, knees, and ankles. The toxins of these lesions can enter into the joints and create psoriatic arthritis.

**Rheumatoid arthritis** (*āma vāta*) is an autoimmune disorder that is more common in elderly people. Long-lingering systemic āma (toxins) goes into the *sthāyi asthi dhātu* and majjā dhātu and covers the cell membranes of the synovial tissue. Neighboring cells send a signal, but those cells in the synovial membrane (part of majjā dhātu) that are covered by āma cannot give a response. As a result, the immune system treats those cells in the synovial membrane as foreign bodies and tries to destroy them. Therefore, the immune system attacks the articular surface of the joints, which leads to rheumatoid arthritis.

**Juvenile arthritis** starts under the age of 16, in the extra-articular tissue of the joints. It is a form of rheumatoid arthritis that affects about 1 in 1000 children. It is the most common form of arthritis in children. Babies with rheumatoid factor are prone to get this disease, due to genetic predisposition. Lack of aseptic measures during the cutting of the placental chord during delivery can also be a factor. Placental toxins can enter the bloodstream and result in arthritis. However, more than 50% of children with juvenile arthritis will enter remission. Their recovery depends upon the responsiveness of *asthi agni* and *majjā agni*.

## Rheumatoid Arthritis (Āma Vāta)

Rheumatoid arthritis is an autoimmune disease affecting the connective tissue of the joints. It is a chronic systemic disease, marked by inflammation, stiffness, muscle soreness, and pain in multiple synovial joints.

Rheumatoid arthritis usually creates bony erosion that can be clearly seen on an x-ray. The wrists, elbows, and shoulders are often affected in the upper extremities, and the knees, ankles and hip joints in the lower extremities.

It typically affects the same joints on both sides of the body, such as either both ankles or both knees. It is an inflammatory, destructive and deforming polyarthritis (arthritis affecting multiple joints), associated with systemic disturbances and a variety of extra-articular lesions.

The pattern of the joint involved is characteristically symmetrical and peripheral—in the sense of a smaller joint going into the bigger joint.

Serum antiglobulin, which is rheumatoid factor (Rh factor), is increased in most patients. In Ayurveda, this is described as tejas is burning ojas. It is a cytogenetic āma that circulates throughout the body.

There is *rasa dhātu dushti* due to an increased number of plasma cells. There is also inflammatory granulation tissue (pannus), with fibrous adhesions spread over the cartilage, creating limited joint space. That causes stiffness of the joints, along with joint pain and swelling.

Rheumatoid arthritis is caused by long-lingering āma (toxins) going into the articular tissue, resulting in tejas burning ojas, which means the immune system attacks the bodily tissues. This is a book picture of *vyāna vāta* pushing āma into the joints. The disease affects both asthi and majjā dhātus.

Āma is thick, sticky, and static, so it causes pain and stiffness in the joints. It is similar to kapha in terms of its qualities. Morning and evening are kapha times, so the patient typically complains of stiffness in the early morning and early evening (after sunset).

Increased kapha at these times causes increased plasma and platelets, which in turn creates more joint pain and stiffness at those times. Increased humidity and cloudy conditions also induce more āma around the joints, resulting in worse pain and stiffness.

Rheumatoid arthritis occurs throughout the world, in all climates and all ethnic groups. All over the world, this disorder is growing and it occurs in about 3-4% of females and less than 1% of males, so the ratio is at least 3 to 1.

Some ethnic groups have a higher rate of the disease. These include Native Americans and South Asian people. The disease may begin in the third or fourth decade of life, but it can happen in any age group. It presents higher than expected in identical twins, because there is a strong genetic predisposition.

We carry the cellular memory of our great grandparents' illnesses within the deep connective tissue of our respective organs. In rheumatoid arthritis, there is a genetic predisposition that creates a khavaigunya (defective space) in the joints. This has been confirmed by tissue-typing studies that show HLA DR4 is the human leukocyte antigen (*rasa gata āma*) that is linked to R.A. These days, they can identify the specific strand of DNA linked to certain genetic diseases. DR4 is the strand that, when affected, causes a predisposition to rheumatoid arthritis. According to Ayurveda, this is due to impaired functioning of pīlu agni and pithara agni at the cellular level in the great grandparent's body, which then produces HLA.

## Causes of Rheumatoid Arthritis

The specific causes of rheumatoid arthritis are obscure. However, ancient Ayurveda talks about this disease being common in people with vāta prakruti or vāta vikruti. Eating too many black beans, pinto beans, adzuki beans, chickpeas, raw vegetables, and other vāta-aggravating foods is one likely cause. Other etiological factors are excessive jogging, jumping, trampolining and straining the joints with exercise or heavy weight lifting, or occupational use and abuse of the joints, which all disturb vāta dosha.

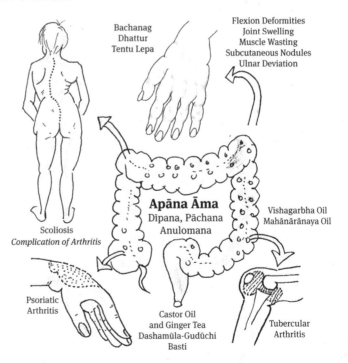

Bachanag Dhattur Tentu Lepa

Flexion Deformities
Joint Swelling
Muscle Wasting
Subcutaneous Nodules
Ulnar Deviation

**Apāna Āma**
Dīpana, Pāchana
Anulomana

Vishagarbha Oil
Mahānārānaya Oil

Scoliosis
*Complication of Arthritis*

Psoriatic Arthritis

Castor Oil
and Ginger Tea
Dashamūla-Gudūchi
Basti

Tubercular Arthritis

The illness can also be triggered by a diet with large amounts of difficult-to-digest foods, such as cheese, yoghurt, beer, and so forth. These foods can produce āma and also worsen the severity of the disease in someone who already has rheumatoid arthritis.

Rheumatoid arthritis may be caused by trauma and is also linked to rheumatic fever. Rheumatic fever involves strep throat, tonsillitis, and pharyngitis and is due to a staphylococcus infection. It often occurs in children, producing an immune response to the bacterial antigen in staphylococcus that can result in rheumatism.

It is believed that a previous infection is the initiating factor for rheumatoid arthritis, although no specific causative organism has yet been detected. There is a good deal of evidence of persistent immune overactivity and antigenic stimulation in a genetically predisposed person, with the presence of immune complexes at the site of articular and extra-articular tissues.

---

**SIGNS & SYMPTOMS OF RHEUMATOID ARTHRITIS**

Joint pain

Stiffness (especially early morning)

Swelling

Small joints are affected first, then bigger joints

Joints look like a spindle shape

**Complications:**

Scleritis (āma in majjā dhātu)

Peripheral Neuropathy (āma in majjā dhātu)

Reynaud's syndrome (vascular, āma in rakta dhātu)

Lymphadenopathy (āma in rasa dhātu)

Hepatosplenomegaly (rakta vaha sroto dushti)

Muscular atrophy (māmsa vaha sroto dushti)

Pleurisy (prāna vaha sroto dushti)

Pericarditis, effusion, or aortic regurgitation (prāna, rasa, and rakta vaha sroto dushti)

---

There is a presence of circulating immunoglobulins IGM, IGG and IGA rheumatic factor, as well as anti-collagen and anti-nuclear antibodies. That will create inflammation, irritation, and depression of the synovial fluid, leading to inflammation of the joints associated with activation of both classical and alternate pathways. There are increased numbers of plasma cells (kapha molecules), lymphocytes, and monocytes in the synovial membrane, associated with local production of rheumatic factor.

Some individuals have local rheumatic factor in the synovia (synovial fluid). This will not show up if you do a serum examination, so that condition is known as atypical rheumatoid arthritis. The presence of serum factor inhibits suppressor T-lymphocyte activity, which involves phagocytes. Amyloidosis is a complication in some cases of rheumatoid arthritis, in which unprocessed protein becomes fibrous tissue, which deposits under the joint space. This leads to shortening of the joint space and contracture.

The etiology and pathology occurs at a deep cellular level, involving pīlu agni and pithara agni. Pīlu agni affects the serum that goes from the extracellular into the intracellular component. Because of low pīlu agni, cytotoxic āma is produced within the cell. This āma covers the cell membrane and inhibits cellular communication. This is a trigger for autoimmune disorders.

Ayurveda says that rheumatoid arthritis is due to long-lingering systemic āma caused by low agni. Vishama agni will create vāta type of rheumatoid arthritis, tīkshna agni will cause pitta type of rheumatoid arthritis, and manda agni will create kapha type.

The earliest changes are inflammation, swelling and congestion of the synovial membrane and overlying connective tissue. The inflammation creates granuloma formation and then slowly starts to destroy the joint. The plasma cells, macrophages, and lymphocytes infiltrate into the synovial membrane. Then effusion of the synovial fluid into the joint space takes place, which causes stiffness of the joints. This is a *shleshaka kapha* disorder.

Shleshaka kapha is released from the synovial membrane (*sleshma dhāra kalā*). This shleshaka becomes more sticky, due to the dry quality of vāta, and this stickiness causes joint stiffness. Phagocytic changes in the synovial fluid are *kapha dushti*. *Rasa dushti* is also involved, with an increased number of plasma cells.

Inflammatory granulation tissue pannus is formed, spreading under the articular cartilage. Later, fibrous adhesion takes place, so the joint space is reduced and there is deformity of the joint.

The individual can get subcutaneous nodules. A central area of cellular debris and fibroid material creates swelling.

Clinically, the onset is insidious, with joint pain, stiffness, and symmetrical swelling of a number of peripheral joints. Initially, pain is only experienced upon the movement of the joints.

Cold is the quality of vāta and kapha, and it causes stiffness and pain. Early morning stiffness is a characteristic feature of rheumatoid arthritis, because morning is kapha time. As the sun rises higher during midday and throughout the afternoon, the person feels better and there is less pain. Then later in the evening, when the atmosphere cools down again, the pain increases.

There is a tendency for the pain to spread from the smaller joints to the wrists, elbows, and shoulders in the upper extremity, and to the knees, ankles, and subtalar midtarsal joints. The hip joints are rarely affected.

The pain can spread to the intervertebral joints, with neck pain and stiffness in the cervical spine being common symptoms. The mandibular, acromioclavicular and sternoclavicular joints are sometimes affected.

Slowly, slowly, the patient develops multiple joint pains. This pain radiates from joint to joint, and ultimately the joint pain, swelling, and stiffness cause the articular surface and articular spaces to be limited.

This is the typical picture of āma vāta or rheumatoid arthritis. The disease can attack at any age. It is a polyarthritic connective tissue disorder due to an autoimmune response, where the body attacks its own tissue. It can damage the heart, lungs, nerves, and eyes.

Due to āma in majjā dhātu, the patient can also get scleritis and peripheral neuropathy. Peripheral neuropathy creates sharp, lightening pain in the nerves of the arms or legs. Because of the pain, the person often uses his or her muscles less and less, so there can be muscle atrophy related to the inflamed joints.

# Treatment Protocol for Rheumatoid Arthritis

*Langhanam svedanam tiktam*
*Dīpanāni katu nīcha*
*Virechanam snehapanam*
*Bastaya cha āma marute*

This sūtra says that patients with rheumatoid arthritis should undergo dīpana (kindle agni), pāchana (burn āma), snehana (application of oil), svedana (sudation), and anulomana (maintain flow of doshas) therapies.

We have to kindle agni by using dīpana chikitsā and burn āma with pāchana chikitsā. Use bitter herbs, such as guggulu, neem, and mahasudarshan. These will burn āma in rasa dhātu.

Anulomana is given in the form of ginger tea and castor oil. Chop one inch of ginger into smaller pieces and boil it in a cup of water to make fresh ginger tea. Add one to two teaspoons of castor oil into the ginger tea. This mixture will burn āma, help to remove the rheumatic factor, improve circulation, and relieve inflammation.

In cold, damp weather, we have to use dry heat, such as a sandbag or water bag. Keeping the patient in a closed room and applying dry heat is an effective way to burn the āma. One can even use a room heater as the form of dry, radiant heat. Dry heat will relieve inflammation, as it caused by āma.

## Shamana Chikitsā

Choose one or two of the following types of guggulu, according to doshic involvement.

Simhanad guggulu   300 mg (anti-rheumatic)
Yogarāja guggulu   200 mg (for skeleton-muscular arthritic pain, for vāta type)
Kaishore guggulu   200 mg (anti-inflammatory, pain relief in smaller joints, for pitta type)
Rasnadi guggulu   200 mg (anti-inflammatory, pain relief in bigger joints, for kapha type)

The following herbal remedies should be taken three times daily with warm water:

Dashamūla           500 mg (specifically for vāta dosha)
Simhanad guggulu   250 mg (specific for āma vāta)
Āma pāchaka vati   200 mg tablet (detoxifies and relieves sroto rodha)

In the early stage of neuropathy, add ashvagandhā or sarasvatī.

Ashvagandhā         300 mg (to strengthen muscles and relieve pain)
Sarasvatī           300 mg (for neuropathy)

In the initial phase of pericarditis, give arjuna and shringa bhasma.

Arjuna              200 mg (to support the pericardium)
Shringa bhasma      200 mg

In the first stages of pleurisy, use the following:

| | |
|---|---|
| Pushkaramūla | 200 mg (to maintain lubrication of pleura and prevent pleuritis) |
| Sitopalādi | 300 mg |
| Talisadi | 300 mg |

Topically, one can apply vishagarbha tailam. It is deeply penetrating, anti-inflammatory and burns āma in the connective tissue. This helps the toxins to move back into the gastrointestinal (GI) tract, making the tongue appear heavily coated.

Panchakarma is contraindicated until the āma has moved out of the deep tissues and into the GI tract. Once the āma is burned away, the pain, swelling and inflammation are reduced and the tongue shows a clear appearance. We can then use mahānārāyana tailam. This relieves the pain and helps to prevent joint destruction. Once the intensity of pain and stiffness is reduced, begin panchakarma using snehana, svedana, anulomana, virechana, basti, and *rasāyana* treatments.

Rheumatoid arthritis often begins in the colon, so we have to detoxify the large intestine with dashamūla-gudūchi basti. Boil 1 tablespoon each of dashamūla powder and gudūchi powder in 1 pint of water for 3 minutes, then cool and strain. Don't put oil in the basti, because this is āma vāta. This basti treatment is most effective, and will help to remove the āma. However, this is a complex disease that takes a long time to heal.

Also give castor oil with ginger tea as anulomana therapy. Additionally, a bachanaga dattura tentu lepa, a green paste, is applied to the affected joints to relieve pain and reduce swelling.

## Rasāyana Chikitsā

Take 4 teaspoons of dashamūla arishta with equal parts of water after lunch and dinner (rasāyana to skeletal-muscular system, calms down vāta dosha).

Take 4 teaspoons of maharasnadi kvātha with equal parts of water after lunch and dinner (specific to rheumatism).

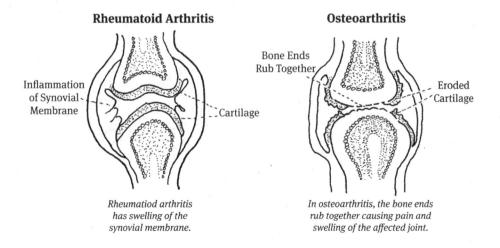

**Rheumatoid Arthritis**

Inflammation of Synovial Membrane

Cartilage

*Rheumatiod arthritis has swelling of the synovial membrane.*

**Osteoarthritis**

Bone Ends Rub Together

Eroded Cartilage

*In osteoarthritis, the bone ends rub together causing pain and swelling of the affected joint.*

259

## Osteoarthritis (Sandhi Gata Vāta)

Osteoarthritis is the most common type of arthritis. It causes progressive deterioration and degeneration of the cartilage ("baby bone") in the synovial joints and vertebrae. This becomes an especially significant risk factor in an aging patient.

Osteoarthritis is a classical book picture of vāta in asthi and majjā dhātus. *Asthi* is the bone and *majjā* is the nerve endings in the articular tissue. In most cases of arthritis there is inflammation of the joints causing pain, swelling, and deformity. However, in osteoarthritis there may be pain but no swelling, with slow degenerative changes due to aging. Typically, only one joint is affected, such as a knee, ankle, hip or knuckles joint.

Etiological factors that can result in sandhi gata vāta include occupational overuse and abuse of a joint such as from a strenuous occupation or from vigorous sports such as football or other athletics.

Generally, osteoarthritis with degenerative changes goes together with aging. Note that rheumatoid arthritis is also common around the age of 55 or 60. However, osteoarthritis shows a definite history of trauma.

Ayurveda states that the samprāpti (pathogenesis) of osteoarthritis has its origin in the colon, the seat of vāta dosha. Vāta from the colon undergoes sanchaya (accumulation) and then prakopa (provocation). After the prasara (spreading) stage, the excess vāta deposits within the khavaigunya (defective spaces) in the joints, which may result from previous trauma and occupational use and overuse of the joints. Once in asthi dhātu and majjā dhātu, this produces the various symptoms of sandhi gata vāta.

## Signs and Symptoms of Osteoarthritis

Generally, osteoarthritis is due to excess vāta, whereas rheumatoid arthritis is due to āma. After the age of 55 (vāta stage of life), excess vāta dosha can create dryness in the synovial membrane and the joints begin to crack and pop. That is why osteoarthritis is uncommonly common in elderly people.

There is often a gradual wearing away of cartilage by age 60. The cushion of the intra-articular tissue is decayed because of trauma, causing the articular surfaces of the bone to rub against each other. That causes pain, swelling, stiffness and permanent damage to the joint. This picture is suggestive of inflammatory changes and degenerative changes within the articular tissue.

### Treatment Protocol for Osteoarthritis

Exercise balanced with rest
Snehana (application of oil)
Svedana (application of heat)

To calm down asthi gata vāta, one should give abhyanga (warm oil massage) using mahānārāyana tailam or visha garbha tailam. Mahānārāyana tailam is used for *nirāma vāta* (without āma), while visha garbha tailam is indicated for *sāma vāta* (with āma) conditions. The application of oil penetrates through the skin, the superficial and deep fascia. It can go into the nerve endings, where it helps to reduce the pain.

Then do svedana (sweating therapy) using localized application of heat. These treatments will produce remarkable pain reduction for the patient of osteoarthritis.

Internally, the person should take the following herbal formula:
Ashvagandhā     500 mg (analgesic and nervine tonic)
Yogarāja or maha yogarāja guggulu 300 mg (vyādhi pratyanika specific to osteoarthritis)
Balā             200 mg (dosha pratyanika to pacify vāta )
Tagara           200 mg (analgesic)

What is the difference between maha yogarāja guggulu and yogarāja guggulu? Yogarāja guggulu is given for asthi gata vāta, whereas maha yogarāja guggulu is more penetrating and thus better for majjā gata vāta and degenerative changes. Maha yogarāja guggulu is a powerful medicine that helps to reduce wear and tear of the cartilage. It is more anabolic, so can help to repair damaged tissue.

If a person with osteoarthritis is obese, they have to do a weight reduction program by using the following herbal remedies:
Ārogya vardhini 200 mg
Chandraprabhā  200 mg
Kutki            200 mg
Chitrak          200 mg

These will scrape away excess fatty tissue.

Rest is also important, so as not to do more damage to the joint by excessive activity. So rest, read and relax, and reduce weight if applicable. These measures are all necessary for controlling the pain.

Nowadays people do joint replacement therapy, depending upon the involved joint. I think that in cases of severe damage to the cartilage, individual joint replacement therapy can produce miraculous changes. However, only kapha people can generally handle that surgical intervention. Vāta or pitta people who get joint replacement therapy may end up getting more stiffness and pain. After all, it is a foreign body that is placed in the body, so the person has to take immune suppressant and anti-inflammatory drugs throughout the rest of their life.

Support should be offered to the patient to assist with mobility. Physical therapy, yoga and specific exercises are based upon the person's prakruti and vikruti, and can prevent muscle wasting. Maintenance of correct body weight and posture is also helpful.

Another important line of treatment is to keep the colon clean, so give **gandharva harītakī,** which is harītakī roasted in a cast iron pan with castor oil. Castor oil has anti-arthritic properties, while the harītakī kindles agni, removes āma, and does anulomana. Hence, gandharva harītakī detoxifies the colon, the main site of samprāpti for osteoarthritis.

Half to one teaspoon of gandharva harītakī with warm water at bedtime will calm down vāta from the GI tract, so that any excess vāta from the joints will head back to its home in the large intestine.

Dashamūla tea basti with tagara or gudūchi added, depending upon the symptoms, is also beneficial. Gudūchi acts as a rasāyana, while tagara is analgesic.

For osteoarthritis of the big joints, such as the knee and elbow joints, a ginger and baking soda bath is helpful, preceded by application of mahānārāyana oil around the affected joints.

## Complications

If the patient is not properly treated, osteoarthritis can lead to calcium deposits and a reduction of the joint space. That will result in restrictive movement and deformity.

Generally, osteoarthritis is due to the entry of vāta into the articular tissue. The increased vāta often comes from extra space created from porosity of the bones. So osteoarthritis and osteoporosis frequently go together.

> **GANDHARVA HARITAKI**
>
> To make gandharva harītakī, heat a small amount of castor oil in a cast iron skillet until it begins to bubble. The heat should be medium low.
>
> Then add and stir in enough harītakī to absorb the castor oil.
>
> This ratio will vary from 4 to 8 parts harītakī to 1 part castor oil.
>
> Stir this mixture constantly with a wooden spoon until it is done. This is indicated by the smell being a combination of both ingredients, with a slight roasted quality.
>
> It will look darker than the uncooked harītakī, but not black or burned.

Osteoporosis-induced osteoarthritis is called degenerative arthritis. In such cases, we have to give vitamin D, calcium, magnesium, zinc, and other minerals to support the bones. In degenerative arthritis, the overuse of a joint can lead to a spontaneous medical fracture, so the patient needs to take care.

## Rasāyana Chikitsā

Finally, rasāyana therapy is given. Give 4 teaspoons each of dashamūla arishta and maharasnadi kvātha with an equal quantity of water after lunch and dinner. This will help to maintain optimal nutrition of asthi and majjā dhātus.

# Chapter 31

# Osteoporosis
## Asthi Saushirya

Fall 2017, Volume 30, Number 2

ACCORDING TO AYURVEDIC KNOWLEDGE, the *pākvāshaya* (colon) is the main site of vāta dosha. *Asthi gata vāta* (high vāta in asthi dhātu) is a principle cause of *asthi saushirya* (increased porosity in the bone tissue).

The mucosal layer in the colon is called *purisha dhara kalā*. The colon mucus membrane absorbs minerals that are carried to the periosteum, which is known as *asthi dhara kalā*. It is from there that those minerals nourish the bones; bone tissue is called asthi dhātu.

The immature bone is matured by the process of *asthi agni*. When this bone-building process is hampered, the result is poor nutrition to the bones. As a result, one disease that can occur is osteoporosis, which is known as asthi saushirya. This causes the bone density to become less and less and the person becomes susceptible to a spontaneous medical fracture.

> *Asthi gata vāta (high vāta in asthi dhātu) is a principle cause of asthi saushirya...*

## Etiology of Osteoporosis

Osteoporosis is a relatively common disorder in older age and is characterized by diminished bone density due to malabsorption of minerals. It is an uncommonly common illness in the Western world, where people tend to live a more sedentary life.

Osteoporosis is a disease of the middle-aged and elderly. Anyone can get osteoporosis, but women are more likely to develop this disease. They have lighter bones than men do, and they lose their bone mass rapidly after menopause.

Age is a key factor in osteoporosis. Women of menopausal age and men over age 65 are much more likely to get osteoporosis. That is the age of vāta dosha and osteoporosis is a vāta disorder. So the vāta phase of life is one of the causative factors of osteoporosis.

. . . . . . . . . . . . . . . . . . . . . . . . . . . . . . . . . . . . . . . . . . . . .

Application of mahānārāyana oil on the skin over the long bones can be very helpful. This medicated oil penetrates into the asthi dhātu and helps to pacify vāta dosha. Kati prushtha basti with mahānārāyana oil is also effective...

. . . . . . . . . . . . . . . . . . . . . . . . . . . . . . . . . . . . . . . . . . . . .

**THE RISK FACTORS OF OSTEOPOROSIS**

Advanced age

Female at menopausal age

Of white or Asian descent

Thin, small body frame (vāta type)

Genetic predisposition; definitive family history of osteoporosis

Low calcium intake

Sedentary lifestyle

Excessive consumption of alcohol or caffeine

Prolonged history of smoking

Nulliparity (a woman who has never given birth or never had a pregnancy beyond 20 weeks)

High protein intake

Excessive phosphate intake

Long-term usage of glucocorticoids, phenytoin, thyroid medication and certain other medical drugs

Endocrine disease, such as hyperthyroidism

Cushing syndrome (hypercortisolism)

Acromegaly

Hypogonadism

Hyperparathyroidism

Osteoporosis often results from reduced levels of the female hormone estrogen, which is responsible for maintaining calcium metabolism of the musculoskeletal system. During the postmenopausal age, which is after the cessation of the menstrual cycle, the body's production of estrogen is reduced and that function is hampered. That may lead to osteoporosis. Almost one third of women over the age 60 are prone to developing osteoporosis.

Ārtava dhātu is the female reproductive tissue. Estrogen is a manifestation of ārtava agni and ārtava agni stimulates asthi dhātu agni (the digestive power in the bones) to utilize calcium and other minerals and thereby nourish the bones. When a woman goes through menopause, estrogen is depleted, so that affects the asthi dhātu agni. This is an Ayurvedic interpretation and it explains why we may have to support asthi dhātu agni by giving estrogen.

In the case of men, the male sex hormone testosterone is also a source of estrogen in the body; it is converted into estrogen in the fat cells. Even at the age 80, men can have enough testosterone that they are less likely to have osteoporosis compared to women of the same age.

Osteoporosis is more likely to affect white people and Asian women and men, and less so African-American people. The reasons for this are not entirely known. In addition, women with a thin body frame, especially those with fair skin, run a higher risk of osteoporosis than women with a larger body frame. These slender women have a predominance of vāta dosha in their prakruti and are more likely to have a greater bone loss.

People who are physically inactive, either by choice, by profession, or by confinement due to illness, are more susceptible to osteoporosis. Osteoporosis can also occur as a result of other medical conditions that result in the surgical removal of both ovaries (oophorectomy), at which point there is no longer any estrogen production.

Chronic arthritis, which is inflammation of the joints, may also lead to osteoporosis. In that condition, there is long lingering vāta dosha in the bony structure. By nature, vāta is dry, light, and cold. Those qualities can lead to depletion of the bone tissue.

A diet that is deficient in nutrients such as calcium, magnesium, zinc and other essential minerals may result in osteoporosis. Osteoporosis is also more common in places where there is less sunlight, such as Seattle, Washington or Ireland. There may not be enough sunlight to produce sufficient vitamin D under the skin. Also, in Australia, New Zealand and parts of South America people avoid the sun because there is so much ultraviolet light from the sun, that it causes higher instances of skin cancer. After many years of avoiding the sun, those people don't absorb enough vitamin D and are more likely to get osteoporosis.

Finally, people who drink heavily, smoke, or take steroid therapy are much more likely to get osteoporosis. This is particularly the case for post-menopausal, white women who smoke and drink heavily.

## Signs and Symptoms of Osteoporosis

Depending upon the strength of the bone tissue, osteoporosis may initially cause no symptoms or it can result in extreme pain. If there is pain, it is most commonly in the lower back area. The disease is not life threatening, but it may lead to a fracture. That can cause deterioration of the intervertebral disc so that the person's height is reduced.

When there is progressive bone loss, it may result in fracture, loss of mobility, disability, hair loss, brittle nails that easily break, deformities of the skeleton, such as kyphosis or dowager hump, weight loss, vertebral compression, and fracture of the vertebrae.

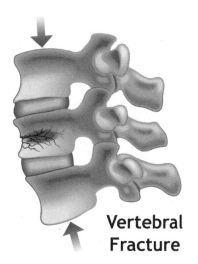
**Vertebral Fracture**

Sudden backache can be caused by a fracture of a spinal vertebra. The pain from the fracture itself may subside, but discomfort from the osteoporosis can continue. Pain in the bones from osteoporosis is due to weakness of the bones and vertebrae. Because of this pain, people don't walk or do other exercise, and the osteoporosis becomes worse as a result. Hence, various cycles develop where pain leads to inactivity and inactivity further encourages the osteoporosis.

Generally, osteoporosis progresses along the spinal column. It can eventually decrease the person's height by several inches, or the spine may become curved, with scoliosis, kyphosis or hump. These are signs of advanced osteoporosis, the result of compression fractures of weakened vertebrae. These spinal deformities can be exacerbated by the restrictive movement of the bones that happens in osteoporosis.

In Ayurveda, the *mala* (waste by-product) of asthi dhātu is *nakha* (nails) and *kesha* (hair). So when a person's hair becomes brittle and easily breaks, or the individual starts losing their hair, it can be an early sign of weak asthi dhātu. Similarly, if the person gets ridges and white spots on his or her fingernails, that is also a sign of depleted asthi dhātu and a deficiency of magnesium, calcium or zinc. Teeth are an upadhātu (superior by-product) of asthi and with osteoporosis the person can have receding gums, fractured dental enamel and cavities in the teeth.

### Diagnosis of Osteoporosis

Often osteoporosis progresses undetected until the bone is fractured and x-rays are taken. At that time, the physician may notice the thinning of the bones on the x-ray. Nowadays, it is more common to do a bone density test, which is an important diagnostic tool to find out about osteoporosis. In Ayurveda, we can use pulse diagnosis to assess the strength of asthi dhātu, and also assess the hair and nails.

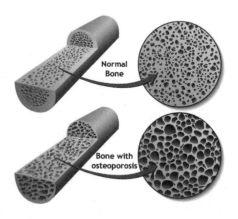

Osteopenia is an early sign of osteoporosis. Osteopenia means a significant decrease in bone mineral density as well as a diminished number of bone cells (osteoblasts) in the blood plasma. People who are prone to osteoporosis or have any of the risk factors listed should get a bone density test done after age 55.

## Management of Osteoporosis

A major part of the treatment protocol for osteoporosis is a gentle weight-bearing exercise program. That will help to strengthen the muscles and thereby support the weakened bones. Swimming, cycling, walking, jogging, power walking, dancing, climbing stairs, and non-jarring aerobic exercise (cardiovascular exercise without jumping) are all good for bones. If you have already had a fracture or you are overweight, then walking in chest-deep water for 30 minutes will be a particularly good form of exercise to strengthen the bones.

To compliment cardio exercise or water walking, do some easy muscle-stretching exercises in a chair or on the floor. One good exercise is back extensions. To do these, lie on the floor on your

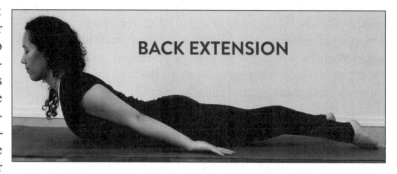

**BACK EXTENSION**

stomach with your arms at your sides. Raise the upper part of your body a few inches off the floor. Use only your back muscles to lift up, not your arms. This is a great exercise to strengthen the spine.

To protect the bones in the spinal column, one should do gentle weightlifting, but avoid heavy weightlifting or vigorous exercise, because that increases the chance of bone fracture. For advanced cases, a back brace or back support can help.

Exercise must be tailored according to the specific individual. Some people with osteoporosis need to use crutches or a walker to assist their walking, so their exercise regimen will be very different from someone who can walk and run unaided.

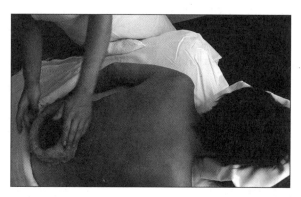

Application of mahānārāyana oil on the skin over the long bones can be very helpful. This medicated oil penetrates into the asthi dhātu and helps to pacify vāta dosha. *Kati prushtha basti* with mahānārāyana oil is also effective. This is done by having the patient lie face down and applying warm mahānārāyana oil. The illustration shows kati basti; kati prushtha basti is higher up the back along the thoracic area.

At one time, women who had reached menopause were helped with estrogen replacement therapy. They were prescribed conjugated estrogen[46] by their medical doctor.[47] An alternative is to take evening primrose oil (500 mg once daily), which supplies a natural estrogen precursor. This gives sufficient estrogen and progesterone to the woman to prevent bone loss. In some cases, women may be prescribed the male hormone testosterone, which can also stimulate the growth of the bones. However, a side effect of this treatment is the development of facial hair, with moustache and beard.

We should give osteoporosis patients a balanced diet, rich in vitamins and minerals, particularly calcium and vitamin D. Ayurveda suggests foods such as milk, yogurt, cottage cheese, coconut, carrots, radish, sesame seeds, and sunflower seeds. The person should use mineral rock salt, because table salt, especially in large amounts, can result in calcium being excreted from the bones.

We usually give a calcium supplement, with something like 1,000 mg per day, or at the menopausal age, you can even use 1,200–1,500 mg per day. It is important also to improve the absorption of minerals into the body. Calcium carbonate is a good source for absorption of calcium. Supplemental calcium and regular exercise help to boost the bones and reduce the rate of bone loss.

However, bones are not made from calcium alone. They contain many other minerals too, so magnesium, zinc, boron, copper and other minerals and trace minerals should be taken on a regular basis. Additionally, ensure the person receives sufficient exposure to the sunlight to get a good level of naturally-sourced vitamin D.

---

46. Brand name is Premarin®.
47. Hormone therapy is now considered controversial because of the risks of increased breast cancer, strokes, blood clots, and cardiovascular disease.

Consider giving a vitamin D supplement, perhaps 400 international units per day, taken 200 IU twice daily. A cup of warm milk contains calcium and in the USA, a cup of fortified milk contains about 100 IU of vitamin D. This traditional Ayurvedic remedy can be taken nightly before bedtime.

*Yogāsana* can be an important part of the therapeutic management of osteoporosis. Beneficial *āsana* for most people with this condition include gentle, slow sūrya namaskāra with deep breathing, along with *ustrāsana* (camel), *bhujangāsana* (cobra), *gomukhāsana* (cow), *paripūrna nāvāsana* (full boat), *dhanurāsana* (bow), *setu bandha sarvāngāsana* (bridge), *salabhāsana* (locust), *padmāsana* (lotus) and *simhāsana* (lion) poses. These are all good for strengthening the muscles and supporting the bone tissue. (see yoga poses page 450)

If you are taking ongoing steroid therapy and you start to develop osteoporosis, you may wish to go to the doctor and request to reduce the dose, because steroids affect the thyroid gland and that can create or worsen osteoporosis.

Man is as old as his bones. According to Sushruta, author of ancient Ayurvedic texts, even though a man dies, still his bones remain. So take care of your bones. Emphasis should be placed on prevention of bone loss through a healthy diet, use of calcium and Vitamin D, and gentle weight bearing exercise. High impact aerobic exercise may create too much stress on the bones of elderly people, so that should be avoided after middle age.

## Ayurvedic Herbal Protocol to Support the Bones

Take this mixture, 1/2 teaspoon, three times daily with an anupāna of warm milk. Additionally, take one teaspoon of triphala at night.

| | |
|---|---|
| Dashamūla | 500 mg |
| Ashvagandhā | 400 mg |
| Balā | 300 mg |
| Praval pañchāmrit | 200 mg |
| Kama dudhā | 200 mg |

The person can also chew a handful of sesame seeds each day. One tablespoon of sesame seeds contains 88 mg of calcium.

Chapter 32

# Headache
## Shirah Shula

Summer 1998, Volume 11, Number 1

AYURVEDIC ANATOMY DIVIDES the body into six parts: the head, trunk and four extremities. *Shira* means head, *shākhā* means extremity, and *madhyama* means the trunk. The head is also called *uttamānga*. *Uttama* means noble or great, while *anga* means a part of the body. The greatest part of the body is the head, because a person is identified by it: if the head is covered, we don't know who the person is.

The head is the seat of the four of the five doors of perception: eyes, ears, nose, tongue, and mouth. It is also the seat of the brain and it is connected to the trunk by the spinal vertebrae. The head and the face together express emotions and most of the srotāmsi (bodily channels), are related to the head.

## Types of Headaches

Shira shūla means headache and it is a complex disorder. Ayurveda classifies shira shūla according to the dosha involved: vāta, pitta, or kapha type. Although headaches are quite common, this disorder can be distressing and may have serious significations. A headache is also classified according to whether it relates to majjā or asthi dhātu (nervous or bone tissues) and is considered to be a disorder of mano vaha srotas, the pathway of the mind. The gastrointestinal and respiratory tracts may also be involved.

*Doshic Headache.* The three doshic types of headache are discerned by the nature and structure of the pain. A vāta headache is throbbing, shooting, and vague. It comes during the vāta times of day, which are dawn and dusk, and it is more common during fall (vāta season). A vāta headache is associated with constipation, indigestion, and abdominal discomfort. It is usually present in the occipital area at the base of the skull. Muscular pain in the neck and misalignment of the cervical spine can also cause an occipital headache. Stagnation of chronic āma in the colon is another cause, and traumatic accident and injury, such as whiplash or cerebral concussion, can also create a vāta type of headache. A vāta headache may also be due to too much exercise or insufficient sleep, or even a change in one's pillow or bed.

A pitta type of headache is due to excessive exposure to sunlight. It is usually located in the temporal area and is usually caused by hyper-acidity and acid indigestion. A pitta headache is associated with nausea, so vomiting can relieve that type of pain. The pain of a pitta headache is intense, sharp and penetrating and it makes the person irritable. This type of headache is more common during midday and midnight and during the summer season.

A kapha headache is slow, dull, and aching. It is located in the front of the head. It may be associated with kapha type of allergies, a cold, or congestion. A kapha headache often occurs during kapha times, which are mid-morning and mid-evening as well as spring season. Gravity plays an important role in a kapha headache. If you bend down, the headache is more intense.

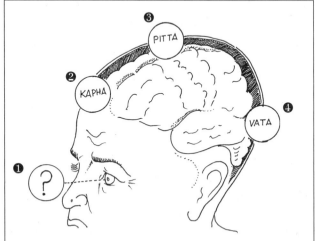

**❶ OBSERVATION of difficult situation or unpleasant sight.**
**❷ KAPHA aggravation has tamasic quality and can lead to sinus congestion.**
**❸ PITTA aggravation has excess sattva, producing acid indigestion or righteous indignation.**
**❹ VĀTA aggravation has rajasic quality and can generate anxiety or constipation.**

### Emotional Headache.

Emotional headaches are often located in the frontal areas of the head: the superior, middle and inferior frontal gyrus. Vāta emotions, such as fear, anxiety, and insecurity create a headache in the superior frontal gyrus. The middle frontal gyrus area is related to pitta and associated with anger, hate, envy, judgment, and intense stress. Pain in the inferior frontal gyrus is related to kapha and associated with depression, attachment, greed, and possessiveness.

**Pathological Headache.** The central top of the head is called the vertex. When this area is aching, it might be due to high blood pressure, cerebral vascular accident, or a space-occupying tumor of the pineal or pituitary gland.

**Referred Headache.** A referred headache may be due to a tooth or gum infection. This type of headache will go from the cheeks to the temple to the parietal area. Trigeminal neuralgia is a typical pain along the track of the trigeminal nerve. It also goes from the cheeks to the temple to the parietal area. Rhinitis or an infection in the throat, nose, or tonsils can also create a headache in the parietal area. A person who has influenza and fever may get a bitemporal headache.

**Allergy and Chemical Toxicity and Sensitivity.** Exposure to toxic chemical substances, such as insecticides or disinfectants, or even to certain pollens, may produce a pitta headache. Foul air, poor ventilation, carbon monoxide poisoning and some drugs, including tobacco and alcohol, can also create a headache. Some people are sensitive to wine, chocolate, or hard cheeses and these substances may cause a headache.

*Eye Problems.* Increased intraocular pressure, which is associated with glaucoma, and refractory errors may result in an intraorbital headache. Toxins in the liver (rañjaka pitta) can disturb allochaka pitta in the eyes and create photosensitivity and pain when the eyes are moving. This kind of headache falls under the pitta category.

*Ear Infection.* Ear infection and mastoiditis can create both temporal and parietal headaches.

*Osteoporosis.* Asthi dhātu is a seat of vāta dosha. When vāta is increased and asthi dhātu is decreased, this leads to osteoporosis, which may be responsible for ringing in the ears. This is a vāta disorder and can cause headaches in the supramastoidal area.

*Metabolic Disorders.* Headaches can also be produced by poor digestion, absorption and assimilation. These may be due to a deficiency of $B_{12}$ or other vitamins or minerals, such as calcium, magnesium, and zinc, which will create changes in the plates of the skull and cause muscle stiffness, creating a headache. Metabolic disorders that can induce headaches also include hypoglycemia or hyperglycemia, sprue syndrome (chronic malabsorption), and obesity.

*Systemic Headache.* When there is a dysfunction in a srotas or system, it can create a headache. Nephritis, uremia, biliary tract disease, liver diseases such as hepatitis, rheumatism, diabetes, and severe anemia are systemic conditions that are all connected to mūtra vaha srotas (the urinary channel). Gastrointestinal tract disorders include hyper-acidity, pyloric stenosis, chronic constipation, acidosis, and alkalinosis. These conditions are associated with anna vaha srotas (the food channel) and are due to metabolic disorders of the digestive fire. Cardiovascular disease, such as congestive heart failure, myocardial infarction and edema, may increase pressure in the vascular system and cause a headache, while endocrine and pituitary tumors can create increased intracranial pressure. Hormonal dysfunction, leading to amenorrhea, polycystic ovary, increased prolactin secretions and pituitary adenoma, can also create headaches.

*Migraine Headache.* A migraine headache is caused by vāta pushing pitta in the hematopoietic system. This imbalance is responsible for disorders of the cranial blood vessels. It will create either artitis (inflammation of the arteries) or dilation of the carotid artery, along with visible pulsations in the temporal artery, leading to a migraine. There is alternation of the pain of a migraine headache. It often intensifies during pitta time (10 to 2 AM and PM) and then gradually subsides. Migraine headaches can create pitta type of depression, which can be serious. This kind of headache is also quite common in meningeal diseases, encephalitis, arteriosclerosis, and intracranial vascular disease.

*Miscellaneous Causes of Headache.* Headache may be due to fatigue, exhaustion, sunstroke, misalignment of the spine, prolonged strain of the neck muscles, or even cerebral metastasis of cancer. Withdrawal from any addictive substance, histamine toxicity, carbon dioxide retention, hypertensive encephalopathy, meningeal irritation or a history of posterior cranial fossa fracture can also create a headache. Headaches may also be due to a local skull lesion and the involvement of the trigeminal, glossopharyngeal, and vagus cranial nerves; the fifth, ninth, and tenth respectively.

***Sattva, Rajas, and Tamas.*** Intense sattva is characterized by righteous indignation and being unnecessarily discriminatory, judgmental, and fanatical. This can lead to temporal headache and is best treated with tagara. Rajas makes the mind hyperactive and nervous, inducing insomnia and leading to occipital headaches. Shankha pushpī will help in this condition. Overindulgence in tamasic activities, such as eating meat, sleeping for several hours during the day, and having a dull and monotonous lifestyle, can all create a sinus headache. The best remedy in this case is the herb brahmī.

## Management of Headaches

With such a vast picture of headaches, one must find the underlying causes and then treat accordingly. During an attack, use essential oils, pastes, nasya, and marma point therapy to alleviate the pain. Then follow up with more long-term management, using the herbs and procedures suggested in "Doshic Management of Headaches" on page 273.

***Essential Oils and Pastes.*** For a vāta headache, gently apply nutmeg paste or oil to the temples and frontal area. Hina, musk, cinnamon, garlic, and sesame oils are also effective.

For pitta, apply sandalwood paste or oil to the site of the pain. Jatamāmsi, jasmine, khus. and coconut oils are helpful as well.

For kapha, apply ginger or vacha paste. Camphor, eucalyptus, clove, cinnamon, or cardamom oils can also help to relieve kapha headache.

***Nasya.*** For vāta, use plain ghee or Sidha Soma® oil. For pitta, use brahmī ghee. For kapha, use vacha oil or dry vacha powder.

***Marma.*** Apply the appropriate oil according to the doshic disorder to the marma points shown in the illustration at right. Other points for headache

**GUIDELINES FOR LEARNING THE SOURCE OF HEADACHES**

Temporal headache — TMJ, migraine, hyperacidity and cerebral vascular accident.

Facial pain — dental infection, nerve involvement and electrical pain.

Instant onset of pain may be due to ruptured aneurysm and is a severe condition.

Cluster headache — peaks over three to five minutes, migraine.

Pain during lifting heavy load or coughing or sneezing may be due to fractured posterial cranial fossa or skull injury.

Accentuation of pain by environment. If pain is increased by head bending back or from side to side, it may be due to meningitis, which is serious.

Pain during ovulation — PMS, hormonal imbalance.

Pressure headache: increased intracranial tension, consider a tumor. This headache wakes the person at midnight.

Local pain and tenderness — frontal and paranasal sinusitis.

When the person sleeps with no pain, but gets a headache the moment he wakens, that is emotional.

When headache is increased by movement of the eyeball, there is involvement of the meninges, which may lead to meningitis.

include *Ūrdhva Skandha* (mid-point along top of shoulders, between neck and arm) and *Hasta Kshipra* and *Pāda Kshipra*.[48]

*Yoga.* Someone with a headache should not do inverted yoga poses. Simple āsanas, such as camel, cobra, cow, boat, bow, bridge, and spinal twist are helpful, as is ujjāyi prānāyāma. Empty Bowl meditation is also effective. (see yoga poses page 450)

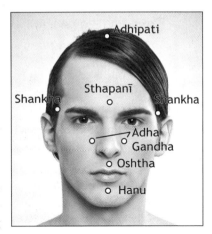

*Diet.* If headaches are caused by food allergies, one should generally avoid sour foods, peanuts, mushrooms, tomatoes, cheese, chocolate, fermented foods, and leftover food.

If the cause of the headache is emotional, try to resolve the issues triggering the headache. Use meditation and non-judgmental watchfulness. Counseling may also be useful in helping to determine the root cause.

One should be aware of the time when the headache is present and its relationship to food, emotions, and environmental or emotional stress. These simple Ayurvedic recipes, although not a quick fix, will eradicate the doshic cause and make the person's life free from headache. One should always consult with experts and have proper medical treatment if the problem persists.

## Doshic Management of Headaches

The herbal treatments that follow are for simple conditions. Other conditions we have mentioned, such as tumors or aneurysm, are more serious and require medical intervention.

| FOR VĀTA HEADACHES | FOR PITTA HEADACHES |
|---|---|
| 1) Use ½ teaspoon of the following mixture three times a day (TID) after food, with warm water: | 1) Use ½ teaspoon of the following mixture TID after food, with warm water: |
| Dashamūla 500 mg<br>Ashvagandhā 400 mg<br>Balā 300 mg<br>Tagara 200 mg | Shatāvarī 500 mg<br>Gulvel Sattva 400 mg<br>Shanka Bhasma 200 mg<br>Kāma Dudhā 200 mg |
| 2) Take 1 teaspoon of harītakī an hour before sleep, with warm water. | 2) Take 1 teaspoon of āmalakī an hour before sleep, with warm water. |
| 3) Massage neck and shoulders with Mahānārāyana Oil. | 3) Massage with coconut oil at the site of pain. |

---

48. Illustrations shown in the appendix on page 456.

## FOR KAPHA HEADACHES

1) Use ½ teaspoon of the following mixture TID after food, with warm water:

| | |
|---|---|
| Sitopalādi | 500 mg |
| Mahāsudarshan | 300 mg |
| Trikatu | 200 mg |
| Abrak Bhasma | 200 mg |

2) Take 1 teaspoon of bibhītakī an hour before sleep, with warm water.

3) Massage with eucalyptus oil or Tiger Balm® at the site of pain.

## FOR HEADACHES CAUSED BY ALLERGIES

Use bee pollen, which helps build immunity.

## FOR TOOTHACHE

Apply clove oil to the affected tooth, or swish warm sesame oil in the mouth.

## FOR TONSILLITIS OR SORE THROAT

1) Use ½ teaspoon of the following mixture TID after food, with warm water:

| | |
|---|---|
| Tālisādi | 500 mg |
| Mahāsudarshan | 400 mg |
| Tikta | 200 mg |
| Goldenseal | 200 mg |

2) Gargle with salt and turmeric at bedtime and in the morning.

## FOR EAR INFECTION

1) Use ½ teaspoon of the following mixture TID after food:

| | |
|---|---|
| Goldenseal | 200 mg |
| Echinacea | 200 mg |
| Osha | 200 mg |
| Turmeric | 300 mg |
| Neem | 300 mg |

If ear infection persists, see your doctor.

## FOR EMOTIONAL HEADACHES

Use ½ teaspoon of the following mixture TID after food:

| | |
|---|---|
| Jatamāmsi | 300 mg |
| Brahmī | 300 mg |
| Shankha Pushpī | 300 mg |

## FOR SUNSTROKE

1) Rub Bhringarāja Oil® onto the soles of the feet and the scalp at bedtime.

2) Use Brahmī Ghee® nasya, five drops in each nostril, twice daily.

3) Take sarasvatī, ½ teaspoon TID with water.

4) Avoid the sun.

## FOR EYE PROBLEMS

1) Use ½ teaspoon of the following mixture TID after food:

| | |
|---|---|
| Punarnavā | 500 mg |
| Brahmī | 300 mg |
| Jatamāmsi | 300 mg |

2) Put 1 drop of castor oil in each eye at bedtime.

3) Rub soles of feet with castor oil at night.

## FOR MIGRAINES FROM VĀTA PUSHING PITTA IN MAJJĀ DHĀTU

1) Use ½ teaspoon of the following mixture TID after food:

| | |
|---|---|
| Ashvagandhā | 500 mg |
| Gudūchī | 400 mg |
| Jatamāmsi | 300 mg |
| Tagara | 300 mg |

2) Use Brahmī Ghee® nasya, five drops in each nostril, twice daily.

3) Have an early breakfast. Then an hour after breakfast, eat a banana with one teaspoon of ghee, a pinch of cardamom and half a teaspoon of sugar.

Chapter 33

# Migraine Headaches
## An Ayurvedic Perspective

Summer 1991, Volume 3, Number 1

MIGRAINE HEADACHES FALL into one of three categories: vāta, pitta, or kapha type. Kapha headaches are congestive and, strictly speaking, do not fall in the category of migraine. Vāta types of migraine headaches are more common at vāta time, which is 2 to 6 AM and PM, or pre-dawn and dusk. A vāta-increasing diet and incompatible food combinations such as milk with yogurt, bananas, or fish aggravate vāta migraines. Such headaches commonly occur on the left side of the head and are associated with light-headedness, constipation, gas, and tightness in the neck and shoulder area.

Pitta type of migraine headaches is associated with the sun. The moment the sun rises, with its heat and light, the headache starts. When the sun moves to its zenith at noon the headache is greatest, and at sunset the headache subsides. This type of headache is commonly on the right side and is sometimes diagnosed as sinusitis. Associated symptoms may include nausea, vomiting, heartburn, and sensitivity to light.

Kapha type headaches are due congestion in the system. The pain of this type of headache usually increases when the person bends over, while a more upright posture is found to relieve this pain.

To remedy vāta-type migraines, it is necessary to follow a vāta-pacifying diet. Basti (enema) is also indicated. In this case, five ounces of warm sesame oil, followed by one pint of strained dashamūla tea, is injected into the rectum and retained for thirty minutes, before being expelled. Then apply warm oil and heat to the temporal area of the forehead. Finally, nasya (nasal administration) of vacha, balā, or ashvagandhā oil is usually effective.

To deal with a pitta migraine, use virechana (purgation therapy). For this, ½ to 1 teaspoon of triphalā should be given at night with warm water. It is also important to follow a pitta-pacifying diet, with no sour food, citrus fruits, or acid-producing foods. Nasya is also good for pitta migraines. The best substances are brahmī or jatamāmsi ghee or even plain ghee.

Kapha headaches respond well to vamana (therapeutic vomiting). First apply warm sesame oil to the chest and back, and then drink a cup of licorice tea. Next, rub the tongue to stimulate the gag reflex. The resultant vomiting helps to relieve congestion from the chest, bronchi, lymphatics, and sinuses. Nasya is effective here too, using vacha powder or a combination of vacha, brahmī, and jatamāmsi. This will help to improve clarity of perception and relieve the congestion associated with a kapha type of headache.

During the period of most intense pain for vāta and kapha headaches, take one teaspoon of ginger powder, make it into a paste using warm water and apply it to the forehead. Kapha headaches can also be relieved by applying a paste made from calamus root powder (vacha). For intense pitta headaches, make a paste of sandalwood powder and apply this to the forehead.

Super Nasya Oil® is a nasya that contains sandalwood, eucalyptus, rose, and basil oils. Even when it is uncertain which dosha is causing the migraine, this balanced nasya oil is frequently effective. Administration consists of three to five drops in each nostril, followed by vigorous sniffing.

Gemstones can be of some help in relieving headaches. They work principally on the astral level and the electromagnetic field of the physical body. For pitta type of migraine, a red coral necklace with a pearl at the center can be effective. A pearl necklace is also excellent. Vāta headaches may be reduced by the use of pink or blue quartz, whereas a darker quartz or medium quality ruby, both of which are heating, is indicated for kapha headaches. Rudrāksha is effective for vāta and kapha headaches. Soak the rudrāksha beads in a cup of water overnight and in the morning drink the water. This will help to relieve an emotional migraine. During the pre-menopausal period, hormonal changes in a woman may create a migraine. Rudrāksha water is also useful in this case, as is wearing tulsi beads.

According to Ayurveda, there is no disorder without disturbance of the doshas. Hence, by balancing these energetic elements, the body can maintain a state of health.

Chapter 34

# Parkinson's Disease
## Vepathu or Kampa Vāta

Spring 1997, Volume 9, Number 4

PARKINSON'S DISEASE IS a condition of disturbed systemic vāta dosha, which has gone into majjā dhātu (the nervous system.) Ayurvedic literature contains a complete description, etiology, symptomatology, pathology, and management of this condition, which is called *vepathu* or *kampa vāta. Kampa* means tremors. *Vepathu* means 'to go out of track' and it comes from the Sanskrit word *pātthā,* meaning passage.

James Parkinson, a British physician (1755-1824), studied vepathu and discovered where the pathological lesion takes place. Centuries before Dr. Parkinson's work, Ayurvedic literature described this disease in exactly the same way as Dr. Parkinson and called it kampa vāta. There is currently no satisfactory treatment for Parkinson's disease in western medicine. This article will present the views of both modern science and Ayurveda as they pertain to Parkinson's, in order to provide a complete picture for the reader.

Old medical books describe Parkinson's disease as paralysis agitans or shaking palsy. These names suggest neurological agitation. Ayurveda says that psychologically, the person with Parkinson's tends to be controlling or aggressive. When such a person loses control over a situation, majjā dhātu (the nervous system) becomes tense and performs under stress.

The initial and most debilitating physical feature of Parkinson's disease is absent or slowed movement. This poverty of movement results in the classic, masked-face appearance of a Parkinson's patient. Cogwheel rigidity may accompany this and the Parkinson's tremor is usually the most conspicuous feature of the illness. The tremor has a regular rate and primarily involves the hands and feet. Because the tremor is most evident when the person sits quietly with arms supported, it is called a resting tremor.

Patients of Parkinson's disease often lose their postural reflexes, which are the compensatory mechanisms that alter muscle tone in response to a change in position. This reflex loss, in combination with slowed movement and rigidity, results in a gait impairment characterized by shuffling, short steps and a tendency for the gait to accelerate in an attempt to catch the center of gravity. In addition, the voices of these people often become tremulous and low in volume, lacking normal fluctuations in pitch. Their handwriting also becomes small and tremulous.

As this illness progresses with the patient's age, dementia is a common complication. In addition, some people exhibit psychotic thought and behavior, manifesting as visual hallucinations, delusions, and chronic confusion. The sleep-wake cycle becomes disturbed and depression is also common.

## An Ayurvedic Understanding

How does Ayurveda describe this condition? A khavaigunya (defective space) is present within the area of the basal ganglia, which is in the deep core of majjā dhātu. Vāta dosha from the colon undergoes sanchaya (accumulation), prakopa (aggravation), and prasara (spread) and then in the fourth stage of disease—sthana samsraya (localization)—it lodges in this defective space in the basal ganglia. Vāta, because of its subtle quality, enters the extrapyramidal system and inhibits its functioning, affecting the person's coordination, gait, balance, and maintenance of posture. Prāna vāta, which works with sādhaka pitta in the cerebral cortex and tarpaka kapha through the basal ganglia, has an important function in coordination. Coordination is synchronization between prāna and apāna subtypes, with prāna providing sensory input and apāna providing motor function.

Classically, Parkinson's is found in a pitta-predominant person; a powerful person who has hundreds of people working under him or her, who is controlling and then loses that control. Loss of control creates fear, which causes a desire for control. They go together. A person who is pitta-predominant and vāta secondary is most vulnerable. One in every thousand of the population is particularly prone to Parkinson's disease and I have seen hundreds of Parkinson's patients in India. These pitta people have an overpowering and controlling nature, and they always come from the space of confidence, courage, and aggressiveness. Then suddenly they lose something of value, such as a job, and they feel they have lost control. Or there may be some vatagenic factors, such as age. From 55 onward, the person is in the age of vāta and is more prone to Parkinson's. Divorce may also be the precipitating factor. In the first 25 years of marriage, there may have been a good relationship with understanding, sharing, and caring. Then suddenly a mid-life crisis may lead to divorce. A combination of stresses creates a vāta derangement and increased vāta dosha enters into the majjā dhātu, creating movement disturbances and involuntary movements, along with a lack of coordination, rigidity and tremors.

The defective space in the basal ganglia mentioned above is the cause of the Parkinson's lesion. The nuclei are affected and the nucleus itself contains sādhaka pitta. Between two nuclei, the communicating system is affected, which is tarpaka kapha. The neurotransmitter dopamine becomes deficient. Neurotransmitters are the product of sādhaka pitta, which manifests as tryptophan, serotonin, acetylcholine, melatonin, and dopamine. In Parkinson's, there is a deficiency of dopamine, as if sādhaka pitta is unable to perform its function because it is dried out by the excess vāta.

Paralysis agitans also results from a slow viral infection present in other conditions. Many times Parkinsonism comes as a complication of encephalitis, which is a pitta-related disease. In general, encephalitis, which is viral, creates a khavaigunya (defective space) in majjā dhātu. Later, at the age of 55 or 60, in combination with other etiological factors, vāta undergoes sanchaya, prakopa, prasara, and then sthana samsraya (deposition) takes place in the basal ganglia. In that way, encephalitis can lead to Parkinson's disease.

The presence of a brain tumor is another causative factor for Parkinson's. A tumor that is either lodged within the extrapyramidal system or in the meninges (meningioma) can be the innermost cause in this type of Parkinsonism, where vāta is pushing kapha.

Venereal disease—gonorrhea and syphilis—can also be a factor. If not properly treated, the syphilitic bacilli move through the blood and can create a meningovascular syphilitic lesion. This type of lesion creating Parkinson's is from vāta pushing pitta.

Looking at these modern concepts with an Ayurvedic interpretation can give great insight. We have seen that psychological causes are important to consider. A person with pitta-predominant and vāta secondary who tends to be aggressive, competitive, successful, and a workaholic can suffer a shock if he or she suddenly loses a job. Similarly, if a person who is quite dominating has a relationship break up during a mid-life crisis, that creates trauma and fear and can affect majjā dhātu. Depression can also be a precipitating cause.

Drug poisoning can also create kampa vāta. Drugs such as LSD, amphetamines, or marijuana affect the nervous system. Copper and lead poisoning is another possible factor, as is exposure to pesticides. Copper, manganese, lead, and carbon monoxide poisoning should also be considered. Carbon monoxide affects the brain, especially the extrapyramidal system, and a person can get Parkinson's from over-exposure to carbon monoxide.

The etiology of Parkinson's involves systemic imbalanced vāta and chronic āma, toxins, circulating in the body. Vāta and āma move throughout the body in the circulatory systems and then go into the rasa, rakta, māmsa, meda, asthi, and majjā dhātus. In majjā dhātu, vāta may push pitta or vāta may push kapha. If vāta pushes kapha, it can create a tumor in the extrapyramidal system of the brain, resulting in Parkinson's disease. If vāta pushes pitta, it may create a syphilitic meningovascular lesion within this area, which can also lead to Parkinsonism.

Within the fifth decade of life, between 50 and 60, the person becomes more prone to vāta disorders. Vāta may enter majjā dhātu by its subtle, dry, and rough qualities and create depigmentation and atrophy of the globus pallidus in the brain, which is involved with muscle movements and motor control. This may lead to depleted majjā dhātu and affect the coordination between prāna and apāna, thus creating tremors.

Generally, the patient comes to the practitioner because of tremors, and many conditions can create tremors. One must take a history and find out if the person has a great deal of anxiety, insecurity, or fear, which can all create tremors. Also, if the person has a toxic thyroid goiter, that will create tremors. Tremors are also present in an alcoholic patient, so one must ask about a history of alcoholism.

However, Parkinson's tremors have certain characteristics. They show up in the hand as fine tremors. If you place a piece of paper on the back of the person's outstretched hand, the tremors become visible. The Parkinson's patient has typically slow, rhythmic tremors, especially noticeable on the thumb. Then the tremors from the thumb move to the proximal parts of the extremity, moving to the wrist and then to the elbow.

In the earlier stages, vāta is mobile and irregular. Because of these qualities, the tremors are more accentuated by stress and embarrassment, although lessened during activity. Yet there is also rigidity, which means tremors with increased tone. Tone is a sustained state of contraction that is maintained by prāna and apāna vāyus and coordinated at the spinal cord through the reflex arc. In kampa vāta, tremors are associated with rigidity and jerky sensations and gradually the fine tremors become more coarse. Flexion of the neck, elbow or knee is also a problem and the patient walks in short steps, as if walking downhill. Because of the tremors, most skillful actions are affected. The patient's handwriting becomes disturbed, he or she cannot thread a needle, and even fastening a button becomes challenging. Turning over in bed or rising from a chair is difficult, as if the person becomes like a statue.

In the classic picture of the Parkinson's patient, there is loss of the normal swinging of the arms while walking. The person walks with small steps, as though walking downhill. The face is without expression and even the eyes blink slowly and are without expression. Speech is slurred and talk is heavy and monotonous. The person's body becomes stiff and the gait looks like a statue walking. Ankles and knees are flexed; elbows and wrists are flexed, with the fingers making a pill-rolling movement. To compensate for *prāna vāta dushti*, bodhaka kapha is over-secreted, resulting in over-salivation, with saliva sometimes drooling down the face. Swallowing is slightly difficult and the facial muscles become rigid and masked, with no emotional expression of sadness, happiness, or joy.

We have discussed how in the sthana samsraya or deposition stage of samprāpti, vāta dosha lodges in a defective space in majjā dhātu. Later, māmsa dhātu is also affected because of the *majjā dhātu dushti* created by vāta. Rasa and rakta act as carriers for vāta dosha and once māmsa dhātu is affected; muscle tone is increased, leading to hypertonia, rigidity, and stiffness. It is as if patients of Parkinsonism are drowning in their own rigidity, both mental and physical. How we think and how we behave are bound to affect the nervous system. Fear, which is associated with vāta, creates emptiness. Therefore, the muscles become rigid to occupy the space of emptiness. Parkinson's rigidity, tremors, and spasticity frequently have their cause in psychological emotions.

One of my patients in India was bright and brilliant and he used to tease me. I was in Ayurvedic school at the time. He said to me "Come on, tell me my problem." I said to him, "Your problem is high pitta. You are controlling." "How will it manifest?" he asked. I told him that if he didn't drop that old habit, one day he would get Parkinson's disease. When I went to India recently, he saw me and he cried. He said that what I had told him long ago was now true. He had developed Parkinson's. I asked him how it happened. He told me an interesting story.

He had a high position in a governmental office. Under him there were two hundred people, which is a typical position for such a pitta-predominant man. He had some kind of dispute with a higher authority and they transferred him from one state to another. Because of that, he was in a state of shock and then developed Parkinson's. So shock or fear can create the trauma that precipitates Parkinson's—the shock of divorce, losing a job, or losing your residence.

## Chikitsā

How can Ayurveda help such a patient? Modern medicine uses drugs such as dopamine that can have drastic effects. Most of these drugs create more dryness, which is a vāta symptom. The person gets dry skin, dry mouth, dehydration, and blurred vision. In addition, dopamine is toxic to the liver, so it provokes pitta as well. It may also produce cardiac arrhythmia, so the heartbeat becomes irregular in some patients, and it increases systolic blood pressure. The person requires increasingly higher doses, but the higher the dose, the worse the pitta symptoms, such as nausea, vomiting, high blood pressure. It becomes a vicious circle.

Ayurveda looks at every individual according to his or her prakruti (constitution) and vikruti (current state). First determine the prakruti and vikruti. (see 'Eight Steps of Ayurvedic Healing') There is no doubt that kampa vāta is a vāta disorder, but there are three types—vāta pushing pitta, vāta pushing kapha, and vāta alone. Ayurvedic treatment is different for each of these three types.

In the absolute vāta type of Parkinson's, the patient has cold hands, cold feet, extreme rigidity, the skin becomes rough and dry, and there is difficulty swallowing. The patient looks stiff and has problems with constipation. In my book,

> **THE EIGHT STEPS OF AYURVEDIC HEALING**
>
> There are eight components in the traditional Ayurvedic program of healing that distinguish it from other systems of healing. They are:
>
> 1. Determine the person's prakruti (constitution)
> 2. Determine the vikruti (the present altered state of the doshas in the body)
> 3. Find out the cause or causes of the illness, such as wrong diet, lifestyle, emotional patterns, quality of relationships, genetic predisposition, etc.
> 4. The first line of treatment: removal of the cause or, if not possible, minimizing the effects, such as putting on a coat in cold weather.
> 5. Provide the proper regimen: diet, exercise, prānāyāma, etc., according to prakruti, vikruti, seasons, climate, etc.
> 6. Detoxification: either shaman (palliation) or shodana (elimination) such as panchakarma
> 7. Provide therapies which are (a) antagonistic to the provoked dosha and (b) antagonistic to the disease, based on the principle that opposite qualities balance
> 8. Rasāyana (rejuvenation) for the body in general, to increase immunity and to strengthen specific organs, tissues, and the mind

*Secrets of the Pulse,* there is a specific pulse described for the Parkinson's patient, in chapter 5, page 85. On the fifth level, when you feel the majjā dhātu pulse, there is a vāta spike that is hard and slender, with a slow rise and fall. If you feel this pulse, you will never forget it.

In the vāta pushing pitta type of kampa vāta, the vāta spike goes to the pitta site and the pulse is full and bounding. The person has profuse sweating of the palms and the skin feels hot and looks flushed. The sclera have a yellowish tinge and the patient has nausea, vomiting or loose stools. There is angular stomatitis, which is inflammation of the oral mucous membrane. Additionally, the systolic blood pressure tends to become high. These are typical characteristics of L-dopa toxicity.

In the vāta pushing kapha type of Parkinsonism, the vāta spike goes to the kapha site under the index finger on the majjā dhātu pulse, which is at the fifth level. The person has a slightly puffy face, anorexia, and low appetite. There is over-salivation, the person looks drowsy, and the skin is cold and clammy. These symptoms indicate a tumor in the extrapyramidal system.

## The Role of Panchakarma

**Snehana.** The first treatment is snehana, which is oil massage. The skin is the door to the internal pharmacy. The application of massage oil aids in healing the doshic imbalance that is present. When we apply oil, it releases certain neuro-peptides within the subcutaneous tissue. These are the same neuro-peptides released in the nervous system that help to create a balance between serotonin, melatonin, and dopamine, thus pacifying vāta dosha and eliminating stiffness and tremors. For the pure vāta type, use sesame oil; for the pitta type, sunflower oil; for kapha type, corn oil. The entire body should be massaged and the oil should be warm.

**Svedana.** Svedana means hot steam therapy and nirgundī svedana is used for vāta. The leaves of nirgundī are boiled and that steam is used for treatment in a steam box. Nirgundī minimizes atherosclerotic changes. It is anticholinergic and relaxes the muscles, relieves spasms, pacifies vāta and eliminates pitta and kapha molecules from the system. For pitta and kapha, use eucalyptus in the steam therapy.

With panchakarma, snehana and svedana may do half of the job, as they relax the muscles and remove rigidity, so that the tremors begin to minimize.

**Shirodhāra.** Shirodhāra is the continuous flow of warm oil onto the third eye, which stimulates the secretion of serotonin and melatonin. The release of these neurotransmitters helps to relax the muscles. Shirodhāra also stimulates tarpaka kapha and pacifies prāna, udāna, and apāna vāta. It brings tranquillity and relaxation.

**Nasya.** For vāta, the classical prescription is to use a vacha oil nasya. It is an herb that has been used safely in India for thousands of years. Unfortunately, the FDA has placed restrictions on the use of vacha in the US, so it cannot be used internally. However, using vacha aromatically and topically is legal. If there is pitta involvement, use brahmī ghee nasya. For kapha, use dry vacha powder for sniffing, called virechana nasya. Vacha oil is also good for kapha as well as vāta. Super Nasya Oil® nasya is balancing for all three doshas. Use of nasya for the nasal mucous membrane stimulates the basal ganglia, which is involved in the extrapyramidal system and performs the functions of equilibrium, maintenance of posture and proper gait. Hence, these functions may be helped by nasya.

### Ayurvedic Internal Medicine

Hypothyroidism is one causative factor in Parkinson's disease. In this condition, tarpaka kapha is blocking prāna vāta. Sometimes tarpaka kapha blocks both prāna and sādhaka pitta, leading to hot flashes or heat. If the patient of Parkinson's also has hypothyroidism, which is a kapha condition, you can use 300 mg each of shilājit and kukti TID.

*Dashamūla Tea.* Dashamūla tea is used for all three doshas and is literally a combination of the roots of ten herbs. Some roots work on vāta, some on pitta, and others on kapha. Give dashamūla tea two or three times a day. To make the tea, place one teaspoon of dashamūla in a cup of hot water for 10 to 15 minutes, strain, and then give to drink. As a sweetener, add honey for kapha and vāta, or maple syrup for pitta.

*Garlic Milk.* Lasuna is garlic. Take one clove of garlic, chop it into small pieces, put it in a cup of milk and bring to the boil. This brings tranquility and acts like melatonin. Milk is also an effective source of tryptophan and induces relaxation. Garlic milk is used for kapha and vāta types of kampa vāta.

*Triphalā.* Triphalā is not only a laxative; it also acts as a rasāyana. It is a superfine food that eliminates free radicals from the system and it rejuvenates all seven dhātus. To rejuvenate majjā dhātu, use ½ to one teaspoon of triphalā daily at night. It keeps the colon clean, burns āma, and removes toxicity.

*Basti.* Dashamūla tea basti (enema) with oil removes toxicity and creates negative pressure in the colon, so that vāta in the majjā dhātu starts coming back to the GI tract. This helps to relieve one of the causes of kampa vāta.

*Gold Water.* Gold water or colloidal gold rejuvenates the nerve tissue. To use gold water, take one teaspoon twice a day on an empty stomach, or 10 drops of colloidal gold diluted in one teaspoon of water twice a day. Mahāyogaraja guggulu is a useful remedy that contains gold. If mahāyogaraja guggulu is unavailable, use yogarāja guggulu with gold water as an anupāna for vāta type of Parkinson's. Use kaishore guggulu for pitta type and punarnavā guggulu for kapha type.

*Other Measures.* People with Parkinson's need general supportive measures. Because of rigidity, they may fall and while cooking they may burn themselves. Family support is important to prevent injury.

Dietary restrictions should include no nightshades, such as potato, tomato and eggplant, and no beans. They should strictly follow a vāta-pacifying diet.

Because people with Parkinson's have disturbed vāta, their agni is vishama, so they need small but frequent meals, with sufficient calories and liquids. They tend to become easily dehydrated, so include water, relaxing herbal teas, and fruit juices to combat the dehydration.

Following a daily routine and an Ayurvedic lifestyle is important for patients of Parkinson's. The patient should practice gentle yoga stretching with support as required, including the camel, cobra, cow, boat, bow, and bridge poses. It is my observation that these are effective in relaxing the muscles. See yoga poses in Appendix page 450.

The person can also benefit from So'Hum meditation, which is powerful yet relaxing. Breathing and sound have great effect upon the extrapyramidal system. The best mantra in this case is pronounced 'hreem.'

We are fortunate to have the knowledge of both Ayurveda and modern medicine available to us. All medical systems have value. A healer's heart should be open to all systems and all possibilities. Ayurveda is a living system that embraces all life and all medical systems. Ayurveda looks at each individual, disease and imbalance specifically, and then recommends a treatment regimen particular to the cause or causes, the unique individual and the presenting symptoms. The treatment regimen may include components from several medical systems, such as herbology, yoga, meditation, counseling, and even pharmaceutical drugs and surgery when necessary. In this way, we can bring a complete and holistic approach to a patient of Parkinson's.

---

**FOR VĀTA-TYPE PARKINSON'S**

| | |
|---|---|
| Ashvagandhā | 500 mg |
| Ātma Guptā (Kapikacchū) | 300 mg |
| Vidārī | 300 mg |
| Balā | 300 mg |
| Tagara | 200 mg |

Tagara is a tranquilizer and muscle relaxant. Balā has anticholinergic action, which relieves muscle spasm, gives muscle energy, regulates normal muscle tone, and relieves rigidity. Vidārī inhibits tremors and ātma guptā is a specific remedy for Parkinson's disease. Ashvagandhā helps to heal the lesion in the extrapyramidal system.

**FOR PITTA-TYPE PARKINSON'S**

| | |
|---|---|
| Shatāvarī | 500 mg |
| Ātma Guptā (Kapikacchū) | 300 mg |
| Gudūchī | 300 mg |
| Balā | 300 mg |
| Vidārī | 300 mg |

Balā and vidārī are specifically antagonistic to the disease. Shatāvarī and gudūchī are used to pacify pitta.

**FOR KAPHA-TYPE PARKINSON'S**

| | |
|---|---|
| Punarnavā | 500 mg |
| Ātma Guptā (Kapikacchū) | 300 mg |
| Gokshura | 400 mg |
| Vidārī | 300 mg |
| Balā | 300 mg |

Punarnavā is a cerebral diuretic. Again we are using vidārī, ātma guptā, and balā to treat the disease.

---

# Chapter 35

# Epilepsy

Spring 2014, Volume 26, Number 4

AYURVEDA CLASSIFIES DISEASE as physical and psychological. Physical and psychological ailments are classified according to the majority of symptomatology. If there are more pathophysiological changes, that disorder falls under the physical classification. Whereas if there are more psychological symptoms, the disease is a psychological or psychiatric illness, in which the mind (mano vaha srotas) is mainly affected.

For example, *unmād* (psychosis) is described as a psychiatric illness. Whereas *apasmāra* (epilepsy) is categorized as a physical disease.

The mind has three qualities: sattva (clarity), rajas (activity), and tamas (inertia). The mind is made from sattva, while excessive rajas and tamas are the root cause of all psychological problems. *Dhi* (buddhi or intellect), *dhruti* (retention of information), and *smruti* (memory) are the major faculties of the mind. In apasmāra, there is a sudden depletion of memory (smruti), which then affects dhi and dhruti.

Epilepsy is called apasmāra, because *smara* means memory (smruti), and *apa* means sudden blockage or break. *Apaya* means to go away or to lose. Hence, apasmāra is a sudden blockage or break to the memory pattern. This causes the person to have a seizure, producing epilepsy, with sudden loss of memory of the surroundings and a loss of understanding (dhi).

Although it is a physical illness, apasmāra can be triggered by intense fear, anxiety, worry, grief, sorrow, shock, or anger, or a surge of any emotion. It can even be provoked by chanting the wrong mantra and mistakes in *tantric* practice. These factors all disturb the doshas and provoke rajas or tamas qualities. The aggravated doshas enter majjā dhātu, causing *sroto rodha* (blockage) of the mind and consciousness.

Epilepsy is a brief disorder of cerebral dysfunction. It is an altered state of consciousness, with sudden changes of sensory and motor functions. The symptoms vary from an almost imperceptible alteration of the person's consciousness to a dramatic loss of consciousness.

Epilepsy is relatively common, being found in at least 2% to 3% of the population. Its incidence is highest in children between 4 years old up to puberty, and in elderly people over age 65.

Charaka's description of apasmāra states that the person enters into darkness, with loss of consciousness. In some types of apasmāra, the mind becomes inactive and the body performs terrifying actions, such as clenching and grinding of the teeth, emitting froth from the mouth, shaking of the hands and feet, and seeing non-existent things. There may be a typical epileptic cry, the eyes are rolled upwards, the tongue is bitten, bloody froth comes out of the mouth, and the person collapses on the ground, then passes urine and goes into deep sleep. The individual will wake up in a drowsy and disoriented state.

In Ayurveda, epilepsy is regarded as a disorder of both majjā dhātu and māmsa dhātu, along with their related bodily channels: *majjā vaha srotas* (the nervous system) and *māmsa vaha srotas* (the muscular system), as well as mano vaha srotas (the channel of the mind). It is marked by abnormal electrical (or *prānic*) discharge within the brain and recurrent fits or seizures that last for between a few minutes and a few hours.

## Nidana: Etiology

Ayurvedic literature states that apasmāra begins with a systemic increase of vāta dosha. The main site of vāta is the colon, from where vāta undergoes sanchaya (accumulation), prakopa (provocation) and then prasara (spread). During the prasara stage, vāta spreads into the hematopoietic system (*rasa-rakta*) and seeks a place to hide.

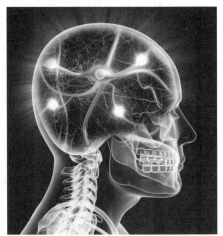
Epileptic Event in the Brain

Vāta deposits in a particular tissue or organ due to genetic predisposition or defective space (khavaigunya) in that tissue or organ. In epilepsy, vāta deposits in the main site of majjā dhātu—the brain—where it also affects the mind (mano vaha srotas).When vāta dosha enters into mano vaha srotas, it unduly stimulates the neuronal activity and therefore affects the person's memory and cognitive faculty.

The brain is a big neuronal battery. Each neuron generates its own electricity, which is prāna. That electric current passes from the head (axon) to the tail (dendron) of the neuron. If a specific neuron creates an electric current, then the other neurons either get excited or inhibited.

When groups of neurons get excited, it creates a strong electrical storm in the brain. The excited neurons produce abnormal brain waves and this can result in seizures. When there are generalized seizures with tonic and clonic phases, including biting the tongue and straining muscles, it is tonic-clonic or grand mal epilepsy. In some children aged 4 to 14, there are no seizures and the child has a vacant stare. This is called petit mal epilepsy or Absence Seizures. Idiopathic epilepsy, where the cause is not known, is regarded as a psychiatric illness.

Not every seizure is epilepsy. For example, a head trauma can also cause seizures. However when there are repeated spontaneous seizures which are not caused by any trauma, that is epilepsy. Epilepsy is a brain disorder, a physical illness.

Epilepsy can result from congenital or acquired brain disease. Infants born with lipid storage disease, tuberous sclerosis, cortical dysplasia, intracranial hemorrhage, or cerebral anoxia of the brain can develop epilepsy. Other common causes of epilepsy in children include being born after a prolonged obstructed labor or a forceps delivery due to cephalo-pelvic disproportion, which causes the baby's head to be traumatized and can result in an intracranial hemorrhage or hypoxic brain injury. Apasmāra can also be due to toxins from the placenta entering into the brain of the fetus. An infection or high fever that causes febrile seizures or convulsions can also result in apasmāra.

An adult can develop epilepsy as the result of a stroke, tumor, abscess or brain infection, head injury, brain trauma, concussion, compression, or contusion. It can be due to inflammation of the meninges—meningitis or encephalitis. If there is kidney failure, the uremia can affect the brain and cause epileptic symptoms. Epilepsy can also be due to a metabolic disorder that affects the liver, resulting in toxins from the liver changing the neuroelectrical brainwaves. These are all important etiological factors to consider in epilepsy.

The symptoms of epilepsy are due to a sudden, excessive neuroelectrical discharge. These kind of abnormal brainwaves occur in majjā dhātu, due to vāta "pushing" pitta or kapha in the nervous system.

Etiological factors that can affect the brain and create apasmāra include:

- inflammation of the brain (meningitis or encephalitis)
- bacterial, parasitic, or viral infection
- recurrent paroxysmal (convulsive) disorder of the brain
- accumulation of poisonous or toxic substances, such as lead, arsenic, mercury and other heavy metals
- buildup of other non-infectious agent (āma) in majjā dhātu
- head injury
- brain tumor
- childbirth trauma
- reaction to vaccination
- psychological factors, such as worries, anxiety, anger,
- vāta-provoking diet, or food that strongly aggravates the doshas
- viruses
- encephalitis
- infection, e.g., mosquito-borne infection causing cerebral malaria
- measles, mumps, rubella (German measles), or chickenpox
- cerebral palsy

## Pūrva Rūpa: Prodromal Signs and symptoms

For a couple of days before an epileptic attack, the person's mood changes, there is a feeling of emptiness, dizziness, and optical, auditory, and olfactory hallucinations. There may be abnormal movements of the eyes, increased perspiration, excessive salivation and drooling, disturbed appetite, and gurgling noises in the abdomen due to hyperperistalsis. These are prodromal symptoms that occur before the person is about to get an epileptic attack.

### Rūpa: Signs and Symptoms
- palpations
- a feeling of emptiness
- perspiration
- worry
- fainting
- delusion
- memory loss
- insomnia and loss of sleep
- tremors
- grinding of the teeth
- biting of the jaw and tongue
- frothy vomitus
- rapid respiration
- violent bodily convulsions
- red flushed face, or purplish colored face
- staring look
- violent movements of the eyeballs
- urinary and fecal incontinence
- amnesia
- alteration of sensory perception
- change in consciousness
- mood changes
- typical epileptic cry
- aura of epilepsy, which is auditory, visual, or olfactory hallucinations

## Clinical Categories of Epilepsy
Although it is primarily a vāta disorder, there are several categories of apasmāra. These are the four main clinical types of epilepsy:

**1) Simple Partial Seizures (*vāta-kapha* type) = Absence Seizures or Petit Mal (little illness) Epilepsy.** This is caused by kapha blocking vāta dosha. It is confined to the temporal area of the brain. The patient remains conscious during the seizure, which typically lasts for less than 20 seconds. There is a feeling of numbness and tingling in the arms, fingers, and feet. The person perceives an unpleasant smell or flashing lights, and speaks unintelligibly. The symptoms are relatively mild. The person is motionless and drops articles from the hands, there is a vacant look, the eyes blink, nose runs, and saliva drools from the mouth.

**2) Complex Partial Seizures (vāta-kapha type).** Also confined to the temporal area of the brain, but due to vāta pushing kapha. The patient loses consciousness, with abnormal gesturing and automatic movements. These seizures happen because *prāna vāta dosha* is overly active and is pushing *tarpaka kapha dosha* in the temporal area.

**3) Generalized Convulsive Seizure (vāta type) = Tonic-Clonic or Grand Mal (big illness) Epilepsy.** Tonic-clonic epilepsy was formerly known as grand mal epilepsy. It causes vigorous epileptic convulsions and there are many symptoms.

In the tonic phase, which happens first, the muscles become tense and the body stiff. Typically, the person cries out, falls down to the ground and loses consciousness. The patient loses urinary and bowel control, has muscle spasms and thrashing movements of the limbs, jerks and spasms of the jaw, and the person typically bites his or her tongue.

Then in the clonic phase, there are generalized convulsions. After the convulsions, the patient falls down in a deep sleep and awakens dazed, with a headache and no recollection of what happened.

Before the attack, a warning sensation may precede the seizures, called an "aura of epilepsy"[49] with visual, auditory, or olfactory hallucinations that last for a few minutes. The person may also have headaches, sleeplessness, and tingling and numbness in the arms. Then the person cries out with a typical epilepsy cry and falls down on the ground, losing consciousness.

**4) Generalized Non-Convulsion Type (pitta-kapha type).** There is an absence of seizures, but periods when the patient stares into space, with rhythmic blinking of the eyelids. It looks like the person is day-dreaming. The individual remains conscious and is totally unaware of the seizure. This is quite common in children, when it may be mistaken as the child having a short attention span or learning disability.

## Doshic Types of Apasmāra

### Vāta Apasmāra

The root cause of vāta epilepsy is due to āma in the colon. There are tremors all over the body, memory loss, epileptic cry, eyes rolled up, breathlessness, vomiting, shivering, grinding of the teeth, violent convulsions, dryness of the mouth, bluish-reddish discoloration of the face, person falls down with a cry.

### Pitta Apasmāra

The root cause of vāta-pitta epilepsy is due to āma in the small intestine. There may be high fever, nausea, vomiting, loose stools, and a red flushed face, and it is generally worse during midday and midnight. This is a form of febrile convulsions. Pitta type of epilepsy is due to fever and inflammation, and is common in children. It results in yellowish discoloration of the froth, the face is flushed, eyes look red, the urine and skin have a yellowish tinge, and the symptoms are aggravated during summer season, in a hot room, or even by

---

49. F. A. Davis Company. *Taber's Cyclopedic Medical Dictionary, 20th Ed.*, Philadelphia, 2005. "A subjective, but recognizable sensation that precedes and signals the onset of a convulsion…the aura may precede the attack by several hours or only a few seconds. An epileptic aura may be psychic, or it may be sensory with olfactory, visual, auditory, or taste hallucinations."

looking at a fire. The person can faint just by looking at blood or watching violent things such as people fighting.

### Kapha Apasmāra

The root cause of vāta-kapha epilepsy is due to āma in the stomach. The person usually remains awake, but there is excess salivation, a staring vacant look and the person loses track of memory, not knowing what he or she was doing. This is a book picture of petit mal epilepsy.

## Diagnosis

The diagnosis of epilepsy can be carefully done through a thorough assessment of the patient's personal history, family history and history of previous illnesses. Get a thorough medical history and note all the signs and symptoms Typically, one has to do blood tests and magnetic resonance imaging (MRI) to find out if there is a lesion, as well as an electro-encephalogram (EEG) to observe the electrical activity of the brain, showing any abnormal brainwave patterns. Note that a normal electro-encephalogram does not rule out epilepsy.

### Differential Diagnosis

We have to differentiate epilepsy from other medical conditions with similar signs and symptoms. For instance, the person may have loss of consciousness for reasons other than epilepsy, including pseudo seizures, syncope, transient ischemic attack, hypotension, severe low blood sugar, or narcolepsy. Common forms of neurological disorder that need to be differentiated from epilepsy include:

**Narcolepsy.** This is an irresistible attack of sleep from which the patient can be aroused immediately. The person may go to sleep at work or in other situations, such as driving a car, and several attacks may occur in a day.

**Catalepsy.** Due to sudden emotion, the person loses power in the limbs but remains conscious.

**Sleep Paralysis.** On waking or falling asleep, the person is unable to move, although mentally the patient is awake. The person may also have hallucinations, sometimes terrifying, just as he or she is falling asleep

**Jacksonian Epilepsy.** The cortical area is affected. The symptoms are related to a circumscribed part of the body and they slowly spread to adjacent areas. There is involuntary twitching and chronic movement that starts in the extremities and then spreads all over the body, unilaterally or bilaterally. There may or may not be loss of consciousness.

In all these disorders, the treatment protocol is aimed at majjā dhātu and majjā vaha srotas.

## Chikitsā: Treatment Protocol

To prevent injury during a seizure, the patient should be kept in a comfortable lying posture with loosened clothing and a pillow under the head. The patient should be turned to the left lateral position, so any vomit is not swallowed. Otherwise, the patient might choke. Ideally, apply tongue forceps to the tongue, so the patient won't swallow his or her tongue and suffocate. Never insert any other object into the mouth, such as a spoon or screwdriver. After the person has had a convulsion, don't open the patient's mouth or the convulsion can reoccur.

It is unwise for children with a history of convulsions to cycle in busy public places or swim in the sea, unless someone is watching closely. Parents are often overprotective of an epileptic child. The child should be educated in a normal school, or he or she will probably feel intellectually deficient.

In modern medicine, drugs are used to control epileptic seizures. The Ayurvedic approach involves dietary and lifestyle changes, as well as herbal remedies and pancha-karma therapy, all in the periods between attacks.

Ayurveda says to eat wholesome food to balance the doshas, and not to restrain natural urges such as sneezing and flatulence, as this can aggravate vāta dosha.

The main herbal remedies are vacha, brahmī, jatamāmsi, gokshura, smritisagara ras, brahmīprash, and brahmī ghee.

Within the medulla, tarpaka kapha maintains an oily quality, while excessive prāna vāta causes dryness and roughness in the medulla. These qualitative changes cause an electrical brainstorm. Brahmī ghee or vacha ghee nasya (nasal drops) are beneficial for treating this condition by balancing the oily and dry qualities. Maha panchagavya ghrita may also be prescribed. This medicinal ghee includes panchamūla (balances vāta), triphala (a rasāyana to the nervous system), kutaja (balances tarpaka kapha), saptaparna, (strength-ens medulla activity) and apāmargā (a nervine tonic), and it balances vāta dosha and elim-inates the khavaigunya in majjā vaha srotas.

*Dhūmana* (smoke therapy) involves the burning of certain herbs and this treatment can also help epileptic patients. Vacha, brahmī, jatamāmsi, shankha pushpī, and neem are all used for this purpose.

Marma chikitsā is used for epilepsy. Mūrdhni, Sthapanī, Brahmarandhra, Oshtha, Hanu, Jatru, Agra Patra, and Pāda Kshipra marma points are treated, often using nutmeg essential oil. See illustrations of these points on page 456.

During an epileptic attack, one should give strong nasya (nasal administration of herbal remedies), such as vacha powder blown into the nose, or onion juice dropped into the nose. That kind of shock treatment can suddenly stop convulsions.

Once an attack is over, one should treat the underlying condition, according to whether it is vāta type, pitta type, or kapha type of apasmāra.

If the patient is taking anti-epileptic medication, tranquilizers, or other medical drugs, do not stop those. We can add the following remedies to this Ayurvedic protocol to supple-ment the person's other medical treatments:

- For vāta type, vacha mishran (mixture)
- For pitta type, smritisagara ras
- For kapha type, gajakesari ras and brahmīprash

## Table 9: Herbal Remedies

| Vāta Type Apasmāra | Pitta Type Apasmāra | Kapha Type Apasmāra |
|---|---|---|
| Herbal protocol, given 3 times daily:<br>Ashvagandhā 500 mg<br>Balā 400 mg<br>Vidārī 300 mg<br>Sarasvatī 200 mg | Herbal protocol, given 3 times daily:<br>Shatāvarī 500 mg<br>Gudūchī 400 mg<br>Shankha pushpī 300 mg<br>Brahmī 200 mg | Herbal protocol, given 3 times daily:<br>Punarnavā 500 mg<br>Sarasvatī 300 mg<br>Tagara 200 mg<br>Trikatu 200 mg<br>Vacha 200 mg |
| Each night, the person should take a teaspoon of gandharva harītakī<br>Vacha tailam nasya<br>Abhyanga with sesame oil<br>Dashamūla tea basti<br>Shirodhāra | One teaspoon of bhumi āmalakī nightly as virechana<br>Brahmī ghee nasya (and orally)<br>Abhyanga with sunflower oil<br>Shirodhāra with brahmī oil | Vacha powder nasya or vacha tailam nasya<br>Abhyanga with sesame oil<br>Shirodhāra with bhringarāja oil<br>Sometimes vamana therapy is indicated, using licorice (yashthi madhu) tea or vacha tea to induce vomiting. |

# Chapter 36

# Stroke
## Cerebrovascular Accident

Fall 2014, Volume 27, Number 2

IN AYURVEDIC LITERATURE, stroke is called *paksha ghāta* or *paksha vadha*. *Paksha* means side of the body, while *ghāta* means partial loss of power and *vadha* is total loss of power. So paksha ghāta and paksha vadha refer to the sudden loss of power to either the right or the left half of the body.

In Charaka Samhitā and Sushruta Samhitā, they mention a group of eighty diseases under the category of *vāta vyādhi*. If we closely observe these disorders, they fall under skeletomuscular, neuromuscular, or neurological disorders. Amongst the 80 vāta diseases, they have mentioned paksha ghāta (partial loss of power, or paresis) and paksha vadha (total loss of power, or paralysis).

Like most neurological diseases, paksha ghāta is due to aggravation of vāta dosha in majjā dhātu (the nervous system). Vāta in majjā creates neurological symptoms, such as tingling, numbness, loss of power and function, and lack of coordination.

According to the broad classification of the human body, there are four extremities: arms and legs, and the head and the trunk. When one extremity is affected, it is called *eka paksha vadha,* which is **monoplegia**. When the right or left half is affected, it is called *ardhānga vāyu,* which is **hemiplegia**. When both lower extremities are affected, it is known as *pāngullya,* which is **paraplegia**. If all four extremities are affected, it is *sarvānga vadha,* or **quadriplegia**. These are all different varieties of stroke, according to the parts of the body that are affected.

## Samprāpti: The Disease Process

Before the development of a stroke, apāna vāyu from the colon undergoes sanchaya (accumulation), prakopa (provocation), and then prasara (spread). After this prasara stage, vāta enters the dhātus (tissues) and in the case of stroke, it deposits in majjā dhātu, the nerve tissue.

Stroke is a central nervous system disorder and it is abrupt in nature. Its sudden onset is caused by an interruption of the blood supply to an area of the brain. In Ayurvedic terms, this is *sroto rodha* in rasa and rakta dhātus. There is loss of function in the parts of the body related to the affected areas in the brain.

Each side of the brain controls motor and sensory functions in the opposite side of the body. The precentral gyrus is the motor area and the postcentral gyrus is the sensory area. For example, movement of the left upper extremity or left lower extremity is governed by the right side precentral gyrus, and vice versa.

Depending upon how much of the blood supply is stopped, and whether there is ischemia (restricted blood supply) or even infarction of the lesion (tissue destruction due to lack of blood supply), there may be a partial or complete loss of power. When there is a partial loss of power, it is called paresis (ghāta). Where there is total loss of power, it is known as paralysis (vadha).

One should clinically distinguish between two types of paralysis. The first is lower motor neuron paralysis, due to *dhātu kshaya janita* (depletion of the tissues). The other type is upper motor neuron paralysis, due to *mārga rodha janita.* In this condition, vāta dosha is blocked by kapha, pitta, or āma (toxins). Even meda dhātu (excess fatty tissue) can block vāta.

If the lesion is in the upper motor neuron, there is increased tone (hypertonia). This causes rigidity. If the stroke affects the lower motor neuron, there will be loss of tone (called atonia), with flaccidity and loss of power.

In upper motor neuron type of paralysis, there is neurological damage to the corticospinal or pyramidal tract in the brain or spinal cord. This results in hemiplegia, paraplegia, or quadriplegia, depending upon the location and extent of the lesion. Clinical signs of this type of paralysis include loss of voluntary movement, increased rigidity, hypertonia, exaggerated reflexes, and sensory loss.

In lower motor neuron type of paralysis, there is neurological damage to the anterior horn cells, peripheral nerves, or peripheral muscles tract in the brain or spinal cord. Clinical signs include loss of power, hypotonia, poor muscle nutrition, rapid muscle wasting and flaccidity, and topical changes (such as purple coloring of the skin).

Sādhaka pitta, tarpaka kapha, and prāna vāta govern functional activity in the brain. Prāna vāta governs sensory activity, while apāna vāta governs motor functions. Increased tone (upper motor neuron lesion) is caused by *prāna vāyu dushti,* while diminished tone (lower motor neuron lesion) is due to *apāna vāyu dushti.*

## Nidāna: Causative Factors of Stroke

The first etiological factor is genetic predisposition to hyperlipidemia, diabetes, high blood pressure, and/or obesity. However, this factor is less important than those that follow.

A second factor is cerebral vascular embolism (known as sirā granthi). If there are varicose veins in the calf or elsewhere in the lower extremities, blood clots can form and if they are set in motion, it causes an embolism. A cerebral vascular embolism is a small blood clot that goes into the cerebral blood vessel, or into the coronary artery where it

## Table 10: Types of Paralysis

| Upper Motor Neuron Lesion | Lower Motor Neuron Lesion |
|---|---|
| Mārga rodha (blocked channel) | Dhātu kshaya (depleted tissues) |
| Increased tone (hypertonia) | Decreased tone (hypotonia) |
| Rigidity | Flaccidity |
| Reflexes are exacerbated | Reflexes are abolished |
| Slow muscle wasting | Rapid muscle wasting |
| Passive exercise may help | Exercise doesn't help maintain tone |
| Affected extremities are warm | Affected extremities are cold |
| Fewer changes in color, temperature | More changes in color, temperature |
| Bedsores and ulcers can be avoided with proper care | Bedsores and ulcers are common |
| Gradual recovery is possible | Recovery is difficult |
| Mainly affects movement | Mainly affects muscle/s |
| Cyanosis and edema may result from underuse of muscles | Skin often cold, blue, shiny |

creates a sudden heart attack, or into the carotid artery and then the cerebral artery where it creates a stroke. Because of this, one should do a thorough examination of *rasa* and *rakta vaha srotas* (the hematopoietic system), with special focus on the person's lipids profile, cholesterol, blood sugar, and blood pressure.

A third cause is an interruption of the blood flow, due to atherosclerosis (sirā kāthinya). If a person has long-standing hyperlipidemia, then fat can deposit on the blood vessels and create thickening of those vessels and hardening of the arteries. That can cause cerebral atherosclerotic changes, localized anemia (ischemia), and an interruption of the blood flow to the brain (infarction), which is a form of stroke.

A fourth causative factor is cerebral hemorrhage. Some people have an abnormality of the cerebral blood vessel, which may have a kink, curve, embolism, or aneurism, or an anatomical disposition of the blood vessel. An aneurism is a balloon-like deformity of the cerebral artery. This can rupture and cause a cerebral hemorrhage, which is when a deformed artery in the brain bursts.

A fifth cause is long-standing chronic hypertension. Hypertension plus atherosclerosis in a person over the age of 60 (which is vāta age), can cause hardening of the artery, then stenosis, thrombosis, and that leads to ischemia in the brain tissue, which causes infarction (death of the brain cells). Stenosis is narrowing (*kāthinya*), thrombosis is clotting (sirā granthi), and ischemia is lack of blood supply (localized *pāndu*).

A sixth causative factor is a space-occupying lesion or cerebral tumor.

The seventh possible cause is chronic smoking. People who smoke have a higher risk of getting a stroke.

Race is the eighth factor that can play an important role in the risk of stroke. Those of African descent experience about twice the rate of stroke compared to those of European descent; and the rate for Hispanics and Native Americans falls somewhere in between those other two groups.

Etiological factor number nine is a transient ischemic attack (TIA) to the brain, which creates a mild stroke or "mini-stroke". With proper treatment, recovery is possible within 24 hours, leaving some residual effects.

According to Ayurveda, the underlying root cause of strokes is aggravated vāta dosha in majjā dhātu. The samprāpti of stroke varies according to the individual, but generally vāta from the colon undergoes prasara (spread) and moves into majjā dhātu, where it can create ischemia, infarction, and so forth.

A person with long-lingering vāta imbalance who is eating a vāta-aggravating diet of black beans, pinto beans, aduki beans, chickpea flour, and so forth, and doing lots of jogging and jumping, and having recurrent sex, is likely to aggravate vāta in the nervous system.

## Signs and Symptoms of Stroke

The moment that vāta goes into majjā dhātu, it can cause mild headaches and malaise, drowsiness, loss of consciousness at the onset of a stroke, and tingling and numbness on the affected side.

A severe headache is unusual, but may occur in some pitta individuals. Epileptic fits can occasionally occur. Loss of power, hyperreflexia, and hemianesthesia (loss of sense of touch) may result on the same side as the hemiplegia.

The main signs and symptoms are:

* loss of power, called paresis
* increased tone (hypertonia) or decreased tone (hypotonia)
* lack of coordination
* memory loss
* loss of speech
* walking is affected
* emotional control is lost, which is why a stroke patient easily bursts into tears
* paraplegia, in which the whole body is paralyzed
* hemiplegia, in which half of the body is paralyzed

If the infarction is in the area supplied by the anterior cerebral artery, hemiplegia can be seen more in the legs on the opposite side of the body. It may be associated with urinary incontinence.

If the lesion is in the area supplied by the posterior cerebral artery, it is contralateral homonymous hemiplegia. This means the hemiplegia is seen on the same side of the body. Depending on the part of the posterior cerebral artery affected, it may affect the arms, legs, or the whole side.

Majjā dhātu is divided into major areas: the cerebrocortical, extrapyramidal, internal capsule, brain stem, and the cervical, thoracic, and lumbar spine. If vāta is lodged in the cerebrocortical area, only one extremity is affected.

The region from the cerebral cortex, extrapyramidal area, internal capsule, brain stem and spinal cord up to the posterior root ganglia is called the upper motor neuron. This is a prānic pathway.

The anterior horn cell to the peripheral nerves, including the reflex arc and individual muscle fibers, is called the lower motor neuron. This is the field of apāna vāyu.

In upper motor neuron lesions, there is rigidity, because of the disturbance to prāna. In lower motor neuron lesions, the motor actions are totally abolished, due to the affliction of apāna vāyu. Hence, there is flaccidity.

If the lesion is in the mid-cerebrocortical region, it will only affect the upper extremities, causing monoplegia on the opposite side. If it is in the internal capsule, the entire opposite side will be paralyzed.

If the lesion is in the thoracic spinal area, there will be monoplegia in the lower extremity on the opposite side of the body.

Major signs of stroke include:

- sudden weakness in the extremities and facial muscles of expression
- tingling and numbness in the extremities and facial muscles of expression
- slurred talk
- unexplained unsteadiness, due to changes in the muscle tone, power and coordination—a paralyzed patient persistently falls on the affected side.

Generally, if a person is right-handed, the speech center is on the left side. If there is right-sided paralysis, there is usually aphasia, which is loss of the power of speech. Whereas if there is left-sided paralysis, a right-handed person's speech may not be affected at all. The opposite applies to left-handed people.

Paralyzed stroke patients often have difficulty in understanding others. The affected individual hears the other person's words, but does not know their meaning. This is called word deafness. Or the patient can read words but not know their meaning, which is known as word blindness.

## Diagnosis

Diagnosis is done by taking a thorough medical history and by physical examination.

An experienced clinician and physician should do a thorough examination of the patient, by doing a systemic sensory and motor examination, taking superficial and deep reflexes, and examining the muscle tone, power, nutrition, and coordination.

One must test both superficial and deep reflexes. Superficial reflexes are the conjunctival, corneal, jaw, abdominal, cremasteric, and plantar reflexes. Deep tendon reflexes are triceps, biceps, brachioradialis, knee-jerk, and ankle.

For stroke, one should test the triceps, biceps, and brachioradialis for the upper extremities; the abdominal reflex; and reflexes for the lower extremities, including knee-jerk, ankle-jerk, and plantar reflexes. After a stroke, the reflexes are exaggerated and sometimes there is ankle clonus and patella clonus. If you pull the patella down there is a jerky up-and-down movement to the patella. That is a sign of hypertonia. This examination helps to determine the exact site of the lesion. It takes great clinical skill to decide the affected site without an MRI.

If you look at a paralyzed patient, the paralyzed side often shows muscle wasting. When you hold the hand at the person's wrist and try to flex it or extend it, there is increased rigidity.

There are two types of increased rigidity. One is cogwheel rigidity, which is present in Parkinson's Disease and causes tremors. Whereas in stroke paralysis, there is clasp knife rigidity. If you try to open the blade of a clasp knife, the blade opens suddenly. Similarly, a paralytic patient will have sudden jerky movements of the affected extremity. Tremors are absent in this type of rigidity.

If you compare the right and left upper arms, you will see that the muscles on the affected side are wasted. This is rapid in upper motor neuron disorders, and slower in lower motor neuron disorders.

Ask the patient to move his or her affected arm, and see if the person can touch the index finger to the tip of the nose. This can be tested with eyes open and then with eyes closed. If the patient cannot perform this test, it indicates coordination is affected in the upper extremity on that side of the body. A similar test for the lower extremity is the heel-to-knee test, whereby the patient is asked to place the heel of one foot onto the knee of the opposite leg.

When a group of muscles is working together, it is called coordination. When someone has a stroke, coordination in the upper extremity or lower extremity is affected.

The next point is that the affected side feels cold. Test this by placing your hand on the patient's right and left cheeks, shoulders, upper arms, forearms, belly, thighs, and feet.

If you feel the person's pulse, you will notice that the fifth level (dhātu) pulse shows a spike indicating high vāta in majjā dhātu.

The face can also be involved. You have to observe whether the patient can frown, raise the eyebrows, or close the eyes, and test if they can whistle. If not, this indicates facial paralysis.

If there is right-sided facial paralysis and paralysis of the right arm and leg, it is called **complete hemiplegia**. Whereas, if there is right-sided facial paralysis and paralysis of the left arm and leg, that is called **ipsilateral paralysis**. The same is true for the other side of the body. Complete hemiplegia is more common than ipsilateral paralysis.

Diagnosis is also done by angiography, a modern medical technique in which dye is injected into the veins and then x-rays are taken. Because normal x-rays don't show the soft tissues, radioactive dye is injected for that purpose. Another technique is computer thermography, which provides a cross-section image that may indicate whether a stroke was caused by a hemorrhage or blocked blood vessel or tumor. Finally, one can do MRI (magnetic resonance imaging).

In Ayurveda, the diagnosis does not depend upon specific techniques. The primary diagnosis is to understand clinically whether a particular stroke is vāta, pitta, or kapha type. Also, by assessing the person's body frame, size, and other factors, we can detect the doshic constitution. In Ayurveda, we always treat the underlying cause of the disturbance to the doshas and dhātus, so it is important to know both the person's prakruti (constitution) and vikruti (current imbalance).

Stroke is a vāta disease. However, vāta can be disturbed by pitta (vāta pushing pitta or pitta blocking vāta), or sometimes by kapha or even meda dhātu (fat tissue) blocking vāta dosha. If we see three stroke patients, we will see three different pathogeneses. One may have a pure vāta disorder, a second may have vāta pushing pitta, while a third could have kapha blocking vāta. Due to the permutations and combinations of the doshas, there will be three unique disease processes.

We also have to find out if the condition is due to sāma vāta (vāta with toxins) or nirāma vāta (vāta without toxicity). Sāma vāta is indicated by a heavily coated tongue and foul smelling urine and feces, whereas in nirāma vāta conditions, the tongue looks clean and the urine and feces have a regular smell. Sāma vāta is linked to mārga rodha (blocked channels), whereas nirāma vāta conditions are linked to dhātu kshaya (depleted tissues) and wasting.

. . . . . . . . . . . . . . . . . . . . . . . . . . . . . . . . . . . . . . . . . . . . . . . . . .

### Snehanam sneha sam yuktum paksha gate virechanam...

This sūtra states that snehana (application of oil) and oily virechana (purgation) are the best lines of therapy for stroke.

. . . . . . . . . . . . . . . . . . . . . . . . . . . . . . . . . . . . . . . . . . . . . . . . . .

## Stroke Management

Snehana (applying oil) and svedana (sweating therapy) are important protocols to deal with any vāta disorder. If there is sāma vāta, we can do an oil massage with visha garbha tailam, whereas if it is a nirāma vāta condition, we will use mahānārāyana tailam, balā tailam, dashamūla tailam, or just plain sesame oil.

The application of oil is effective in improving the circulation, maintaining normal muscle tone and coordination, and preventing muscle wasting. As part of snehana therapy, we can do shirodhāra or shiro basti using dashamūla oil or balā oil, and also nasya (nasal therapy) with vacha oil nasya.

Snehana will calm down the dry quality of vāta throughout the body. Shirodhāra or shiro basti are part of the snehana treatment for stroke.

Svedana is done after oil massage. The patient is put into a sweat box and nirgundī essential oil is added to the steam. Nirgundī penetrates into majjā dhātu. Svedana improves circulation, promotes perspiration, and enhances neuronal communication.

After three or four days of snehana and svedana, *āma* in the deep tissues starts to move back into the gastrointestinal tract. At that moment, virechana is given, using gandharva harītakī. This helps to remove the toxins from the system.

Paralysis is a vāta disorder, and generally basti is the main panchakarma therapy for vāta diseases. However, in the case of a stroke, virechana is the therapy prescribed. In the pathogenesis of a stroke, rasa and rakta vaha srotas (the hematopoietic system) are involved, with symptoms such as high blood pressure and blood clots. Therefore, rañjaka pitta in the blood and sādhaka pitta in the brain are affected.

Virechana is the treatment for excess pitta. It acts on the small intestine, creating negative pressure in the microvilli, thereby allowing sādhaka pitta and rañjaka pitta to be removed from the body. If you do virechana, it will remove excess pitta from the circulatory system and improve circulation in the cerebral blood vessels. Hence, virechana can eliminate the pathophysiological causes of a stroke.

Even though stroke is a vāta disorder, Charaka did not specifically mention basti as a primary treatment. Basti is given only if there is absolute constipation, because repeated basti may create mineral loss and the paralyzed muscles will be fatigued.

However, virechana also works on apāna and samāna vāyu, and even activates prāna vāyu, helping to regulate the coordination between the sensory and motor systems. Hence, virechana works on the *crown chakra* via samāna and prāna vāta.

Nasya is actually an important treatment protocol for stroke patients. The nose is the doorway to the brain, and the stroke lesions are in the brain. Appropriate nasya calms down vāta dosha, and also balances pitta and kapha. Nasya helps to produce stem cells and those stem cells start healing the lesion in the brain.

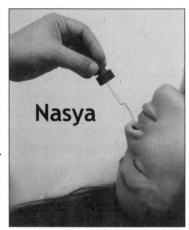

When a blood vessel is damaged, a special enzyme in the rakta dhātu is produced, called angiogenic enzyme. This has rakta agni, and helps to create a new network of blood vessels and capillaries, to continue the blood flow to affected areas. This healing process is called anastomosis.

Along the same lines, some studies show that the axons and dendrons can create new ramifications. This is called neuronal anastomosis. This term is not accepted by modern medicine, which says that nerves cannot be repaired. However, in an Ayurvedic practice, one can see remarkable improvement in the sensory stimuli and motor responses. Thus, we can call this neuronal anastomosis.

Based upon clinical evaluation, if the person is emaciated and there is wasting of the tissues, it shows the stroke paralysis is due to dhātu kshaya. These people need more *bruhana* (anabolic, nutritive therapy), snehana (application of oils), and *tarpana* (nourishing and energizing treatments). Examples include massage with balā oil and nutritive herbal remedies.

Whereas if we find there is sāma dosha (with toxins), it indicates mārga rodha. In that case, one needs to use dīpana therapy to kindle the digestive fire and pāchana (digestive) therapy to burn toxins, along with *anulomana chikitsā* to maintain the normal vector of vāta dosha.

## Herbal Protocol

An effective base formula for someone recovering from a stroke is:

| | |
|---|---|
| Dashamūla | 500 mg (rejuvenative, healing to damaged nerve tissue) |
| Ashvagandhā | 400 mg (improves tone, power and coordination) |
| Balā | 300 mg (maintains vigor and vitality, prevents muscle wasting) |

To this formula, add guggulu in the form of:

Yogarāja guggulu for vāta prakruti

Kaishore guggulu for pitta prakruti

Triphala guggulu for kapha prakruti

If the stroke patient is older and the muscles are wasting, one can give mahāyogarāja guggulu and maha vāta vidhvamsana rasa (which improves communication between the axons and dendrons and enhances neuronal anastomosis).

For virechana, a vāta person can use gandharva harītakī, while someone with pitta prakruti is better with āmalakī. A kapha person may be given bibhītakī, while in all cases you can just close your eyes and give triphala. For any of those medicines, it is good to use ghee and warm water as an *anupāna* (carrier): add one teaspoon of the herb and one teaspoon of ghee into one cup of warm water and drink it.

Many times, a patient of paralysis has urinary incontinence or incontinence of feces. Vacha oil or dashamūla oil basti can be used for these conditions, to improve the tone and coordination of the sphincter muscles of the urethra and the anal sphincter. This can help patients retain their urine and feces.

In men, the cremaster muscle (related to the testicles) can be affected. In that case, he can have ātmaguptā added to his formula to improve the cremasteric reflex.

Along with snehana, svedana, shirodhāra, and virechana, supportive therapy is also beneficial. One important treatment option is physiotherapy. Another is speech therapy, which can retrain patients how to pronounce words.

You can ask the patient to hold a rubber ball and try to squeeze it. This trains the muscles to improve their tone and power. Similarly, you can throw the ball and they can try to catch it.

Other herbal remedies can help to supplement these treatments. For instance, to improve the power of speech, we can rub akarakarabha paste on the person's tongue, in order to stimulate the speech center in the brain. In some cases, this can enable a stroke patient to talk.

If there is word deafness, one can put vacha oil drops into the ears (*karna bindu*). If the person has a speech disorder, one can give orally brahmī, sarasvatī, and vacha to improve their power of speech.

## Important Guidelines for Dealing with Stroke Patients

Stroke patients usually have a speech disorder, so these people cry because they can feel unhappy or miserable. Because they can't express their emotions, they get overwhelmed and then frustrated.

We should pay attention to these emotional factors and give the person tender loving care. I used to work with stroke patients in a hospital. I would write a letter to the patients' family, who often neglect the patient, saying they need more love because they are dependent and need constant care. We should pay attention and give them courage and support. Stroke is a long, lingering disorder. It happens quickly, but it takes a long time to heal.

## Prevention of Stroke

Certain precautions can be taken to prevent strokes and transient ischemic attacks. Angiography and arteriography can be used to find out the condition of the cerebral blood vessels, and whether there is a small aneurism, kink, or blood clot. Then one can implement a proper preventative protocol.

If a person has hypertension, we need to monitor the blood pressure and also control triglyceride and cholesterol levels. If the patient is diabetic, then we must manage the person's blood sugar as well.

Every person over age 60 should regularly check their cholesterol, triglyceride and sugar levels. Anyone concerned about stroke should stop smoking or drinking hard liquor, although a glass of wine is fine for vasodilatation.

There are alternatives to the prescription drugs used in modern medicine. To regulate blood pressure, one can use punarnavā, passion flower, hawthorn berry and sarpagandha. If there is high cholesterol, one can take flax seed oil or other omega 3 fatty acids as well as triphala guggulu, shilājit, neem, and kutki. For diabetes, Ayurveda suggests gurmar, vasant kusumakar ras, neem, and turmeric to regulate the blood sugar.

So we can deal with these different disorders with an Ayurvedic protocol, but it is always advisable to do this in conjunction with your medical doctor.

## Chapter 37

# Restless Legs Syndrome

Winter 2015, Volume 28, Number 3

RESTLESS LEGS SYNDROME or restless foot syndrome is called *nakte pada chaltvam* in Sanskrit. This means "shaking the legs at night", which refers to the characteristic nocturnal jerking movements.

According to Ayurveda, restless legs syndrome is due to increased vāta. In particular, it is caused by an increase in the mobile (chala) and irregular (vishama) attributes of vāta dosha. Because the legs are the main site affected, it indicates the disorder is due to disturbed apāna vāyu.

In restless legs syndrome, vāta dosha from the colon undergoes accumulation (sanchaya), provocation (prakopa), and then spreads (prasara). During this prasara stage, vāta moves into the rasa and rakta dhātus, which are the plasma and hematopoietic system. It can then circulate throughout the body, and in this case, it deposits into the musculoskeletal system, disturbing the lower extremities. The māmsa and majjā dhātus (the muscle, bone marrow, and nerve tissues) are most affected.

*V→ R/R→ mamsa/ majjā*

### Causes

Though the precise cause of this condition is still unknown in modern medicine, we can understand the disorder from an Ayurvedic point of view. Anything that aggravates vāta can be a causative factor. This includes vāta-provoking diet and lifestyle. A person whose diet and lifestyle is vāta aggravating is more likely to get restless legs syndrome.

Vāta is mobile, so elevated vāta often results in twitching and restlessness. This increased mobile attribute causes the restlessness that is typical in the syndrome, affecting the legs and feet. The vishama attribute of vāta causes the symptoms to come and go. Because of vāta's cold quality, there may be constriction of the blood vessels, resulting in decreased blood supply to the lower extremities.

Some authorities consider this syndrome to be brought about or intensified by poor circulation. This is *rasa-rakta gata vāta,* in which increased vāta affects rasa and rakta dhātus. If circulation is poor in the lower extremities, the feet feel cold and to get rid of that feeling, the person moves the legs.

Some authorities believe that restless legs syndrome is more common in hyperactive patients. Excessive exercise, or exercising at the wrong time, can severely aggravate vāta dosha. People who do intense physical activity just before going to bed are especially prone to this disorder.

Other authorities believe a lack of physical activity is a key trigger. The human body needs movement. Anyone who does not do much physical activity, just sitting at home and watching TV, or doing sedentary work, is also more likely to suffer from restless legs syndrome. In that case, the body demands more action, and if the person tries to sleep after a day of inactivity, the legs can be restless from this unfulfilled desire of the body to move.

A number of other etiological factors can also activate the mobile and irregular attributes of vāta in māmsa and majjā dhātus, thereby resulting in restless legs syndrome. These include:

- Chronic constipation
- Diverticulosis
- Iron-deficiency anemia
- Irritable bowel syndrome (IBS)
- Kidney stones or a stone in the bladder or ureter
- Pregnancy
- Renal colic
- Side effects of medications (drug-induced)
- Stimulants, such as caffeine, tobacco or psychotropic drugs

Additionally, this syndrome may be due to an itching or creeping sensation in the lower extremity, which can be so powerful that there is an irresistible urge to move the legs.

## Symptoms

This syndrome produces a number of symptoms. These include:

- restless legs when lying in bed at night, especially the thigh and calf muscles
- twitching of the muscles
- shakiness
- difficulty falling asleep at night because of uncomfortable feeling or jerky sensations within the legs
- subjective feeling of uneasiness

Movement often relieves the discomfort, because movement increases circulation and helps the muscles to relax. However, as a result of moving the legs, normal sleep is disrupted and in some cases there is hardly any sleep at all. Consequently, the person is often excessively tired the next day.

Most of the time, someone with restless legs syndrome will suffer from insomnia. Being unable to fall asleep or stay asleep is almost always the result of this being a chronic condition, but the insomnia can also aggravate the symptoms. Effect becomes cause; cause becomes effect.

The symptoms occur mainly at vāta times (dawn and dusk, and early morning hours) or at the end of the day when someone goes to bed feeling excessively tired or fatigued. The condition is worse in cold climates. Restless legs syndrome most commonly affects middle-aged women.

## Diagnosis

Diagnosis can be generally made by doing a thorough physical examination, and taking a proper medical history and family health history, pinning down every sign and symptom that the patient is going through. A physician should rule out other neurological disorders that may be an underlying cause, such as thyroid disorders, renal colic, and anemia.

# Management

Internally, the person should take the following herbal remedy to calm down vāta dosha.

| | |
|---|---|
| Dashamūla | 500 mg, specific to vāta dosha |
| Ashvagandhā | 400 mg, relaxes the muscles |
| Tagara | 200 mg, tranquilizer |
| Mustā | 200 mg, muscle sedative |

This mixture should be given three times a day before food.

Take ½ teaspoon of gandharva harītakī at bedtime, to maintain the normal movement (*anuloma*) of vāta dosha.

Before bedtime, the person can drink a cup of *Tranquility Tea* or *Goodnight Sleep Tea*.[50] This will create a mild sedative effect and relax the muscles, which can help to lessen the symptoms. They are natural alternatives to valium; a drug often prescribed that has multiple side effects.

Since the syndrome is connected to the circulatory system, any herbs or other treatments that will increase the circulation will be beneficial.

Don't eat a big meal late at night. Eating a heavy meal will create nightmares, disturb your sleep, and trigger other symptoms.

Avoid coffee, because it is a strong stimulant. Coffee is bitter and astringent and will provoke vāta dosha. Drinking coffee in the late afternoon or evening will definitely worsen the symptoms of Restless Legs Syndrome.

Snehana (oil massage) is an important first-line treatment. Rub and massage mahānārāyana oil or visha garbha tailam (oil) onto the feet and lower legs up to the knees or thighs. Doing this before going to bed will help to relax the legs. If you don't have either of those oils available, use plain cold-pressed sesame oil, or even a 50:50 mixture of mustard oil and vacha oil. Warm the oil before applying it to your legs and feet, especially in cold weather.

---

50. Vasant Lad's formulas, available in our store and online at www.ayurveda.com.

Svedana (steam therapy) is another important therapy. After massaging with mahānārāyana or visha garbha oil, soak both feet up to the calves in a bucket of hot water to which mustard seeds have been added. Place two tablespoons of slightly crushed mustard seeds in a piece of cheesecloth and add to the hot water. Alternatively add baking soda to the warm water. Soak the feet for about 10 to 15 minutes before going to bed to relax your muscles and improve circulation, and it will help reduce the symptoms of restless legs syndrome.

One should do an appropriate amount of exercise to prevent restless legs syndrome. Exercise improves circulation and helps relax the muscles. People report that if they exercise in the afternoon or early evening, they are less likely to get restless legs syndrome at night. Beneficial yogāsanas for restless legs syndrome include palm tree (tadāsana), tree (vriksāsana), eagle (garudāsana), legs up the wall (viparīta karanī), locust (shalabhāsana), plow (halāsana), easy cross-legged (sukhāsana), accomplished (siddhāsana), and lotus (padmāsana). (see yoga poses page 450)

For best results, one should take a brisk walk after dinner. Swimming is a very good form of exercise that improves circulation and relaxes the muscles. This is especially true if swimming in a pool that uses mineral-based purifiers, such as magnesium. Exercise also helps release endorphins, which are natural painkillers, so the pain caused by this syndrome is also relieved by exercise.

Through clinical observation, it can be seen that iron deficiency and lack of other minerals and vitamins can trigger restless legs syndrome. Hence, a good diet and regular multi-vitamin and multi-mineral supplements will help to buck up the blood and relax the muscles.

Some individuals observe that drinking a glass of wine in the evening improves circulation, relaxes the muscles, and eases the restless legs syndrome. Ayurvedic wine such as *drāksha* can be a helpful alternative.

Smokers are more likely have restless legs syndrome, so anyone with this condition who smokes should quit smoking.

If the condition is due to the side effects of psychotropic drug use, nutmeg can be used an antidote. A good mixture for such a situation is ½ teaspoon of ashvagandhā, ½ teaspoon of jatamāmsi, ¼ teaspoon of mustā, and a pinch of nutmeg. This is best taken after dinner, followed by ½ teaspoon of gandharva harītakī at bedtime. Massaging the legs with mahānārāyana oil will also help.

For pregnant woman with this condition, give one cup of warm milk with a teaspoon of *ghee* (clarified butter) daily at bedtime. Additionally, the following herbal remedy can be taken twice daily with warm water—ashvagandhā (½ tsp.), balā (¼ tsp.), and vidārī (¼ tsp.).

If the restless legs syndrome is due to anemia, the person should take 200 mg each of loha bhasma and abhrak bhasma and/or four teaspoons of loha āsava[51] after food, mixed

51. Drāksha and āsava are two kinds of herbalized wine.

with an equal part of water. Natural sources of iron, such as currants, raisins and beets, can be included in the diet.

If the condition is caused or aggravated by caffeine consumption, eliminate coffee and other caffeinated drinks such as tea and cola. In addition, increase protein and grain drinks, such as kefir, as well as soups made with barley, quinoa, and so forth.

Chapter 38

# Maintaining a Healthy Brain

Spring 2016, Volume 28, Number 4

THE BRAIN IS a vital organ. This major organ is governed by majjā dhātu (nerve tissue) and is fundamental to the central nervous system. According to Ayurveda, the ancient system of medicine from India, three subdoshas–tarpaka kapha, sādhaka pitta, and prāna vāta–are responsible for the organization of the brain. Prāna vāta carries sensory information to the brain and the motor responses, while sādhaka pitta governs higher intellectual function, understanding, and comprehension. Tarpaka kapha is a sensitive film that records all experiences.

Ayurveda teaches that brain health depends upon the functional integrity between prāna vāta, sādhaka pitta, and tarpaka kapha. The brain is the main seat of consciousness, memory, intellect, reasoning, and understanding. The entire personality depends upon the development of the brain. In Ayurvedic philosophy, a balanced brain is made up of pure awareness and is an expression of consciousness through the cerebrum (in Sanskrit, *shiro-brahma*). It maintains equilibrium of the body through the cerebellum (*shiroloma*).

The brain cells are constantly thinking, feeling and evaluating. Thought is a complex biochemical, neuromagnetic, and neuroelectrical response from the memory cells. Due to the constant interaction of thoughts, feelings and emotions, each thought creates a groove in the brain. The brain feels comfortable working along the grooves. In this context, the human brain is somewhat limited.

From the accumulation of these grooves, the brain becomes bruised. This bruising process makes the brain senile, so the brain becomes slow and sluggish in daily life, and the person starts forgetting things. The brain undergoes degeneration and decay and literally starts to shrink. Many neurons simply die, which leads to memory loss and an inadequate response to challenges. This, in turn, leads to faster aging. That is why the brain needs *rasāyana* (rejuvenation), which is an important aspect of Ayurvedic therapy.

The following are three major Ayurveda rasāyana herbs that benefit the brain. Brahmī supports sādhaka pitta, jatamāmsi sustains tarpaka kapha, and shankha pushpī maintains prāna vāta.

## Brahmī

Brahmī (*Centella asiatica*) works on sādhaka pitta by maintaining cellular intelligence, understanding, and comprehension as well as higher cellular intelligence. It is bitter and astringent, cooling, and has a sweet vipāka (post-digestive effect). It pacifies all three doshas. Brahmī is light, oily, and expansive; it enhances memory and promotes intercellular communication and longevity of cellular life.

Brahmī is anti-epileptic and anti-psychotic. It is the best alterative tonic and mental energizer, and it rejuvenates the brain. It is also a well-known antidepressant according to Ayurvedic literature. Brahmī brings clarity of perception and improves the power of speech. It helps to regulate blood pressure, improves cerebral circulation, and prolongs an individual's lifespan.

In Ayurveda, the herbal form of brahmī can be used as a tablet, steeped as a tea, or taken as *brahmī ghee* (a mixture of the herb with ghee) for nasal administration. Brahmī is the primary herb that maintains the functional integrity of sādhaka pitta.

To preserve brain health, use the herbal preparation brahmī ghee for nasya, which is the application of herbalized substances inside the nose. Put five drops of lukewarm brahmī ghee into each nostril. This application will activate the right and left breath cycles, which will work on sādhaka pitta and unfold cellular intelligence, understanding, and comprehension, helping to maintain cellular awareness. Ayurveda teaches in-depth about prānāyāma (breathing exercises) and meditation, and brahmī ghee nasya is of benefit to both of these.

## Jatamāmsi

Jatamāmsi (*Nardostachys jatamamsi*) works specifically on tarpaka kapha and it improves the functional integrity of the three sub-doshas in the brain: tarpaka kapha, sādhaka pitta and prāna vāta.

Jatamāmsi is bitter, astringent and sweet, cooling, and has a sweet vipāka. It pacifies all three doshas. Its *prabhāva* (special effect) is that it improves memory and cellular intelligence. This herb is called *bhūta nashini* in Sanskrit, which means it removes possession by evil spirits.

Jatamāmsi nourishes cellular perception and retains cellular information within the deep matrix of tarpaka kapha. Tarpaka kapha performs nutritional nourishment of cellular perception and sensation. Cellular information and all life experience are recorded on the sensitive field of tarpaka kapha. Jatamāmsi supports access to recent and remote memory, and it works great with brahmī to enhance moment-to-moment awareness.

This herb is a nervine tonic and it improves the cognitive function of brain cells, promotes good color complexion, and is a tranquilizer and an anticonvulsant. It unfolds tranquility, inner peace, and bliss. Jatamāmsi can be used as an herbal tea and as an herbalized oil that is applied to the skin. This application to the skin opens the doors of perception to a deeper level of consciousness.

## Shankha Pushpī

Shankha pushpī (*Evolvulus alsinoides*) works primarily on prāna vāta, which includes coordination between sensory stimuli and motor responses. Prāna is the vital life force and maintains cellular respiration. According to Ayurveda, in the human body, every cell is the center of cellular awareness, every cell is a conscious living functional unit of the body, and every cell has cellular intelligence, cellular memory, and cellular communication. The flow of cellular communication and intelligence is prāna. Therefore, this communication is essential to maintain brain health.

Shankha pushpī is astringent and bitter, cooling, and it has a sweet vipāka (post-digestive effect). A general rejuvenative tonic, it pacifies all three doshas. It maintains cellular respiration, promotes memory, and improves the flow of cellular intelligence. This cellular communication is necessary to maintain brain health.

Shankha pushpī also reduces fever and inflammation, is a liver detoxifier and anthelmintic (treats worms and parasites), and acts as an anti-epileptic. It is acts as an aphrodisiac and mild tranquilizer, and it reduces depression. Finally, it helps to bind the stools, so is commonly used for diarrhea.

Shankha pushpī can be used as an herbal tea, taken as a powder with warm water, or used as an herbalized, medicated oil on the skin. It can also be taken as an herbalized ghee, 1 teaspoon twice a day. This ghee decoction directly nourishes the myelin sheath, helping to prevent multiple sclerosis and Alzheimer's disease.

### Tips for Improving Brain Function

- Regular exercise – over the age of 40, memory starts to decline and the brain starts to deteriorate. Regular exercise improves the blood flow to the brain, which aids the act of thinking and enhances memory.
- Memorize a poem or sūtra by heart – this is a drill or exercise for the memory faculty.
- Tune into television talk shows – this is an easy way to meet new people (via TV), and it stimulates the memory faculty to remember the names of the guests and so forth.
- Read the dictionary to improve your vocabulary.
- Remember rhymes – memory is association.
- Eat foods rich in beta carotene – carrots, dark green vegetables and certain fruits are abundant in beta carotene and stimulate sādhaka agni.
- Walnuts, almonds and cashews support tarpaka agni.
- Sūrya namaskāra (Sun Salutation) is a great form of daily yoga.
- Yogāsana – shoulder stand, plough pose, and many other āsanas are beneficial for memory.
- Bhrāmarī and Ujjāyi prānāyāma are particularly good to improve memory.

# The Use of Ghee

Ghee is clarified butter. It is an ancient formula coming from cow's milk and is the pure essence of the milk. The milk is turned into thick, creamy yoghurt. This is churned into butter and then clarified into ghee. Ghee sustains the myelin sheath.[52] It maintains ojas (immunity), and tejas (cellular intelligence), and the balance of prāna (flow of cellular communication).

> **HOW TO MAKE AN HERBALIZED GHEE**
>
> Take one part of the herb or herbal compound and sixteen parts of water and mix in a pot and cook on medium heat.
>
> Powdered herbs (churna) are best to use but you can use the whole herb.
>
> Stir occasionally, so the herb is not burned. Boil this down until only one fourth of the concoction remains.
>
> Then, add the same quantity of oil or ghee.[1] Cook it, stirring as necessary, until no water remains.
>
> In this slow, time-consuming process, the qualities of the herbs are yielded into the oil or ghee. Strain the oil or ghee, leaving behind the solid residue.
>
> 1  Instructions on how to prepare ghee can be found on our website: https://www.ayurveda.com/recipes/ghee

Ghee is a *yogavāhi,* which means the properties of medicated ghee act as a catalytic agent, carrying the healing qualities of brahmī, jatamāmsi, and shankha pushpī into the subtle cellular level of the connective tissues and nervous system. This is the case whether it is given orally, nasally, or in the form of a medicated oil applied to the skin.

On the cellular level, the cell membrane is well lubricated by ghee. On the systemic level, the bone marrow can be nourished by ghee. The functional aspect of ghee maintains the strength, vigor, and integrity of the myelin sheath, protecting this protective covering, which is so central to brain health.

## Neurotransmitters and Hormones

According to the ancient Vedic system of Ayurveda, brahmī, jatamāmsi, and shankha pushpī improve neural communication. These herbs keep the neurotransmitters and hormones of the brain, such as serotonin, melatonin, and acetylcholine, well balanced. Production of serotonin is stimulated by brahmī, acetylcholine is augmented by jatamāmsi, and melatonin is improved by shankha pushpī. These herbs work on a hormonal level through the three doshas to regenerate the human brain. Used together, they help the brain to become bright, brilliant, and blissful.[53]

# Techniques to Rejuvenate Nerve Function

Panchakarma measures are commonly used in Ayurveda to maintain brain health. The brain is the seat of prāna vāta, sādhaka pitta, tarpaka kapha, and majjā dhātu. Prāna vāta carries sensory information to the brain and the motor responses; sādhaka pitta governs higher intellectual function, understanding, and comprehension and yields into understanding of sensory stimuli into knowledge and experience. Tarpaka kapha is a storehouse of this knowledge and information.

There are twelve cranial nerves. Some serve a purely sensory function, others are purely motor, and the remaining cranial nerves perform both sensory and motor functions. Due to over-stimulation of sensory and motor activities, the brain becomes tired. This yields into stress.

---

52. *Dictionary.com,* "myelin sheath: a wrapping of myelin around certain nerve axons, serving as an electrical insulator that speeds nerve impulses to muscles and other effectors." reference http://www.dictionary.com/browse/myelin-sheath, downloaded April 09, 2016.
53. The Ayurvedic Institute sells a special rejuvenative brain tonic, Medhya Rasayana Intelligence Tea, as well as brahmī ghee.

Ancient Ayurvedic panchakarma therapies are an important way to help maintain brain health. The diagram on page page 314 gives us a relationship between various panchakarma measures according to the twelve cranial nerves. In due course, these therapies yield into perfect brain health.

Nasya works on the olfactory nerve and relieves the stress in the olfactory bulb in the brain through the cribriform plate.

*Netra basti* works on the entire optical pathway, including the optic nerve, optic chiasm, lateral geniculate body, and optic radiation. It goes to the occipital cortex. Oculomotor, trochlear and abducens are motor nerves that govern the eccentric muscles of the eye bulbs. Netra basti works on these motor activities.

The trigeminal nerve has three major branches: the optic, olfactory and lingual. This is sensory to the tongue and motor to the nasal passage and eyeball. Ayurveda suggests *kavala* (swishing oil) and *gandūsha* (gargling) as treatments for the trigeminal nerve. The molecules of sesame or coconut oil used in kavala stimulate the trigeminal nerve and relieve the stress in the related areas to unfold a divine smile on the face.

The facial nerve supplies all muscles of facial expression. Do abhyanga (oil massage) of the facial muscles and stimulation of the facial marma points (Adhipati, Bhrūh, Agra, Apānga, Adha and Ūrdhva Ganda, Oshtha, Chibuka, and Hanu, see page 457). This protocol will relieve facial paralysis, ptosis, and stress on the facial area.

The auditory nerve has two branches: the vestibular and cochlear. Disorders include tinnitus and deafness, which induce stress in the temporal lobe of the brain. *Karna pūrana,* which is filling the ears with medicated oil, enables the subtle oil molecules to travel along the tract of the vestibular and cochlear nerve and relieve stress in the temporal lobe of the brain.

The glossopharyngeal nerve supplies the back part of the tongue and the pharynx and assists with the act of swallowing. Stress can build up in the throat. Ayurveda suggests relieving the stress by doing gandūsha, which is gargling. Do gandūsha with a glass of warm water and half a teaspoon each of sea salt and turmeric. Do not do gandūsha with oil, as you may choke!

The vagus nerve interfaces with the parasympathetic control of the gastrointestinal (GI) tract, lungs and heart. *Vamana* works on the stomach and the lungs, while virechana

---

**NETRA BASTI**

To do netra basti, make a dough of whole-wheat flour or urad dal flour. Shape it like a round doughnut or bagel, and seal it to the skin around the eyes by applying gentle pressure to the skin with wet fingers, so it is leak-proof.

The patient lies comfortably on his or her back, with the head slightly tilted to the opposite side. Then, lukewarm[1] but still liquid ghee is poured into the pool created by the dough, so that the person's eyes and eyelashes are totally covered in ghee. The person then gradually opens and closes both eyes and lies like that for up to 40 minutes.[2]

---

1 **Note:** be very careful of the temperature of the ghee. It should *never be too hot*; not above skin temperature.
2 Lad, BAM&S, MASc, Vasant. *Textbook of Ayurveda: General Principles of Management and Treatment*, Volume Three, the Ayurvedic Press, Albuquerque 2012, p. 176. Excerpted with permission.

works on the small intestine and basti works on the colon. These panchakarma measures remove the stress from the hypothalamus.

The accessory nerve is a motor nerve that supplies the muscles of the neck, shoulders, and trapezius. A disorder of this nerve can cause tension in the neck and base of skull. For that, Ayurveda suggests *manya skandha basti.* This is the application of warm medicated oil to the neck and shoulder area. Using whole wheat dough, create an inverted Y-shaped dam or pool over the neck and shoulders, affixing the dough to the skin. Fill this pool with warm medicated oil. Mahānārāyana oil is commonly used. When there is āma, use vishagarbha oil.

The final nerve is the hypoglossal nerve. Ayurveda suggests scraping the tongue when you get up each morning. Gently scrape the tongue from back to front seven times. That scraping will stimulate the hypoglossal nerve and relieve the stress from the hypothalamus and medulla oblongata. Practice a gentle facial marma massage like the one on page 457.

# Various Panchakarma Measures to Maintain Brain Health

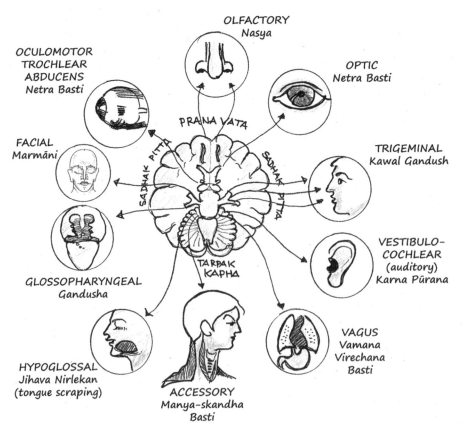

OLFACTORY
Nasya

OCULOMOTOR
TROCHLEAR
ABDUCENS
Netra Basti

OPTIC
Netra Basti

FACIAL
Marmāni

PRANA VATA

TRIGEMINAL
Kawal Gandush

SADHAK PITTA

SADHAK PITTA

VESTIBULO-
COCHLEAR
(auditory)
Karna Pūrana

GLOSSOPHARYNGEAL
Gandusha

TARPAK
KAPHA

HYPOGLOSSAL
Jihava Nirlekan
(tongue scraping)

ACCESSORY
Manya-skandha
Basti

VAGUS
Vamana
Virechana
Basti

# Chapter 39

# Neuralgia
## Sanchāri Vedana

Spring 2017, Volume 29, Number 4

• • • • • • • • • • • • • • • • • • • • • • • • • • • • • • • • • • • • • • • • • • • • • • •

### *Nahi vātādrute shūlam*
There is no pain without disturbance of vāta dosha.

• • • • • • • • • • • • • • • • • • • • • • • • • • • • • • • • • • • • • • • • • • • • • • •

WHENEVER THERE IS DISTURBED SPACE in a srotas (channel or pathway), such as the sinews or nerve tract, there will be pain. Whenever these spaces are clogged by āma or excess kapha or pitta dosha, it can cause congestion, inflammation and pain.

The modern concept of neuralgia is quite closely connected to the Ayurvedic group of diseases called *vāta vyādhi*. Vāta vyādhi means a condition in which vāta dosha is high in majjā dhātu, and often in māmsa dhātu, creating pain along the tract of a nerves, called *sanchāri vedana*. This group of vāta vyādhi diseases is neuromuscular or neurological conditions that are difficult to cure.

In neuralgia, there is severe recurring pain along the course of a nerve. 'Neuro' means a nerve or nerve tissue and 'algia' means pain, so the term neuralgia means pain along the tract of a nerve.

## Causes of Neuralgia: General Signs and Symptoms

Neuralgia pain is caused by either pressure on the nerve trunk or faulty nerve nutrition. This may be because of vitamin $B_{12}$ deficiency or even vitamin $B_6$ deficiency. It can be due to toxins (āma) or to increased vāta pushing pitta in the majjā dhātu, which causes inflammation of the nerves. All these factors are connected to the neuralgia.

In Ayurvedic literature, pain is called *shūla*. A Sanskrit sūtra says, *"Nahi vatādrute shūlam"*. This means there is no pain without disturbance of vāta dosha. Hence, aggravated vāta is the main inner cause of neuralgia. There are two internal causes of vāta disturbance. One is called *mārgava rodha,* which means clogged channels. The other is dhātu kshaya, which means depletion, deterioration and degeneration of the tissue.

. . . . . . . . . . . . . . . . . . . . . . . . . . . . . . . . . . . . . . . . . . . . . . . . . . . . . . . . . . . . .

Whenever there is disturbed space in a srotas (channel or pathway), such as the sinews or nerve tract, there will be pain. Whenever these spaces are clogged by āma or excess kapha or pitta dosha, it can cause congestion, inflammation and pain.

. . . . . . . . . . . . . . . . . . . . . . . . . . . . . . . . . . . . . . . . . . . . . . . . . . . . . . . . . . . . .

The first cause of *vata dushti* is mārgava rodha, which means clogging of the channels or pathways. The five subtypes of vata move in a specific directions or vectors. Prāna vāyu moves downward, apāna vāyu also moves downward in the pelvic cavity, udāna vāyu moves upward, vyāna vāyu moves in a circular direction, and samāna vāyu has a horizontal or linear movement. The vector of vāta dosha is a natural movement in a particular direction. When that movement is blocked, either by pitta, kapha or āma, it usually leads to pain.

Pain is also called *dukha* in Sanskrit. *Du* means disturbed and *kha* means space. Whenever there is disturbed space in a srotas (channel or pathway), such as the sinews or nerve tract, there will be pain. When these spaces are clogged by āma or excess kapha or pitta dosha, it can cause congestion, inflammation and pain. Sometimes increased vāta alone may push āma into the pathway of a srotas and the space gets disturbed. This disturbed space can cause pain.

Bodily tissues are made up of atoms, cells, and connective tissue, so when the atoms are separated, it creates gaps or spaces, causing the tissues to lose their mass. This leads to degeneration, decay, destruction or atrophy. This important internal cause of vāta aggravation is *dhātu kshaya janita vāta prakopa,* which means vāta is aggravated because of degenerative changes in the tissues.

The symptoms of dhātu kshaya will be intimately connected to the attributes of vāta dosha. Vāta is rūksha (dry) and this quality of vāta can create dryness in the tissues. Rasa dhātu can become depleted, resulting in subtle cellular dehydration, leading to dhātu kshaya. This is all due to the dry quality. This kind of neuralgia pain is relieved by oil massage and by giving the person plenty of fluids.

Another quality of vāta is shīta (cold). Cold can create constriction or spasm of the tissues. When the connective tissue, muscle tissue or sinew is contracted, it becomes stiff and hard, which may lead to severe pain. That can be relieved by the application of heat, such as a warm compress or hot bath.

A third important attribute of vāta is khāra (rough). The rough quality of vāta dosha may cause hardness or roughness of the tissue, and these hard, stiff, rough tissues are difficult to move. If the person moves, it causes pain because of the breaking of the tissue. This can be relieved by nourishing herbs, such as ashvagandhā, balā and vidhari, along with milk or ghee.

The last important quality of vāta is chala (mobile). Vāta pain is radiating, fluctuating, shifting and migrating pain or referred pain. It can be shooting, throbbing, pulsating pain, and can also be excruciating, spasmodic or colicky pain. This kind of pain can be relieved by bed rest or resting localized areas by applying a bandage or tourniquet.

Even though the sūtra says there is no pain without disturbed vāta dosha, the qualities of pitta can also be expressed by the pain when vāta is disturbed by pitta dosha. Pitta pain is sharp, penetrating, hot, inflammatory, burning pain. This type of pain indicates that pitta is blocking vāta or vāta is pushing pitta in the nervous system. It will create burning, sucking, pulling, or sharp pain, and pain on pressure, which is tenderness. These are all typical characteristics of pitta (inflammatory) pain. Any kind of neuralgia has radiating, fluctuating, or lightning, which is all due to aggravated vāta. However sharp or burning pain and tenderness are due to the involvement of pitta.

When vāta dosha is blocked by kapha, or vāta pushes kapha dosha, then the pain is localized, static, deep, dull, and/or aching pain. This is because kapha is heavy, dull, static and cloudy.

Āma is a toxic, metabolic waste that can build up at the cellular level, at the systemic level in the dhātus and srotāmsi, and in the gastrointestinal tract. Āma is a sticky substance and when it enters into a tissue it will create āma pain, called *āma shūla.* That pain is similar to kapha pain: local, static, dull, aching pain.

Clinically we can distinguish the type of pain through the application of *upashaya,* which is a therapeutic trial. Generally vāta pain is relieved by warn oil massage, hot baths, nutritive herbs and rest, which will pacify the dry, cold, rough and mobile qualities of vāta dosha. Many times vāta pain can also be relieved by the application of pressure, because vāta is mobile and the pressure helps to bring more stability.

On the other hand, cold compresses and anti-inflammatory herbs, such as sandalwood, turmeric, neem, or camphor, relieve pitta pain. A cooling, calming, anti-inflammatory herbal paste can relieve inflammatory pitta pain.

Kapha pain can be relieved by deep massage, or by movement of the body, such as walking and underwater exercise. Whenever exercise relieves the pain, it indicates kapha pain, because kapha is static and the movement helps to pacify kapha and move excess kapha away from the srotas. Most forms of exercise relieve kapha pain.

Āma shūla can be relieved by dīpana and pāchana therapies, which means kindling agni (digestive fire) and burning āma (metabolic toxic waste). For that purpose, we can give chitrak and trikatu (ginger, black pepper and long pepper). These herbs can increase agni and burn āma, as does āma pāchak vati. Topically, you can apply ginger paste or cinnamon paste or even garlic paste. Those hot, sharp, penetrating herbs will burn the molecules of āma, relieve the *sroto rodha* (clogged channel) and the pain will disappear.

Neuralgic pain is marked by brief attacks of severe lightning or stabbing-like pain. It may disturb one or many branches of the nerve. The attack can last for a few seconds to a few minutes. It can be triggered by touch, cold, chewing, brushing the teeth, smiling, loud laughter or loud talking. It occurs most frequently in persons over the age of 40, which is the pitta age.

## General Management of Neuralgia

The Ayurvedic approach is to deal with the root cause, which is generally vāta pushing pitta dosha in the nerve tissue. We use analgesic herbs such as kaishore guggulu, ashvagandhā, and balā, along with vāta-pacifying herbs such as dashamūla and anti-inflammatory herbs such as gudūchi and kāma dudhā. Other typical treatments include *kavala* (oil pulling or swishing), nasya, abhyanga (oil massage), snehana, svedana, shirodhāra and shiro basti.

Nasya is a particularly useful therapy for trigeminal neuralgia as is netra basti. Gargling is beneficial for glossopharyngeal neuralgia, and application of analgesic paste on the chest area is helpful for intercostal neuralgia.

### Generalized Neuralgic Pain
We have to treat both vāta and pitta. In generalized neuralgic pain throughout the body, we can use the following herbal protocol:

| | |
|---|---|
| Dashamūla | 500 mg (pacifies vāta dosha) |
| Ashvagandhā | 400 mg (pacifies vāta and works on neuromuscular cleft) |
| Kaishore guggulu | 200 mg (anti-inflammatory) |
| Kāma dudhā | 200 mg (anti-inflammatory) |
| Tagara | 200 mg (analgesic and tranquilizer) |

## Trigeminal Neuralgia
Trigeminal neuralgia is facial neuralgia pain and it is common in old age. This is a disease of the trigeminal nerve when systemic vāta dosha pushes pitta into the majjā dhātu. It is marred by brief attacks of severe lightning pain along the tract of the nerve and it can move along the branches of the nerve, such as the maxillary nerve. The attack usually lasts for between two seconds to two minutes and it can be triggered by touch, exposure to the cold, chewing, brushing the teeth, or even smiling and loud laughter.

### The Trigeminal Nerve

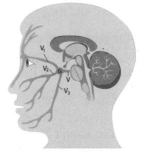

Localized pain or tenderness is present along the passage of the nerve.

The trigeminal nerve has three nuclei and three major branches. These are the nasal, oral, and ophthalmic nerves. In trigeminal neuralgia, the pain from the temple mandibular joint goes to the forehead, eyes, nose, or mouth.

Facial neuralgia symptoms include pain in the facial muscles of expression, muscle pain, muscle spasm and you will see the affected site looks a little dry and cold. The cause may be pressure of the blood vessel on the trigeminal root.

### Trigeminal Neuralgic Pain
In this condition, use this herbal remedy three times per day:

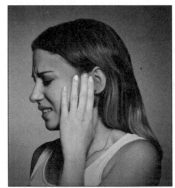

Sudden severe lancinating pain along the tract of the trigeminal nerve. The pain is provoked by touch, cold or movements of the face in eating or talking.

| | |
|---|---|
| Ashvagandhā | 500 mg |
| Balā | 400 mg |

| Vidhari | 300 mg |
| Tagara | 200 mg |
| Yogarāja guggulu | 200 mg |

In modern medicine, strong analgesics and tranquilizers such as carbamazepine are used to treat trigeminal neuralgia. Many times, even though the patient is taking analgesic medication, the pain persists. In those cases, surgical intervention is often advised. In this surgery, the nerve ganglion is cut. That means the pain goes, but it's not usually a good idea to cut the pathway of the nerve. Instead of surgery, we should try Ayurvedic treatments.

Mostly, trigeminal neuralgia is vāta-type radiating pain, so we need to pacify vāta dosha. If there is inflammation and the nerves become tender, use kaishore guggulu instead of yogarāja guggulu to pacify pitta dosha.

In addition, do a gentle facial massage with a mixture of coconut oil and mahānārāyana oil. Also do netra basti with plain ghee and nasya with anu tailam. Holding and swishing a mouthful of sesame oil or coconut oil, called kavala or oil pulling, is another special Ayurvedic remedy for neuralgic pain in the facial area.

Marma therapy is helpful, especially the shankha, apānga, kapola nāsā, kapola madhya, ūrdhva gandha, adha gandha, and kanīnaka marma points. (see page 457)

### Glossopharyngeal Neuralgia

Glossopharyngeal neuralgic pain is due to neuralgia along the course of the glossopharyngeal nerve. It is characterized as pain in the back of the throat and tonsils, and it can be referred to the middle ear. For this kind of pain, we can gargle a glass of warm water with half a teaspoon each of turmeric and sea salt. One can also use khadiradi vati or lavanga vati achusanam (achusanam means lozenges). Using lozenges and also gargling will relieve glossopharyngeal neuralgia pain.

Neuralgia along the course of the glossopharyngeal nerve with severe pain in the throat and middle ear.

### Cardiac Neuralgia

In neuralgia, the pain is along the tract of a nerve. In cardiac neuralgia, it is typical angina pectoris pain from the cardiac area that travels to the jaw, goes to the shoulder, and follows along the tract of the meridian and it can go to the tip of the pinky finger.

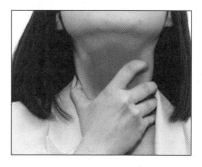

This is a specific herbal protocol for cardiac neuralgia pain, called angina pectoris. Because this can be a serious medical condition, you should consult with your cardiologist or medical professional. You may need to monitor your blood pressure, cholesterol, and ischemia.

### Cardiac Neuralgia

Such cardiac neuralgic pain is relieved by the following herbal formula:

Arjuna              200 mg
Pushkaramūla        200 mg
Kasturi (deer musk) 200 mg or Shringa bhasma (deer horn ash) 200 mg – both these act as a coronary vasodilator.

## Post-Herpetic Neuralgia

This type of neuralgia is a complication of shingles and can occur in a nerve anywhere in the body, wherever the shingles occurred. It can be quite severe and last for months or even years, as the virus lays hidden in the neuromuscular cleft. Even though the shingles may be gone, the pain can remain.

In modern medicine, there is no cure for shingles. The treatment focuses on reducing pain.

In some cases of post-herpetic neuralgia, antidepressant and anti-seizure medications may be given to the patient, as well as electrical stimulation of the affected area and analgesics to reduce the pain. Steroid drugs to reduce nerve inflammation can be effective, but must be taken soon after the shingles occurs. A good Ayurvedic anti-inflammatory formula is the combination of equal parts of licorice, neem, and gudūchi, taken three times daily.

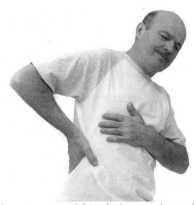

*Herpes zoster (shingles) pain along the track of the intercostal nerve.*

### Post-Herpetic Neuralgia

A useful Ayurvedic herbal painkiller for shingles is:

Shatāvarī            500 mg
Tagara               300 mg
Gulvel sattva        200 mg
Kaishore guggulu     200 mg
Kāma dudhā           200 mg

This formula can be taken three times daily. These are all anti-inflammatory herbs that relieve burning sensations and also act as analgesics.

## Hallucinatory Neuralgia

In this condition, there is an impression of local pain without an actual stimulus that causes the pain. This hallucinatory neuralgic pain is due to *mano vaha sroto dushti*. Mano vaha srotas (the mind) and *majjā vaha srotas* (the nervous system) are intimately connected. The frontal lobe, amygdala, hippocampus, and hypothalamus are all associated with the neuronal pathways of the mind.

When vāta or pitta is high in majjā dhātu, the patient gets a psychological impression of pain along the nerve, without any actual stimulation. Hallucination is a permanent false impression. There must have been previous pain, which creates a khavaigunya in the mind. Then the cellular memory may trigger more of that pain.

The patient subjectively feels pain. However, there is no inflammation, irritation or other physical factor that is causing the pain. It is a psychological impression of pain. Due to a memory, the patient feels pain. Even if you press the nerve there is no pain. The person says, "Oh, the pain came and just now it went".

Actually, there is nothing there that is causing the pain, but the memory of past pain can trigger hallucinatory neuralgic pain in a certain area of the body, depending upon which nerve was affected. It may be a facial nerve, the glossopharyngeal nerve or the optic nerve.

In this condition, we have to treat the mind with 200 mg each of brahmī, jatamāmsi, shankha pushpī, and tagara. These herbs will take care of hallucinatory neuralgia pain.

## Intercostal Neuralgia

This is pain between the ribs. It is frequently associated with the eruption of herpes zoster on the chest and with costochondritis, which is inflammation of the costochondral joint. This pain occurs along the tract of the intercostal nerve. Causes can include hypothermia, infection, diabetes, or rheumatoid arthritis.

A classic example is eruption of herpes zoster or shingles with a rash along the tract of the intercostal nerve. Even when the rash disappears and the herpes zoster is gone, the pain remains for months.

Topically, you can apply red sandalwood and turmeric paste. Red sandalwood is analgesic and both these herbs are anti-inflammatory.

### Intercostal Neuralgia

For intercostal neuralgia, we can use:

| | |
|---|---|
| Kaishore guggulu | 200 mg |
| Kāma dudhā | 200 mg |
| Mustā | 200 mg |
| Tagara | 200 mg |

## Mammary Neuralgia

In some women and girls, there is mammary neuralgia, which is neuralgic pain of the breasts. This is due to vyāna vāyu pushing rañjaka pitta in the rasa vaha srotas and rasa dhātu. The upadhātu of rasa dhātu is rajah (menses) and stanya (lactation), so vāta pushing pitta can result in neuralgia of the breasts. That happens in the pre-menstrual period, due to hormonal changes. The woman gets pain in the breast. It starts at the nipple and goes to the base of the breast. The nipples become sensitive to the touch and the breasts are swollen, tender and painful.

Additionally, doing daily massage of the breasts with coconut oil (for pitta), flax seed oil (kapha), or mahānārāyana oil (vāta) can relieve this pain. This massage can be done for five minutes at bedtime.

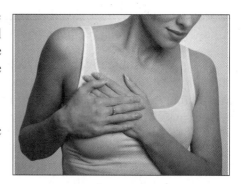

## Mammary Neuralgia

The woman should take the following Ayurvedic herbal remedy:

| | |
|---|---|
| Shatāvarī | 500 mg |
| Gulvel sattva | 300 mg |
| Kāma dudhā | 200 mg |

# Chapter 40

# Multiple Sclerosis

Summer 2017, Volume 30, Number 1

MULTIPLE SCLEROSIS is a book picture of vāta pushing pitta in majjā dhātu, which slowly affects the person's motor functions.

At the cellular level, it [MS] is a condition of tejas burning ojas. In multiple sclerosis, the myelin sheath (containing ojas) has degenerated, after being attacked by tejas, which is part of the body's immune system.

Multiple sclerosis (MS) is also called disseminated sclerosis. It is a demyelinating disorder where vāta pushes pitta in majjā dhātu, the nerve tissue. This is a chronic disease of the central nervous system, including the brain, spinal cord, and spinal nerves. It then goes on to affect māmsa dhātu, the muscles.

At the cellular level, it is a condition of tejas burning ojas. In Ayurveda, we call this disease *māmsa majjā gata vāta pitta,* which is vāta pushing pitta in the māmsa and majjā dhātus.

The protective myelin sheath, which is tarpaka kapha, provides an insulating covering of the nerve fibers. In multiple sclerosis, the myelin sheath[54] (containing ojas) has degenerated, after being attacked by tejas, which is part of the body's immune system. In magnetic resonance imaging (MRI)[55] or a CAT[56] scan, there may be multiple lesions in the medulla or ventricles of the brain and optic nerves.

Multiple sclerosis causes the body's functioning to become impaired, so much so that the person may become a wheelchair user or even die from complications, such as pneumonia or respiratory failure. Alternatively, this disease may only flare up only once in the

---

54. Myelin is a fatty white substance that surrounds the axon of some nerve cells, forming an electrically insulating layer. https://en.wikipedia.org/wiki/Myelin, retrieved March 24, 2017.
55. A technique that uses a magnetic field and radio waves to create detailed images of the organs and tissues within your body.
56. An X-ray image made using computerized axial tomography.

**MULTIPLE SCLEROSIS**

### Healthy

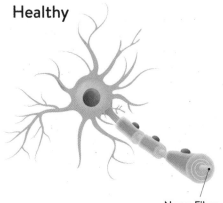

Nerve Fiber

### Nerve Affected by MS

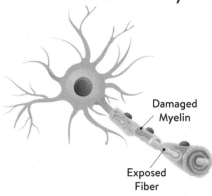

Damaged
Myelin

Exposed
Fiber

person's lifetime, leaving the individual minimally impaired.

### Causes

The exact cause of this disease is not known. Genetic predisposition, indicated by close relatives having multiple sclerosis, is an important factor. Because the person's immune system mistakenly identifies the myelin covering (tarpaka kapha, containing ojas) as a foreign body and tries to destroy it, multiple sclerosis is an autoimmune disease.

Evidentially, it is seen that the nerve cells and nerve sheath play an important role. The immune system treats the nerve tissue as a foreign substance. This is due to long-lingering āma (undigested toxins) in the nervous system. The neighboring cells send a neuroelectrical signal to the nerve cells and there is no response, due to the āma. That makes the immune system attack the myelin sheath.

Secondary etiological factors include:

+ Living in tropical regions, with high temperatures that increase tejas
+ Recurrent exposure to a virus in the brain that can lie dormant in the neuromuscular cleft
+ Persistent measles
+ Infection
+ Stress
+ Exposure to radiation or toxic substances such as arsenic, mercury, or lead
+ Vitamin B$_{12}$ deficiency

Women are more often affected than men are, because ārtava (the female reproductive tissue) is more fiery and supportive of tejas, whereas shukra (the male reproductive tissue) is more cooling and supportive of ojas. The common age of onset is from 20 to 30 years, which is the early part of the pitta period of life.

## Signs and Symptoms
+ Tingling and numbness in the arms and legs
+ Incoordination
+ Difficulty walking and unstable gait
+ Retrobulbar neuritis creating blurry vision, double vision or partial loss of vision
+ Optic neuritis that can cause blindness

- Nystagmus (uncontrolled oscillatory movements of the eyeball)
- Pallor of the optic nerve, due to insufficient blood supply
- Extensive nerve damage
- Facial paralysis
- Trigeminal neuralgia
- Vertigo
- Ataxia (loss of control of body movements)
- Severe muscle fatigue
- Muscle spasms
- Muscle wasting
- Muscle weakness and loss of muscle power and coordination
- Electric shock-like sensations
- Impaired bladder functioning, causing urgency of urination and urinary incontinence
- Recurrent urinary tract infections
- Mood swings, possibly depression
- Impaired speech
- Peripheral itching
- Burning sensations
- Low sex drive
- Staccato stammering speech

| A GOOD HERBAL FORMULA | |
|---|---|
| Dashamūla | 500 mg |
| Ashvagandhā | 400 mg |
| Balā | 300 mg |
| Vidārī | 300 mg |
| Sarasvatī | 200 mg |
| Brahmī | 200 mg |

Take this mixture, 1/2 tsp, three times per day.

The first four herbs are important to improve the muscle functioning, while sarasvatī and brahmī work on the brain and nervous system.

Too much exposure to either heat or cold makes the person tired and debilitated. Multiple sclerosis is a book picture of vāta pushing pitta in majjā dhātu, which slowly affects the person's motor functions. Excess heat aggravates pitta and extreme cold disturbs vāta.

A person with multiple sclerosis gradually becomes disabled, so that he or she is usually a wheelchair user after 10 to 20 years of living with multiple sclerosis.

Diagnosis of MS is done by taking a thorough medical history. Analysis of the spinal fluid shows elevated gamma globulin and more than 70% protein in the cerebrospinal fluid.

## Management

In the treatment protocol, we have to use a muscle relaxant, anti-inflammatory herbs, and passive movement. (see "A Good Herbal Formula" above)

For retinitis, one can use netra basti.

For incontinence, urgency and increased frequency of urination, one can use white sesame seeds (a handful twice a day), which are a good source of calcium and act as a muscle relaxant. This

| IMPAIRED BLADDER FUNCTION | |
|---|---|
| Punarnavā | 500 mg |
| Gokshura | 300 mg |
| Shilājit | 200 mg |

Take this mixture, 1/2 tsp, three times per day.

will help with urinary control. For urinary problems as well as muscle fatigue and incoordination, one can use 200 mg each of vidārī and mustā.

During the early stages of motor disability, one should do regular snehana therapy such as abhyanga (oil massage), svedana (sweating therapy), basti (medicated enema), nasya (nasal administration) and rasāyana chikitsā (rejuvenative therapy). Regular massage can be given with vishagarbha tailam for āma conditions. Vacha oil or brahmī ghee nasya are the best types of nasya for multiple sclerosis.

We have to support the māmsa dhātu, calm down vāta and pitta doshas, relieve inflammation, and support the immune system. One can use chyavanprash as a rejuvenative tonic. Dashamūla arishta, ashvagandhā arishta, and maha rasnadi kvath are other tonics that help to protect the nervous system.

Healthcare professionals should provide supportive therapy and group therapy for multiple sclerosis patients, to improve the quality of their lives. MS patients should also undergo periodic panchakarma detoxification treatments over a two-week program. Finally, they should receive gentle, cooling, calming, soothing treatments, including marma chikitsā therapy that incorporates adhipati (mūrdhni), ājña (sthapanī), shankha, jatru, nābhi, jānu, kshipra and other marma points. (see illustrations on page 458)

Chapter 41

# Glaucoma

Summer 2014, Volume 27, Number 1

GLAUCOMA IS AN EYE DISEASE that is characterized by increased intraocular pressure. In the anterior and posterior chambers of the eyeball, there is a type of kapha called tarpaka kapha, which is clear, transparent, and translucent. In modern medicine, this is known as the vitreous humor.

Normally, there is constant circulation of this vitreous humor from the anterior chamber to the posterior chamber and back. If it becomes stagnant, it causes increased intraocular pressure, resulting in the atrophy of the optic nerve and possibly leading to blindness. Glaucoma is the third most prevalent cause of visual impairment or blindness. Cataracts and macular degeneration are the leading causes of blindness, but they are principally due to aging, whereas glaucoma can happen at any age.

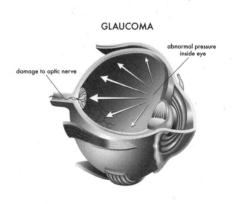

GLAUCOMA

abnormal pressure inside eye

damage to optic nerve

## Nidāna, Causative Factors

In glaucoma, the fluid-regulating mechanism of the eyeball develops a problem. The fluid in the anterior chamber of the eyeball is under a slight degree of pressure, which is normally 14-20mm Hg. If the pressure is more than 20, it is regarded as high. When the pressure has increased, it can damage the sensitive structure of the nerve endings, as well as the optic disc, or it can result in atrophy of the optic nerve.

In this condition, the pressure within the eyeball increases because the fluids are unable to drain away as they normally do. Chronic (open angle) glaucoma occurs when the pressure is increased gradually. There are no symptoms to start with, but there is a gradual blurring of the peripheral vision.

Acute (closed angle) glaucoma is when the pressure suddenly increases. In that case, the sudden increase in pressure blocks the drainage of fluid and causes severe headache or retro-orbital pain. This needs prompt medical treatment—within days.

Both types of glaucoma are common in adults over the age of 40, which is pitta age. In certain families, there is a family history of glaucoma, which indicates there is genetic predisposition to this disease.

Another etiological factor is the long-term use of steroid therapy. Steroids are kapha-type substances, so they can induce increased intraocular pressure. Other causes are cataracts, diabetes, high cholesterol, high triglycerides, and hypertension. These are all kapha-genic factors. Infection can also cause glaucoma.

Ayurveda says our eyes are derived from the pure essence of tejas, which is the essence of pitta dosha. Because of tejas, the eyes look intelligent, penetrating, and lustrous. They are sparkling and attractive organs. The eyes are said to always have a fear of kapha. Kapha can make the eyes dull and the lens opaque. Glaucoma, cataracts, and corneal opacity are all kapha disorders.

## Samprāpti, The Disease Process

Systemic kapha, and in particular kledaka kapha from the stomach, undergoes sanchaya (accumulation) and prakopa (provocation). Then it spreads during the prasara stage, entering into majjā dhātu (the nerve tissue). The eyeballs are a major organ of majjā dhātu.

The increased kapha goes into the vitreous humor of the eye, which is tarpaka kapha. There is an angle between the anterior and posterior chambers. Through that angle, the vitreous humor circulates and drains from the anterior chamber to the posterior chamber and back again. Kapha is sticky, slimy, dense, and thick. In excess, these qualities can create a blockage to the angle, with either a gradual or a sudden increase of pressure.

If the samprāpti is slow, with predominantly increased liquid quality of kapha, it will gradually widen the angle and manifest as chronic, open angle glaucoma. If the disease process is fast, with increased dense, sticky, and slimy qualities, the increased kapha will close the angle and result in acute, closed angle glaucoma.

### Signs and Symptoms of Glaucoma

In the beginning, there are no noticeable signs and symptoms. Thus, chronic glaucoma is also called painless glaucoma. The vision gradually starts to deteriorate. It is a sneaky thief of sight. Loss of peripheral vision occurs first and then slowly progresses to loss of the central vision, which results in blindness. There is often foggy or blurry vision, with difficulty in adjusting to bright light and darkness.

Other symptoms include:
+ Peri-orbital pain, which is pain around the periphery or orbit of the eye
+ Perception of a faint white circle
+ Halos surrounding car headlights when driving at night

Acute glaucoma can bring on sudden severe eye pain, blurry vision, nausea, and vomiting. It can rapidly lead to blindness, possibly within a few weeks or months.

### Diagnosis

Diagnosis of glaucoma is done by checking the eye pressure, field of vision, and visual acuity. If untreated, glaucoma can lead to blindness, so have your eye pressure checked at least once a year.

In Ayurveda, we ask the patient to close the eyes and with the help of the index finger, place a little pressure on the eyeball. Try to feel the elasticity. If the eyeball is dense, that means the pressure is high. If the eyeball is elastic, the pressure is normal. However using a tonal meter provides a more accurate measurement.

Then examine the iris and cornea. A simple clinical test is to examine the field of vision. Sit one foot away from the client, and look into his or her eyes. Tell the client to look into your eyes, and then hold up your index finger. Move your finger across the patient's field of vision, and ask if they can see the finger while looking straight ahead. If the patient does not see your finger at any point, that is called anopsia, loss of field of vision. Check the right side, left side, up and down. This is an important clinical test.

If there seems to be any loss of vision, the patient should see an eye doctor for further investigation, including an eye pressure test.

## Chikitsā, Management

The treatment protocol in modern medicine is to give beta-blockers. Beta-blocker eye drops reduce the pressure in the eyes. They do not alter the size of the pupils, as other treatments can do. However, they have other side effects, such as affecting the person's heart rate and causing narrowing of the bronchial tubes. Hence, they may not be appropriate for asthma patients or athletes.

Another option is surgery, in order to open a new pathway for the fluid to drain. This is usually required if there is acute glaucoma.

From an Ayurvedic point of view, we can maintain intraocular pressure and help in the earlier stages of chronic glaucoma by using an Ayurvedic regimen.

An effective formula for glaucoma is:

Punarnavā 500 mg
Gulvel sattva 200 mg
Yashthi madhu 200 mg
Sarasvatī 200 mg

Eyewash Cup

Take ½ teaspoon of this mixture orally with warm water, three times daily.

*Eyewash Instructions.* Most important is to use triphala and punarnavā eyewash. Boil 1 teaspoon of triphala and 1 teaspoon of punarnavā together in a cup of water for 2-3 minutes. Then cool it, and filter or strain the liquid. Using an eyecup, apply this punarnavā-triphala eyewash at least once a day, preferably in the morning. If possible, give it twice a day: morning and evening.

I've had good results with this punarnavā and triphala eyewash. Those individuals who regularly use it have good results compared to beta-blocker eye drops.

Netra basti is another important treatment. Use a whole-wheat donut around the eye, and pour lukewarm ghee into the eye. That will relax the eye and open the angle, helping with the drainage. (see instructions page 313)

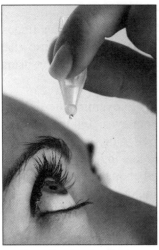

Netra Bindu, eye drops

Netra bindu is Ayurvedic eye drops. It contains rose water, edible camphor, alum, triphala, and honey. This combination will help to reduce the eye pressure. One or two drops are applied directly into each eye.

With each of these external treatments, it is best to apply them to both eyes, whether glaucoma is present in one eye (unilateral) or in both (bilateral).

Eye exercises are also beneficial. One useful exercise involves looking up, then down, side-to-side, diagonally, and then rotating the eyeballs clockwise and counterclockwise. Next, gaze at the tip of the nose, and then up towards the forehead. Finish by holding your palms against your eyes.

Beneficial yogāsanas include camel, cobra, cow, boat, bow, bridge, lotus, locust, lion, and moon salutation. Most importantly, periodically check your eye pressure and, if it is 20 or above, do not do sūrya namaskāra, headstand, or other inverted yoga poses. Inverted poses will further increase the pressure.

Follow an Ayurvedic protocol suitable for your prakruti and vikruti. An appropriate diet and lifestyle, along with the herbal protocol above, punarnavā and triphala eyewash, netra bindu, and netra basti should help to regulate intraocular pressure and manage glaucoma.

Finally, there is an ancient spiritual technique called palming. Sit in any comfortable posture and gently close both eyes. Slowly bring both palms up and place them over each eye. Don't put any pressure on the eyes; just gently touch the eyelashes. Continue looking but with closed eyes, looking into the heart of the palms.

The eyes are extremely active sense organs—outgoing, extroverted. One loses tremendous amounts of *pranic* energy through the eyes. Using this palming technique, this lost energy starts to gather in the third eye.

Keep breathing slowly and deeply into the belly. The accumulated energy in the third eye will start to fall, drop by drop, from the eyes into the heart. In the beginning, there are single drops. By and by, the drop becomes a drip, and then slowly turns into a flow. Gradually the flow becomes a flood. This flood of energy from the third eye into the heart becomes a flame of attention.

The heart is a seat of love and compassion. Increased ālochaka pitta in the eyes causes judgment and divisiveness, and it builds pressure in the eyes. Sādhaka pitta in the heart processes emotions into compassion and love. These emotions unfold in the heart as the flame of awareness.

This simple, non-invasive palming mirror technique relieves eye tension and eye pressure, and unfolds emotion into compassion. Do it; it works.

# Chapter 42

# Macular Degeneration

Summer 2014, Volume 27, Number 1

ONE SŪTRA SAYS the eyes are composed of fire, from the tejas principle (which relates to pitta dosha) but they have 'fear' of kapha dosha. Therefore, the eyes are strongly connected to ālochaka pitta as well as prāna vāyu, vyāna vāyu and tarpaka kapha. However, the eyes are susceptible to kapha disorders, including cataracts, excessive lacrimation, glaucoma, diabetes, lacrimal cysts, and corneal opacity.

The eyes are derived from majjā, rasa and rakta dhātus. Ayurveda talks about the various mandala related to the eyes, shown in the illustration at right.

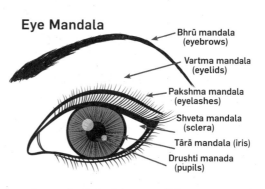

**Eye Mandala**

- Bhrū mandala (eyebrows)
- Vartma mandala (eyelids)
- Pakshma mandala (eyelashes)
- Shveta mandala (sclera)
- Tārā mandala (iris)
- Drushti manada (pupils)

Macular degeneration is the deterioration of the macula, which is the yellowish depression in the central part of the retina of each eye, located at the back of the eye. The macula is the part of the retina with the greatest density of visual receptor cells. It is situated around the central area of the retina, near the optic disk. It's a small but very sensitive part of the retina.

Any light that comes onto *drushti mandala* (the pupils) creates an image on the retina. Then the macula allows us to perceive fine details in the central vision. The image formed on the macula is perceived by the brain. The fovea, in the center of the macula, lets us focus and do things such as read books.

· · · · · · · · · · · · · · · · · · · · · · · · · · · · · · · · · · · · · · · · · · · · · · · · · · · · ·

## *Chakṣuṣ tejomayam tasya...*

The eye is composed of fire...from *Astanga Hridaya Samhita*, Vagbhata

· · · · · · · · · · · · · · · · · · · · · · · · · · · · · · · · · · · · · · · · · · · · · · · · · · · · ·

# Etiological Factors of Macular Degeneration

Macular degeneration is of two types:

Dry type is a vāta disorder in which the visual receptor cells degenerate. This is dhātu kshaya (degeneration of the tissue), due to excess vāta dosha.

Wet type is a pitta or pitta-kapha disorder that occurs because of inflammation and exudation that causes a sudden change in the central vision. This is *dhātu paka* (inflammation of the localized tissue).

Macular degeneration may be due to the hot and sharp qualities of pitta or the dry and rough attributes of vāta.

**Macular Degeneration**

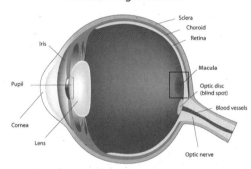

In a normal, healthy condition, the retina has a reddish color, due to the presence of rod cells, cone cells, and rakta dhātu. Degenerative changes in the cells cause loss of color in the macula. Loss of pigmentation in the macular region frequently occurs after age 50-55 years (the beginning of vāta age).

Specific causes of macular degeneration include:

- prolonged exposure to bright sunlight, which can disturb ālochaka pitta
- smoking – nicotine toxicity can disturb both ālochaka pitta and vyāna vāyu
- alcoholism – the hot, sharp, and penetrating attributes of alcohol can cause inflammatory changes in the eyes

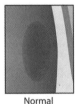

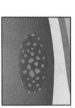

Normal     "Wet" Macular Degeneration     "Dry" Macular Degeneration

- low carotene levels – for the sake of your eyes, you should eat at least two carrots per week
- atherosclerosis – due to high cholesterol, high triglyceride levels, or diabetes

## Signs and Symptoms of Macular Degeneration

Symptoms of macular degeneration include:
- Blurring of central vision
- Straight lines can appear distorted or the central visual field becomes distorted
- Dark areas or white spots appear in the center of the visual field
- Change in color perception

The peripheral vision remains intact.

**Dry type:** Develops slowly and there is gradual blurring of central vision. It is usually painless.

**Wet type:** Blurring occurs rapidly with sudden loss of vision. People with this condition cannot do work that requires good central vision, such as driving, threading a needle, or doing skillful artwork. Attempting to focus can induce pain, due to inflammation.

## Management of Macular Degeneration

In modern medicine, there is no treatment for dry macular degeneration (vāta type). Special powerful eye glasses are sometimes used.

Laser beam surgery can be used for the wet type of macular degeneration (pitta or pitta-kapha). Retinal surgery using laser photocoagulation of the new blood vessel membranes can help to arrest the visual loss.

Doctors sometimes use antibiotics or angiogenesis inhibitors,[57] drugs such as angiostatin or endostatin, which block the formation of new blood vessels.

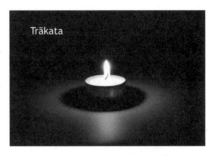

Trākata

The primary Ayurvedic therapy for both types of macular degeneration is netra basti with plain ghee. (see instructions page 313) Doing this at least twice a week will help to promote healthy ojas and balance tejas. In cases of pitta type of macular degeneration, it will help to regulate any inflammatory changes. For vāta type, it will help to arrest the degenerative process.

Watching a ghee lamp flame (*trātaka*) is prescribed in most cases of macular degeneration. *Brahmī ghee nasya* is also beneficial, and triphala tea eyewash can be done every morning. (see page 329 for instructions)

Gentle eye exercises can be beneficial, including:

♦ Looking up, down, sideways, diagonally, and clockwise and counterclockwise

♦ Palming: rub your hands together and then hold the palms over each eye

### Dry Type

| | |
|---|---|
| Ashvagandhā | 500 mg |
| Balā | 400 mg |
| Vidārī | 300 mg |
| Yogarāja guggulu | 200 mg |

Also 1 teaspoon of triphala given orally each evening.

### Wet Type

| | |
|---|---|
| Shatāvarī | 500 mg |
| Gudūchi | 400 mg |
| Kama dudhā | 200 mg |
| Moti bhasma | 200 mg |

---

57. Angiogenesis is the sprouting of new capillary growth from pre-existing blood vessels.

Also 1 teaspoon of bhumi āmalakī in the evening.

These anti-inflammatory herbs can help to pacify pitta dosha in the eyes.

Remember that if you have macular degeneration, you should follow the protocol recommended by your medical doctor. If that does not help, try these Ayurvedic recommendations under the guidance of an expert Ayurvedic practitioner.

# Chapter 43

# Netra Roga
## Eye Disorders

Summer 2016, Volume 29, Number 1 and Fall 2016, Volume 29, Number 2

*Chakshu*
to pay visual attention

*Netra*
the leader of all the senses

*Lochana*
to see or to perceive

These words show the vital importance of the eyes to human beings. According to Ayurveda, the eyes are derived from majjā dhātu. They contain ālochaka pitta, which operates functionally together with the three subdoshas in the brain: sādhaka pitta, tarpaka kapha, and prāna vāta.

THE EYES HAVE many different parts. The eyebrow (*bhrūh mandala*), eyelid (*vartma mandala*), eyelashes (*pakshma mandala*), conjunctiva (*rakta mandala*), sclera (*shveta mandala*), iris (*krishna mandala* or *tārā mandala*), pupil and cornea (drishti mandala), lens (netra bindu) and eyeball (*netra buda-buda*). The junctions between all these different *mandala* are called *sandhi*. There are six sandhi, which are six layers of petals. Hence, poetically, the eye is described as a lotus flower, called *padma lochana* (eye lotus).

The great Ayurvedic surgeon Sushruta described 76 different types of eye diseases. Ten are due to vāta dosha, ten are due to pitta disorder, and thirteen are due to kapha imbalance. A further 16 eye diseases are due to rakta disorders, 25 are due to a disturbance of all the doshas, and the remaining two are due to external causes.

**Eye Mandala**

- Bhrū mandala (eyebrows)
- Vartma mandala (eyelids)
- Pakshma mandala (eyelashes)
- Shveta mandala (sclera)
- Tārā mandala (iris)
- Drushti manada (pupils)

Charaka says that embryologically, the eyes are derived from *sūrya* (the solar principle) and tejas. Hence, the eyes have a fear of kapha dosha and a dislike of too much exposure to the sun. The signs and symptoms of eye diseases are mainly due to doshic imbalance. In common practice, we see pink eye (pitta disorder), dry eyes (vāta disorder), and thick white discharge, glaucoma and cataracts (kapha disorders).

The eyes can be affected by all three doshas. In vāta dushti, the eyes are dry and itching and there is excessive blinking.

There is a deep connection between the eyes and the liver. The liver is the seat of rañjaka pitta and eyes the seat of ālochaka pitta. Hence when there is a pitta disorder, the eyes can look yellow or reddish colored and there is often a yellowish discharge and inflammation.

Kapha disorders can cause sticky, mucous discharge, puffiness, and corneal opacity and deposition of kapha molecules, leading to cataracts.

Charaka has clearly mentioned the detailed symptomatology and treatment protocol in the special branch of Ayurvedic medicine called *shalaka tantra*. In ancient times, there were specialists that are the equivalent of today's eye specialists.

## How the Eyes Work

When we look at outer objects, the eyeball operates like a pinhole camera. The rays of light from the object cast an inverted image onto the retina. Prāna carries that inverted image through the optic nerve, then through the optic chiasma and the external geniculate body to the occipital cortex.

In the occipital cortex is a special type of pitta called sādhaka pitta. Within the retina are cone cells and rod cells. These contain ālochaka pitta. Light particles from the object are absorbed by the cone cells and rod cells, with the help of prāna in the optic nerve. Color perception is done by the cone cells, while rod cells govern the perception of black and white.

> **GENERAL AYURVEDIC EYE TREATMENTS**
>
> Triphala tea eyewash
>
> Fresh organic sliced cucumber on the eyes will cool down burning sensations
>
> Fresh aloe vera gel applied to the closed eyes is calming, cooling and anti-inflammatory
>
> One drop of castor oil in each eye at bedtime is beneficial to the eyes

In due course, prāna vāta with the help of ālochaka pitta carries the light particles through the optic nerve into the occipital cortex, which contains sādhaka pitta. The functional integration of ālochaka pitta from the retina and sādhaka pitta from the brain in the occipital cortex governs correct interpretation of visual perception.

In this article, we shall discuss some common eye disorders that are treatable.

## Amblyopia | Diminished Vision Drishti Māndya

*Drishti māndya* means diminished vision in one or both eyes, without any obvious physical defect. The modern name of this disease is amblyopia.

Amblyopia is not the same as near sightedness (*hrasva drishti*), far sightedness (*dīrgha drishti*), or astigmatism (*drishti dosha*). Those visual disorders can all be corrected by using corrective lenses. That is not the case for amblyopia.

There are two main types of amblyopia: lazy eye amblyopia, which is called *ālasya netra māndya*, and toxic amblyopia, called *visha sāmata drishti māndya*.

Lazy eye amblyopia is quite common in people with *pitta-kapha* or *kapha-pitta prakruti*. It happens most frequently in young children whose eyes do not line up correctly. The eyes are out of focus, because some of the eye muscles are weakened. This specific symptom is called strabismus, which in Sanskrit is called *netra chanchalatva*. This means that the eye is mobile and out of focus.

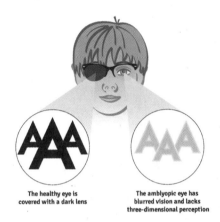

The healthy eye is covered with a dark lens

The amblyopic eye has blurred vision and lacks three-dimensional perception

In amblyopia, the vision of each eye is different. For example, if the left eye is the lazy eye and the right eye is normal, the lazy left eye might only see the top-most letter of the standard vision-testing chart, which is the region of 20/200, whereas the right eye may be able to read the last line, indicating 20/20 vision. There may be such a pronounced difference in this condition.

Unless corrected, the unfocused eye causes double vision, where the patient sees two images of everything. This is confusing and causes dizziness. To compensate for this double vision, the human brain (using sādhaka pitta and tarpaka kapha) suppresses the visual center relating to the lazy eye. This suppresses the sight of one eye, meaning the person sees only with the other eye. This brings about unilateral correct vision, meaning one eye does all the work and the brain suppresses the perception from the other eye. The muscles in the lazy eye become weak, and the optic nerve can be affected. So slowly, slowly the brain functions related to the lazy eye will undergo atrophy. This is a vāta disorder in majjā dhātu.

## Signs and Symptoms

There are usually no obvious signs and symptoms of amblyopia. The child with amblyopia appears to see as well as any other child. By the time the condition is recognized, the eye may be permanently damaged.

However, other times the condition that causes the amblyopia may be very noticeable. The eye may turn either outward or inward, or one eye may look upward when other eye is looking downward. Or the affected eye could have sluggish movement. This is vāta dushti in the eccentric muscles of the eyeball, as vāta is blocked by kapha dosha.

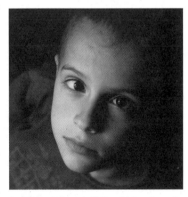

Amblyopia is a unilateral blurring of vision. Early detection can help reduce risk of impaired vision.

Test the vision by holding up your index finger in front of the patient. Move your hand right to left, and then left to right. When you move your finger to the right, a normal eye will follow the movement to the right, while the lazy eye will lag behind. Similarly, when you move the finger up or down, the lazy eye will lag behind. The lazy eye will lag behind in one or more of the directional movements of your finger. The affected eye can also turn either outward or inward. You can also detect this condition when you move your finger upwards and then downwards.

This condition leads to diplopia (double vision). A child with amblyopia may get behind in his or her schooling. They tend to be a slow reader.

## Management

To restore the sight in the lazy eye, treatment must begin before the child is five or six. The age of childhood is the time of kapha dosha. When systemic kapha blocks prāna vāta, kapha dosha makes the eyes slow and sluggish.

This condition may be corrected by wearing special eyeglasses or contact lenses, and by doing eye exercises. Look up and down, side-to-side, then diagonally, then circularly in a clockwise direction, and then again in a counter-clockwise direction. Finally blink the eyes tightly a few times, squeezing them shut then opening them. These eye exercises help to improve the tone, power, and coordination of the lazy eye muscle.

> **AMBLYOPIA**
>
> Herbal formula to support the muscles of the eyeball:
>
> | | |
> |---|---|
> | 500 mg | Shatāvarī |
> | 400 mg | Ashvagandhā |
> | 300 mg | Balā |
> | 200 mg | Dashamūla |
>
> Take ½ teaspoon two or three times daily
>
> Amblyopia is a unilateral blurring of vision. Early detection can help reduce risk of impaired vision.

Netra basti should be done at least once a week to support the muscles of the lazy eye. It should always be done bilaterally, even if only one eye is affected. (see instructions page 313)

Triphala tea or punarnavā tea eyewash will also help. It is very important to strain all the herbs from the tea before using these eyewashes. For punarnavā tea eyewash, for the directions for triphala tea eyewash using ½ teaspoon of punarnavā instead. (Instructions are on page 329.)

Sometimes a patch is used on one eye, to diminish the activity of the normal eye and thereby stimulate the lazy eye to work. (see illustration page 337) Typically, the child wears glasses, with a corrective lens for the lazy eye and a patch for the normal eye. This forces the child to look through the lazy eye. This treatment strengthens the muscles of the eyeball and improves communication between ālochaka pitta and sādhaka pitta, and coordination of the eccentric muscles of the eyeball. The brain center of perception for the lazy eye will become active.

This disorder can sometimes be corrected by eye surgery. This is to correct strabismus (crossed eye) or any squint that has developed.

Whenever there are symptoms of lazy eye, it is important for an ophthalmologist to re-examine the eyes periodically until the child is at least 10 years old. It can be a lengthy procedure to correct the lazy eye, so it is important to keep doing what is needed to fix this condition.

## Myopia | Nearsightedness Hrasva Drishti Dosha

Myopia or nearsightedness is called *hrasva drishti dosha*. It is a common optical defect in which close objects can be seen clearly, but faraway objects look blurred. About one in every five persons is myopic. This condition tends to be hereditary, developing around the early teenage years, which is the beginning of the pitta phase of life. It typically progresses until the person is in his or her 20s, which is the peak period of pitta dosha.

### Causes

Myopia occurs if the eyeball is too long from front to back, making it oblong. Normally, the cornea and the lens (a disc-shaped structure just behind the front part of the eye) refract or bend the light occurring from a distant view, so that the image is focused exactly on the retina. In myopia, the focused image falls in front of the retina, causing the vision to be blurry. This is because of the altered shape of the eyeball.

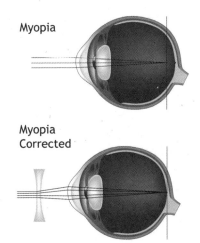

Myopia

Myopia
Corrected

There are several kinds of myopia. Curvature myopia is an extended curve of the cornea of the eyes, which causes light to fall short of the retina. Netra basti with plain ghee is beneficial, along with palming the eyeballs morning and evening.

In index myopia, there is increased light refraction. This is from accumulation of kapha dosha in the vitreous humor and lens. Hence, it can be associated with the future development of cataracts. Index myopia is a pūrva rūpa (prodromal symptom) of cataracts. The best remedy is triphala tea eyewash.

Progressive myopia is an uncommon form of nearsightedness in which the eyeball continues to elongate throughout the person's life. Eventually it leads to the degeneration and detachment of the retina, which is a serious visual disturbance.

Malignant myopia, also called pernicious myopia, is a form of progressive myopia that also is also a disease of the choroid plexus, leading to retinal detachment and blindness.

### Management

Diagnosis of myopia is done by an ophthalmological examination. The ophthalmologist looks inside the eye using an ophthalmoscope. Usually nearsightedness is corrected easily by using concave lenses that help the image to fall correctly on the retina.

A surgical procedure known as radial keratotomy is used to correct myopia. It involves cutting numerous spokes into the corneal surface coming out from the center. The cornea flattens as it heals, which this means the eyeball comes back to its natural shape.

## Hyperopia | Farsightedness Dīrgha Drishti Dosha

Farsightedness is called *dīrgha drusthi dosha*. It is another common optical defect in which faraway objects can be seen clearly, but objects close to the person look blurred.

Hyperopia usually is inherited and children who are hyperopic often become less hyperopic as adults because the eyeball lengthens with normal growth. About one in every five to ten people has hyperopia.

Another form of farsightedness is presbyopia, *drusthi mandhya,* which is due to the aging process. Presbyopia usually begins in middle age, which is the time of transition from the pitta stage of life to the vāta phase. It typically progresses as the person gets further into his or her 60s or 70s.

### Causes

Farsightedness occurs when the eyeball is too short or the cornea is too flat, without enough curvature. In hyperopia, usually the eyeball is smaller than normal. This is due to high pitta in the majjā dhātu. Presbyopia is caused by loss of elasticity of the lens of the eye.

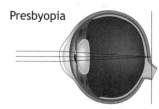

Presbyopia

### Signs And Symptoms

In both cases, the person cannot see small print close up or must hold things far away to read them. Reading or close work results in eyestrain, headaches, fatigue, aching or burning eyes, and/or irritability.

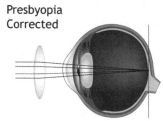

Presbyopia
Corrected

### Management

To help to change the shape of the eyeball back to normal one must balance majjā dhātu agni. Several therapeutic measures are effective. It is not a 'quick fix' and will take at least three months before you may notice changes.

Finally, perform this exercise with a pencil. Fully extend your arm out in front of your eyes with a pencil held upright in your fingers. Have the sharpened tip of the pencil pointing upward. Gaze at the tip of the pencil as you slowly bring it closer and closer until it touches your forehead, on your third eye. During this movement of the pencil, keep gazing at the tip of the pencil. Next gradually move pencil outward to where your arm is fully extended from your face. Repeat this seven times, one for each *dhātu.*

## Astigmatism Drishti Dosha

Astigmatism is a kind of distorted vision caused by a defect in the curvature of the cornea (drishti mandala), lens (netra bindu) and eyeball (netra buda-buda). It affects ākruti, which is the form of the eyeball. Because of the change of curvature, the image is not formed on the retina, but slightly in front of the retina in the anterior chamber.

Some authorities say this prevents the rays of light entering the eyes from being focused on the retina at the back of the eyeball, which is why the person gets blurred vision. Drishti dosha prevents the rays of light entering the eye from being properly focused on the retina at the back of the eyeball. Some rays go forward, some rays backward, and the result is blurry vision.

## Signs and Symptoms

Most people with astigmatism can clearly see objects that are directly in front of them, which means clear central vision. However, their peripheral vision is defective. If a straight line looks curved, it indicates astigmatism.

There may be vertical astigmatism, so that the areas above and below the person's direct gaze are blurred. Other individuals have horizontal astigmatism, in which the areas to the right and left of the central vision are blurred. Vertical astigmatism is prāna vāyu dushti and more of a vāta disorder, while horizontal astigmatism is samāna vāyu dushti and more of a pitta disorder.

## Causes

Most people with astigmatism are born with the tendency towards this condition. A few cases are caused by eye disease or injury. Injury-induced astigmatism can be difficult to correct.

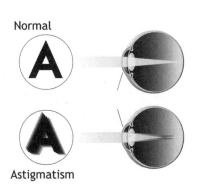

Normal

Astigmatism

Pitta prakruti children are particularly at risk to develop these changes. In pitta children, their tejas is high. High tejas and low prāna can create flattening of the horizontal curvature, while high prāna and low tejas usually causes flattening of the vertical curvature.

## Management

Regardless of the cause, astigmatism should be corrected as early as possible. Fortunately, the defect in the curvature of the cornea or lens is usually uniform, and can be easily corrected with eyeglasses or contact lenses. The fault is usually in the shape of the cornea, the clear window of the eye.

In the front of the iris is the pupil. The cornea is the clear window, the tejas principle. Because of samāna vāyu and pāchaka pitta disorder, the horizontal curvature is disturbed, causing horizontal astigmatism. Because of prāna and apāna vāyu disorder, the vertical curvature gets distorted and that creates vertical astigmatism.

The person needs to wear glasses or contact lenses that are curved to adjust the angle of the rays entering into the eye. That way, this dushti dosha can be corrected and one can get clear vision.

To maintain optimal tejas, one can do netra basti with plain ghee. Internally, the person can take one teaspoon of shatāvarī ghee twice daily.

Rubbing castor oil on the soles of the feet also helps. There are marma points called *pādānguli mūla* at the root of the second and third toes on each foot. Pressing each of these four points for half a minute will give energy to the eyes.

Finally, there is an exercise called *adeshani anguli āgra darshana,* which means gazing at the tip of the index finger. You place your right hand one hand's distance in front of your eyes. Then slowly bring the index finger closer and closer until it touches your forehead, on your third eye. During this journey of the index finger, keep gazing at the tip of the finger. Gradually move your index finger back, positioning it one hand's distance from the eyes. Then repeat this process with the index finger using the left hand.

## PART TWO: Netra Roga, Eye Disorders

In Part One of this chapter, we discussed these eye disorders: amblyopia (diminished vision), drishti māndya, myopia (nearsightedness), hrasva drishti dosha, hyperopia (farsightedness), dīrgha drishti dosha, and astigmatism, drishti dosha. We also covered the ancient origins of Ayurvedic eye treatments and the Ayurvedic understanding of how the eyes work and the anatomy of the eye.

To recap, the great Ayurvedic surgeon Sushruta described 76 different types of eye diseases. Ten are due to vāta dosha, ten are due to pitta disorder, and thirteen are due to kapha imbalance. A further 16 eye diseases are due to rakta dhātu disorders, 25 are due to a disturbance of all the doshas, and the remaining two are due to external causes.

Charaka says that embryologically, the eyes are derived from sūrya (the solar principle) and tejas. Hence the eyes have a fear of kapha dosha and a dislike of too much exposure to the sun. The signs and symptoms of eye diseases are mainly due to doshic imbalance. The eyes can be affected by all three doshas. Charaka has clearly mentioned the detailed symptomatology and treatment protocol in the special branch of Ayurvedic medicine called shalaka tantra. In ancient times, there were specialists that are the equivalent of today's eye specialists.

### Cataracts Moti Bindu

Cataracts are called *moti bindu*. Moti means pearl and, in this condition, there is clouding of the lens of the eye, so the lens looks like an opaque pearl. Cataracts are a kapha disorder of the eyes.

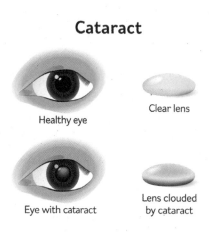

**Cataract**

Healthy eye

Clear lens

Eye with cataract

Lens clouded by cataract

Cataracts cause obscured vision. People with cataracts see their environment as if they are looking through a waterfall. Normally, the lens is clear. Its function is to focus light onto the light-sensitive cells at the back of the eyes, so that the object can be seen clearly. If the lens becomes milky or cloudy, the incoming light is dispersed, resulting in blurred vision.

Clinically, there are two types of cataracts: peripheral cataract and central cataract. In the earlier stages, it depends upon where the kapha molecules lodge. If they are lodged in the center of the lens, the central vision will be blurred. If they lodge at the periphery, the peripheral vision is blurred.

## Cause

The exact cause of cataracts is unknown by modern medicine today. However, ancient Ayurvedic wisdom says that someone with kapha prakruti (constitution) who has kapha vikruti (disorder) is the key causative factor. Even pitta and vāta types with long-lingering kapha vikruti can develop cataracts. Aging plays an important role in the formation of cataracts, although this condition also occurs in some young people, such as newborns whose mother contracted German measles during pregnancy or those with juvenile diabetes.

Other known causes include diabetes, glaucoma, detached retina, and lead, copper or mercury poisoning. These factors can all lead to cataract formation. Extended use of certain drugs, such as steroids, can also cause cataracts, as can prolonged exposure to radiation, such as working in an x-ray department.

Although cataract conditions are usually curable, cataracts can cause blindness. In addition, the lens prevents some of the light from passing onto the retina, which can sometimes lead to other potentially serious problems, such as changes in the retina or damage to the optic nerve.

## Symptoms

The main symptom of cataracts is blurry vision. This usually occurs in one eye first. During the initial stage of its development, cataracts can cause the person to experience glare from bright lights at night, such as car headlights. Since the clouded lens scatters the light rather than focusing it, this creates the glare. As the condition progresses, the lens becomes milky white and vision diminishes.

---

**PREVENTATIVE MEASURES TO AVOID CATARACTS**

- Do twelve or more sūrya namaskāra daily to strengthen the eyes (under the guidance of a yoga teacher).
- Rub castor oil on the soles of the feet and bhringarāj oil on the scalp.
- The juices of pomegranate, cranberry, beets, and carrots are all good sources of vitamin A and antioxidants that benefit the eyes.
- Triphala tea eyewash is beneficial. Triphala contains natural precursors of N-acetylcarnosine and can help to prevent cataracts and macular degeneration.
- Ayurvedic anjana (kohl) is a medicinal combination that was traditionally used as a healing eyeliner. Collyrium (another name for anjana) is a dark eye shadow or medicated eyewash used in India and made from herbal ingredients such as rose, camphor, ghee and coconut oil.
- Bhramārī prānāyāma will reduce kapha in the eyes.
- Ghee lamp trātaka, which is gazing at the flame of a ghee lamp.

---

## Treatment Protocol

Successful treatment begins with the surgical removal of the affected lens. Local anesthetic is given and the procedure is mostly painless. The surgeon opens the area in front of the eye and removes the lens. An expert ophthalmological surgeon does this. Before surgery, the person's blood pressure, blood sugar and any cough or lung infection will need to be treated. The vast majority of cases of surgical removal of cataract go without any complication, and restoration and improvement of the vision is the usual result.

Nowadays, the most common option that doctors recommend is implantation of an intraocular lens following the cataract removal. This lightweight, plastic lens results in vision that is closer to normal than with cataract eyeglasses. It occupies the exact position of the lens.

After the patient has recuperated for a week, special cataract eyeglasses or contact lenses can be prescribed to help correct the vision. These aids are by no means perfect, so an adjustment period may be required.

An Ayurvedic treatment protocol can prevent further cataracts. Triphala tea eyewash is the main remedy. (see page 329) This eyewash can be done every morning and evening for one month. If that proves effective, it can be continued indefinitely, either once or twice daily. There are also special Ayurvedic eye drops that can be used to prevent cataracts. These contain rose, camphor, alum, and roasted palasha root extract. These remedies can even treat cataracts that are in the early stages, but once the cataracts become dense, surgery is needed.

## Blepharitis Pakshma Pāka or Pakshma Sāta

Blepharitis is inflammation of the edge of the eyelid, with redness and swelling. There is formation of scales and a crust or shallow, small eruptions. The disease commonly occurs in children and often affects the upper and lower eyelids of both eyes. There are itching, burning sensations and, commonly, the eyelashes are destroyed. This condition is called *pakshma pāka* in Sanskrit. *Pakshma* means eyelashes, while *pāka* means inflammation. It is also known as *sāta,* which means ulcerations.

### Causes

The principal cause is infection of the eyelash follicles and oil glands by staphylococcal infection. Anterior blepharitis is often associated with staphylococcus. Alternatively, a viral infection can be a cause of either form of blepharitis.

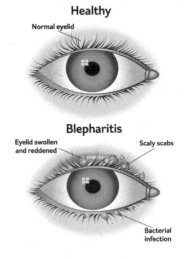

Nowadays pollution is increasing, car and smoke pollution, for example. This dirt and dust, during summer season particularly, can accumulate within the spaces, within the eyelashes, and cause pitta people to have more sweat at the fold of the eyelashes. This becomes the breeding ground for the staphylococcal bacterial infection that causes blepharitis with ulcer. In that case, the hair follicles curl inward, touching the eye and irritating the cornea and conjunctiva, causing severe pain. Then the infection can become well established.

Some people have allergic conjunctivitis and rub their eyes, and that contact of the hands with the eyes can also cause blepharitis. The allergic reaction may be linked to seborrheic dermatitis, which is high pitta in rasa and rakta dhātus. There may also be inflammatory scaling of the scalp or eyebrow. Therefore, eye infection, ear infection and eyebrow infection can go together.

The non-nuclear variety of blepharitis, which means no ulcer and irritation without any initial focused patches of inflammation and infection at the root of the eyelashes, may be due to an allergic reaction along the eyelashes.

Lice irritating the lid margin can also cause the non-ulcerative form of blepharitis.

## Signs and Symptoms

The main symptoms of blepharitis include itching, burning, discoloration of the eyelid with redness on the eyelid margin, irritation of the inside of the eyelid, swollen eyelids and eyelashes, and loss of eyelashes. It feels as if dirt, sand, or some other foreign body has entered the eyes. This creates tears and causes the eyes to become sensitive to the light, which is known as photophobia. Small ulcers can form on the eyelid, forming a tough, dry crust that can bleed and flake off.

Anterior blepharitis affects the outside and front of the eyelid, where the eyelashes are attached. Posterior blepharitis affects the meibomian gland within the eyelid, which secretes oils that mix with the tears to lubricate the eye. It is most common to have a mixture of both anterior and posterior blepharitis.

## Treatment Protocol

An eye specialist will likely recommend washing the eyes with a gentle soap, such as baby shampoo. A natural Ayurvedic soap is also good to use. Eyelid hygiene is very important. For posterior blepharitis, omega 3 fatty acids are commonly recommended. Flax seed oil is a good source of omega 3, which helps the functioning of the meibomian gland.

Ideally, one should wash the affected eye/s at least twice daily with neem soap or sandalwood soap, to keep the eyelashes and eyelid clean. Hold a warm compress, such as a clean washcloth, over the affected area for five or ten minutes. This treatment will prevent the formation of any dry crust around the eyes.

One can also do triphala tea eyewash, using a cotton swab dipped in the strained tea. Triphala tea eyewash has an antibacterial action. Another option is to do an eyewash with goat's milk, taking aseptic precautions. Goat's milk is good for acute inflammation, whereas triphala tea eyewash is best for chronic inflammatory conditions.

Once any crust has been removed, one can apply medicated eye drops to prevent further irritation. Alternatively, one drop of castor oil in each eye is a natural remedy that also relieves inflammation.

Avoid allergenic substances, such as (chemical) cosmetics. If an allergy to a certain cosmetic is the cause of the blepharitis, then discontinue the usage of that particular cosmetic. If there is scaling on the eyebrows and scalp, which indicates seborrheic dermatitis, Ayurveda recommends use of gandhak druti (a special, purified sulphur preparation), or just washing the affected area with natural neem soap or shampoo to control the dandruff.

Pay careful attention to cleanliness of the scalp. If the blepharitis is caused by lice, the lice eggs should be carefully removed with tweezers and steps taken to keep the patient free from head lice. Neem oil or sitaphal seed oil is the best remedy for lice, and can be applied to the scalp and the eyebrows.

A good Ayurvedic antibiotic herbal remedy for anterior blepharitis is 200 mg each of neem, turmeric, osha, golden seal, and echinacea. This can be taken orally three times daily after food.

Posterior blepharitis can create dryness of the eyelashes. Just put a drop of castor oil in the affected eye at bedtime. Then give the eye a good wash in the morning, using appropriate hygiene measures.

There may be pakshma pāka (inflammation of eyelid) and/or *vartma pāka* (inflammation of eyelashes). Either can be caused by bacterial infection and treated by an antibiotic applied topically. Ayurveda suggests the use of ghee with turmeric and neem applied over the eyelid. Modern medicine typically uses an antibiotic ointment.

Non-ulcerative blepharitis causes no permanent damage. However, ulcerative blepharitis can recur, scarring the eyelids and causing loss of eyelashes. The person can even get an ulcer on the cornea, as the eyelashes turn inward, irritating the cornea and creating an ulcer. Those patients should see an ophthalmologist.

An herbal tea of lodhra in water (boiled and cooled) with ghee, can be applied to the eyelid to ease burning and itching sensations. Boil one teaspoon of lodhra in one cup of boiled water for three minutes, cool and strain. To that tea, add one teaspoon of ghee and mix thoroughly. Then wash the eyelashes with this lodhra ghee tea.

Blepharitis is aggravated by a constipated colon, so keep the colon clean by taking one-half to one teaspoon of triphala daily at bedtime. The eyelashes are related to asthi dhātu, and the colon mucous membrane is *purisha dhara kalā,* which is also related to asthi dhātu. Hence, whenever there is constipation or āma in the colon, it can result in blepharitis symptoms. Triphala can be a good remedy for this condition.

Two pinches of pravāl pañchāmrit mixed with one teaspoon of honey can be licked early each morning to prevent blepharitis.

Coconut water is a good remedy for someone with blepharitis, as it cools down pitta.

For crusty blepharitis, rub one chandro daya vati on a sandstone and mix into a paste (with clean fingers) with one teaspoon of honey. Use this as an eyeliner.

For lekhana (scraping) of any scabs, place one drop of pure liquid honey into the eye. It will burn a bit, but will help to soften and remove the scab.

## Color Blindness Ranga Andhatva
Sunrays are full of the seven rainbow colors. When they are blended together, they look white. Leaves are green, roses are red, and the sky looks blue. We perceive all these beautiful colors because there are cone cells and rod cells in the eyes. Cone cells in the retina perceive color and rod cells perceive black and white. There are six to seven million cone cells in the central zone of the human retina, called the macula. This is the area responsible for color perception. An inherited form of color blindness can cause deficiencies in certain types of cone cells.

Rod cells recognize only black and white. The cone cells contain pigments of red, green, and blue. These primary colors can combine to produce all other colors of the spectrum. The pigments become more vivid and fade in response to colors that the eyes see. Changes in the pigmentation produce tiny flashes of electricity and these are carried by means of the optic nerve to the visual center in the brain. Abnormal electrical impulses can interfere with the color perception. The electrical signals normally combine into the full color spectrum. In a colorblind person, some cones are missing, or there are defective cone cells. There is no cure for this condition.

In Parkinsonism, the light sensitive cells in the retina are damaged. As a result, those people can often become color blind. People with epilepsy taking anti-epileptic drugs can get color blindness as a side effect of the medication. Cataracts can also lead to partial color blindness, due to the blurred vision. In patients with optic neuropathy, there is a degree of color blindness. The failure of the pituitary gland can lead to poor development of sexual organs (shukra dhātu), which leads to poor quality ojas—this results in poor color perception. Finally, the aging process damages the retina, causing defective color perception.

## Treatment Protocol

Triphala tea nightly and an herbal formula of equal parts of shatāvarī and punarnavā are the best eye tonic. Do a triphala tea eyewash each day (see page 329) and netra basti with plain ghee weekly. (see page 313) Ghee promotes ojas.

Special colored contact lenses or eyeglasses can help the person to overcome partial color blindness. Eating carrots, beets, broccoli, spinach, red cabbage, pomegranates, and unripe bananas can all help to strengthen the eyesight.

Color blindness is an inability to distinguish certain colors. Total color blindness[58] is rare, but partial color blindness is uncommonly common. The most common type of color blindness is red and green color blindness. Red-green color blindness can either be inherited or acquired. The inherited form of red-green color blindness affects about 8% of men and boys, but only 0.5% of women and girls.

This ālochaka pitta disorder is often due to genetic predisposition, which creates khavaigunya in the retina. *Ālochaka pitta agni* is impaired. When light sensitive cells in the retina fail to absorb and respond accurately to the variations in light wavelength, it may lead to partial color blindness. The longest wavelengths are red and orange, in the middle is green, and the shortest wavelengths are blue. In red-green color blindness the red and green wavelengths are the most difficult to digest for ālochaka pitta.

There are three main types of color blindness.[59] Second most common type is blue-yellow color blindness and third is total absence of color. Disease or injury to the retina is one of the factors of color blindness, as is malfunction of one set of the rods that detect color.

---

58. Monochromacy: those with monochromatic vision can see no color at all and their world consists of different shades of grey ranging from black to white.
59. Deuteranopia - unable to perceive 'green' light, tritanopia - unable to perceive 'blue' light, and protanopia - unable to perceive 'red' light.

Why is red-green color blindness inherited by males more often than females? The reason is that the defective genes that direct the production of defective pigments are carried on one of the pair of chromosomes that determine gender: the X chromosome. Females have two X chromosomes, so the other X chromosome can overcome the defect on one X chromosome. However, males have only one X chromosome, so there is no compensation. Hence, boys can much more easily become colorblind.

Red-green color blindness cannot be passed from father to son. It also cannot be passed to a daughter unless the mother carries the defective genes and the father is color blind. However, if the daughter is carrying the defective genes and produces a son, the son will have a 50% chance of being color blind. Blue color blindness is not carried on the sex chromosomes. So it affects males and females equally.

The seven colors can be split into the three doshas: red-orange-yellow are pitta, green is kapha, and blue-violet-indigo are vāta. There is a relationship between the type of color blindness and the doshas, and taking an herbal remedy to balance the doshic imbalance may help the partial color blindness to some extent.

Color blindness is incurable, but Ayurveda can support color perception in people who are not genetically colorblind. Triphala-punarnavā ghee taken orally and applied topically via netra basti will protect the person's tejas, which is responsible for perceiving color. Good foods for color blindness are high in beta-carotene or vitamin A, which is present in carrots, beets, cauliflower, cabbage, and soaked almonds.

## Night Blindness Nakta Andhatva

Night blindness or nyctalopia is a condition in which a person can see well in bright sunlight, but cannot see clearly in a dim light or at night. The retina contains a layer of photoreceptors, which are specialized light sensitive cells that lie in the interior of the eyeball. These photoreceptors adapt to varying degrees of light. There are two types of photoreceptors: cones and rods. Cone cells perceive color and rod cells perceive black and white.

Cones concentrate in the center of the retina, called the macula. They allow us to perceive distinct, fine details and colors. The rods, which are predominantly located around the edge of the retina, perceive the amount of light. The rods contain a pigment called rhodopsin, which is a kind of ālochaka pitta that adjusts according to the relative brightness or darkness. This adaptation is affected when there is an insufficient supply of vitamin A in the body, causing night blindness.

### Causes

Night blindness is usually caused by either severe deficiency of vitamin A, or from retinitis pigmentosa, which is a rare, inherited degenerative disorder of the retina that causes the cornea to become shortened and the eyes excessively dry. There are several other causes of night blindness, including glaucoma, cataracts, diabetic retinopathy, and retinitis.

## Treatment Protocol

Vitamin A can be given to treat night blindness. However, large doses of vitamin A are not advised without a doctor's recommendation, because it can create other dangers. The best preventative measure is sufficient intake of vitamin A in the diet, in the form of egg yolks, dark green vegetables, leafy greens, carrots, sweet potatoes, apricots, butter, cream, and ghee.

For other types of night blindness, one must treat the underlying condition that is causing the night blindness. For example, one should treat glaucoma, if that is the cause, or diabetes if the condition is due to diabetic retinopathy.

## Sty Pakshma Pitika

A sty is called *pakshma pitika* in Ayurveda. It is an inflamed or infected swelling of subcutaneous oil-producing glands in the eyes. Staphylococcus bacteria commonly cause the infection. An external sty typically appears on the surface of the skin at the edge of the eye. Part of the sty is on the inner surface of the eyelid.

### Symptoms

A sty is often seen as a protrusion or lump on the eyelid, without any visible puffiness or redness. Initially, the sty feels like a foreign object in the eye, causing tearing, redness, swelling, and tenderness in and around a particular area of the eye.

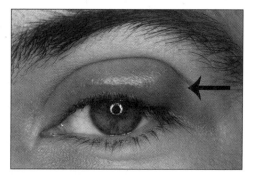

It soon follows that the eye becomes sensitive to light and the eyelid sensitive to touch. In addition, a pustule (a small yellow bump filled with pus) might develop. This causes pain. In most cases, the pustule eventually bursts, releasing the pus and beginning the healing process. Once the pressure from the pus has eased, the pain usually subsides.

### Treatment Protocol

Sty is a common pitta disorder, when a person has excess stagnation of pitta in the rakta vaha srotas. The treatment of a sty often involves antibiotic eye drops and ointment. This may be best if the sty is acutely inflamed. Ayurveda uses a natural antibiotic made from rose, camphor, alum, and turmeric. These are all present in chandro daya vati.

Applying a warm moist compress to the eye for about 5-10 minutes, two or three times a day will help the suppuration, bringing the pus to the surface where it will burst easily. In cases where there is an internal sty, surgical opening may be required. One should never squeeze a sty, as it can create a more extensive infection.

Daily wash the eye with triphala and punarnava tea eyewash—one teaspoon of each in a cup of boiled water, carefully cooled and strained. On the sty, apply a small paste of turmeric right over the sty, and that way it can be healed. People who get a sty tend to have constipation, so they should take one teaspoon of bhumi āmalakī or triphala nightly, with warm water.

# Chapter 44

# Male Health Issues

Winter 2006, Volume 19, Number 3

IN AYURVEDIC LITERATURE, the prostate gland is called *ashthīlā,* round pebble, for its resemblance in structure. Made of muscular tissue, it secretes an alkaline, soft, liquid and slightly dense seminal fluid, in which sperm floats. The gland is located just below the bladder and surrounds the neck of the bladder and the urethra. Both the *shukra vaha srotas,* male reproductive channel, and mūtra vaha srotas, urinary channel, share the common passage of the urethra and the neck of the bladder.

Ashthīlā's function is to act as a pump and during sexual intercourse it helps to ejaculate semen forcefully to reach its goal. This gland, however, may become inflamed, infected, or enlarged. Predominately during old age, or around age 60, this gland may become enlarged, a condition called benign prostatic hyperplasia. However, nowadays this is also manifesting in younger men in their 40s. Though it is not a serious thing, chronic enlarged prostate can create recurring urinary tract infections.

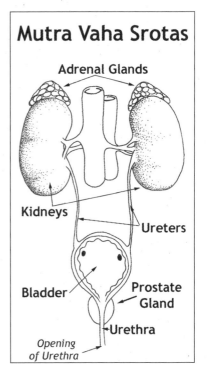

**Mutra Vaha Srotas**

Adrenal Glands

Kidneys

Ureters

Bladder

Prostate Gland

Urethra

Opening of Urethra

## Prostatism and Prostatitis

In old age, the agni of shukra is low and it can lead to undue production of raw shukra dhātu, reproductive tissue, leading to enlarged prostate. The enlarged prostate in turn constricts the urethra and the flow of urine from the bladder; this condition is called prostatism.

Prostatitis is the inflammation of the prostate gland. According to Ayurveda, this is a pitta-type disorder in which the apāna·vāyu pushes pitta into either shukra or mūtra vaha srotas and causes inflammation of the prostate gland, generating prostatitis.

Prostatitis can be uncomfortable, irritating, or painful because it disrupts urine flow. Later, the swelling increases with consequent blockage and retention of urine flow. The urine backs up from the urethra to the ureters and ascends, causing inflammation in the kidneys. When chronic prostatitis occurs, it can lead to bladder or kidney damage and marked malaise of these organs.

## Samprāpti (Etiology and Pathogenesis)

Repeated attempts and prolonged effort to start the flow of urine is the pūrva rūpa (prodromal signs and symptoms) for both prostatism and prostatitis. Gradually there is decreased urine flow and the force of flow is weak or may dribble near the end of the act of urination. At this point, the man feels as if the action is completed but leakage may occur afterwards, wetting the underwear. This contributes to the typical urine odor of these conditions. Additionally, some amount of residual urine remains in the bladder, as the bladder never empties itself completely. The residual urine can become a fertile breeding ground for bacteria to grow and be the cause of bladder infections.

## Nidāna (Causes)

Causes for prostatitis and prostatism are sexual transmitted diseases such as gonor-rhea, syphilis, herpes, urinary tract infections, or low agni of shukra vaha srotas. In cases of low agni, tejas starts burning ojas and there is excessive production of prostate tissue resulting in a high PSA (prostate specific antigen) count.

## Signs and Symptoms

Trouble starting urine flow or reduced flow with dribbling result in increased frequency of urination causing the person to wake up at night to urinate, thus creating insomnia. Burning urination, fever, and chills, caused by the pitta-type inflammation, are other signs of these conditions.

## Diagnosis/Assessment

A doctor does the assessment through a physical examination and, typically, the examination of the prostate is performed by digital rectal examination (DRE). The physician examines the size, feels the condition of the prostate, and massages the prostate. Further findings of pus in the urine on the same day of examination would be indicative of abnormality. In some cases, a urine culture is collected for bacterial examination; in others, an IVP[60] is recommended and, in obscure cases, a rectal ultrasound and prostate biopsy may be performed. In an Ayurvedic assessment, both the shukra dhātu pulse and the bladder pulse would be weak.

---

60. Intravenous pyelogram, an x-ray for the urinary tract using contrast material by injection in the bloodstream.

One should inquire about weight loss as well. If there has been rapid weight loss, then the prostatic hyperplasia may be malignant. If there has been no significant weight change, the prostatic hyperplasia is generally benign. Additionally, one can observe the flow of urine in passing. If the flow goes more to the right side, that is indicative that the left gland is enlarged.

## Chikitsā (Management)

Asthila belongs to both shukra and mūtra vaha srotas. So, one needs to remember always to include in the herbal formulation substances that address the following: the dosha pratyanika (dosha specific), vyādhi pratyanika (specific to disease), ubhaya pratyanika (specific to dosha and disease), dhātu pratyanika (specific to tissue), and srota pratyanika (specific to bodily channel).

In cases of bacterial infection with burning sensation, in India, one would use sūkshma triphalā (triphalā powder that has been potentized by a triphalā concoction several times) and gandhak rasāyana (compound of purified sulphur), 200 mg of each TID with an anupāna (vehicle) of cumin, coriander, and fennel (CCF) tea. In the USA, one would use 200 mg each of goldenseal, shilājit, echinacea, haridrā, and take ½ teaspoon of this mixture TID for a similar effect.

> The PSA count is done by evaluating the nanograms of prostate specific antigen per milliliters of blood.
>
> In the past, most doctors considered PSA values of 4 or below normal. Recent research found prostate cancer in men with PSA levels below 4.0 ng/ml. Many doctors are now using the following ranges, with some variation:
>
> - 0 to 2.5 ng/ml is low
> - 2.6 to 10 ng/ml is slightly to moderately elevated
> - 10 to 19.9 ng/ml is moderately elevated
> - 20 ng/ml or more is significantly elevated.

In cases of fever and chills, have the client take punarnavā 500 mg, gokshura 400 mg, and mahāsudarshan 300 mg with aloe vera gel, ½ teaspoon, TID.

If a person has dribbling urination, they should drink large quantities of water to flush the prostate and gently massage the perineum with castor oil. Also, a bath with 1/3 cup of baking soda (no ginger) would be helpful to relieve dribbling.

In cases of prostatic enlargement, the dosha pratyanika of choice would be ashvagandhā for vāta, shatāvarī for pitta and punarnavā for kapha. Shilājit would be the vyādhi pratyanika, to reduce the enlarged prostate; gokshura, the dhātu pratyanika, to maintain the tone of the prostate tissue; and kutki or gokshurādi guggulu for scraping of the abnormal growth as ubhaya pratyanika.

Other herbal formulas that have been proven to be useful in maintaining health in the area are chandraprabhā vati, gokshurādi guggulu, shilājit, ashvagandhā pills, and the very alkaline ushīra to reduce burning.

When PSA values are high, Ayurveda suggests consumption of a handful of white sesame seeds with jaggery[61] as one's only food for one to two days. Also, take internally a

---

61. Unrefined brown sugar obtained from the sap of the East Indian jaggery palm.

formula comprising equal parts (300 mg each) of punarnavā, trikatu, shilājit, and gudūchī with hot water. Take this for 90 days as a preventative measure and to maintain proper dhātu agni of the prostate gland.

### Āsanas and Kriyā

The best yoga āsanas for prostate are *kukkutāsana,* cock or rooster pose, *vajrāsana,* thunderbolt pose, and *dhanurāsana,* bow pose.

A *kriyā* (action) that is called *Ganesha dhauti kriyā* can be very helpful. After each bowel movement, wash the anal orifice with warm water and apply castor oil to the anal orifice. The technique then is: with a properly clipped and filed nail, put the castor oil on the left middle finger and insert it into the rectum. Breathing by the mouth to relax the sphincter muscle, gently rotate the finger three times clockwise and three times counter-clockwise while pulling forward in an attempt to massage the top of the prostate. This kriyā is quite effective to reduce the size of the prostate gland. You can wear surgical-type gloves for this, available at any drugstore.

Another practice that can be done for self-healing is the *ashwini mudrā,* which means female horse gesture and is done by contracting the sphincter muscles of the anus. This practice improves the circulation in the prostate gland and maintains its tone. The technique is very similar to *mula bandha* (root lock); however, it does not require the breathing technique. This technique is contraindicated in cases of fissures, fistula, thrombosed piles, and prolapsed piles/hemorrhoids.

Recurring sexual intercourse is considered to help maintain the health of the prostate gland. In cases of prostatic problems, therapeutic sex is often advised. However, frequency of intercourse should be maintained at once or twice a month.

# Impotence

The corpora cavernosum penis[62] normally are filled with blood during sexual excitement. *Klaibya,* impotence, is an inability to achieve and maintain an erection, which is necessary for sexual intercourse. The blood in the prostate is rich in ojas, which causes the penis to become rigid, erect, and firm with tone. Impotence is a lack of blood supply to this gland, often due to high cholesterol, high triglycerides, diabetes, and obesity. Impotence is classified as a partial or total impairment of function.

> **BHASMA**
>
> A specialized Ayurvedic preparation alchemically produced by fastidious purification and burning into ash; bhasmas are very potentized, easily absorbable, and release prāna into the system.

There are two types of impotence, primary and secondary. In primary impotence, either kapha is blocking vāta or vāta is pushing kapha in the shukra vaha srotas, creating a block. In this case, the man has never had the ability to have an adequate erection from the onset of puberty. This primary impotence may be due to trauma or intense fear. In secondary impotence, there is an inability to complete the act of intercourse to the fullest satisfaction for both partners, which may be interrupted

---

62. The two columns of erectile tissue on the dorsum of the penis.

by premature ejaculation. In both cases, impotence can create low self-esteem, put a strain on the marriage, and stress the relationship.

## Nidāna

In primary impotence, causes can be varied ranging from a vāta or kapha-provoking diet and lifestyle to physical trauma, psychological trauma, job-related stress, fear of pregnancy, unresolved deep-seated grief, sadness, and/or childhood sexual trauma or abuse.

Secondary impotence may occur in a person who is recovering from a heart attack or has undergone major surgery. In these cases, the fear of death transfers itself to a fear of sex because during orgasm there is a temporary death. Secondary impotence may also occur as a result of antihypertensive drugs, tranquilizers, diuretics, antidepressants, drugs, pituitary surgeries or tumors, alcohol, marijuana, smoking cigarettes, and excessive masturbation, which depletes shukra dhātu.

Structural abnormalities, obesity, chronic consumptive disease, tuberculosis, diabetes, hypertension, stress, trauma, and sexual trauma in previous relationships can be both primary and secondary causes.

The *asthāyi shukra dhātu,* which is raw or unprocessed reproductive tissue, is generally processed by shukra dhātu agni, creating ojas, vigor, and vitality. If the nutritional fire of shukra dhātu is low, it can create imbalanced hormonal changes and diminished testosterone.

## Signs and Symptoms

First, one can notice a lack of interest in sex; this is followed by an inability to maintain an erection. One should understand that this does not mean infertility or the person's inability to father a child when, in general, the sperm count is good.

Normally the inability to maintain an erection causes irritability and low self-esteem. This sexual anxiety leads to abnormal behaviors ranging from seeking stimulation through pornography to extramarital affairs as a proof of manhood. Using romance as a stimulus to maintain an erection is short-lived for the organ that cannot endure. These behaviors cause further conflict in the man's relationships, thus producing more frustration, irritability, and low self-esteem.

## Assessment

Assessment of this disease can be done by darshana (observation), sparshana (palpation), and prashna (questioning) to find out the cause of impotence. In addition, check the blood pressure and the person's weight. Run blood tests for hormone and cholesterol levels. Rule out diabetes and venereal diseases. Perform a urine examination to assess semen-urea content. Often impotence can be a weight-related problem, even when the man is only twenty or thirty pounds overweight.

Modern medical assessment tests include the nocturnal penile tumescence test (NPT) performed by an electronic monitoring device or a snap gauge fitted around the penis. This test can determine if a man is having normal erections during sleep, their duration and stiffness. If there are no erections in the course of two days then there is a definite physical cause and not an emotional cause. Another test is the intercavernosal injection test, in which a medication is injected into the base of the penis to produce an erection and fullness, stiffness, and duration of the erection are then measured.

## Prevention

To prevent impotence, a man should limit or abstain from the consumption of drugs and alcohol. Another preventative measure is to maintain proper weight and, if necessary, embark upon a weight-reduction program. Ayurveda recommends a regular yoga practice that includes sūrya namaskāra (sun salutation) and prāṇāyāma.

The herbal approach to heal this problem would be the use of aphrodisiacs, called *vājīkaranam*. Typical vājīkarana substances are herbs such as ashvagandhā, balā, vidārī, kapikacchū, also called ātma guptā, gokshura, shilājit, pippalī, and spices such as cardamom and bay leaves. Vājīkaranas also encompass the use of almond milk, goat's milk, goat testicle soup, and dates in ghee or date shakes.

> **DATES PRESERVED IN GHEE**
>
> Warm one pound of fresh ghee and pour over 30 unseeded dates in a glass jar. Stir gently to evenly distribute the ghee amongst the dates. Close the container and allow it to sit for at least 15 days. As an aphrodisiac and to promote healthy ojas, consume one date daily for a full month.

A week or two of the cleansing program panchakarma can be very helpful. Typically, the administration of a basti (enema) containing dashamula and ashvagandhā milk will follow the snehana (oiling) and svedana (sudation or sweating) treatments. This combination has a very powerful healing and rejuvenation potential.

To help maintain an erection there is an herbal ointment that can be applied to the pubic bone and penis to enhance circulation and tone. Prepared in a ghee base, use a combination of herbs such as ashvagandhā, vidārī, clove, deer musk, nutmeg, gokshura, and ātma guptā. One can substitute ashvagandhā oil for the ghee. In general, Ayurveda recommends the use of garlic milk, ashvagandhā milk, shatāvarī milk, chyavānaprāsh and, in India, mākaradvāja, to enhance and maintain erectile function.

> **DASHAMULA-ASHVAGANDHA MILK BASTI**
>
> 1 pint of water
> 2 Tbs. of dashamūla
> 2 Tbs. of ashvagandhā
> 1 cup of warm milk
>
> **Option One**
> Bring the herbs to a boil in the water for 3 minutes, turn off heat and allow the brew to cool before straining. Once strained add one cup of warm milk to the brew.
>
> **Option Two**
> Bring the herbs to a boil in the milk and water together. Then strain and allow to cool.

## Surgical Solutions

Some patients may require surgical repair of the artery or vein. Various surgical implantation methods can help to produce a functional erection. Many require training to master the techniques and all have some side effects including but not limited to local bruising, scarring, complications, surgical risks, and penile pain. Psychological counseling by a sex therapist is usually advised as well.

## Conclusion

The male reproductive system is important in the life of every man. For some disorders of shukra vaha srotas are connected with physical causes such as obesity, diabetes, and hypertension. Trauma and emotional issues can be causative factors as well, leading to low self-esteem that may put a stress on relationships. The clinician must always consider both physical and emotional factors when managing male sexual health. Additionally, Ayurveda offers many non-surgical remedies that can support and enhance male sexual function, leading to greater satisfaction in one's life.

**MAKARADVAJA**

Also called cinnabar-gold and known as the best alchemical drug for longevity, is a renowned of mercurial rejuvenator or bhasma, whose main ingredients are mercury, sulphur, and gold. It regenerates vigour and vitality, improves immunity, and assists in body development by increasing metabolic activity. The best forms of Mākaradvāja have gold leaf on the outer surface of the pill as well as gold within.

# Chapter 45

# Impotence
## Klaibya

Summer 2017, Volume 30, Number 1

*Psychological considerations are often causative factors in this condition...*

IMPOTENCE IS THE INABILITY to achieve and maintain an erection, which is necessary for the penis to penetrate into the vagina during sexual intercourse. The corpus cavernosum of the penis normally fills with blood during sexual excitement, which causes the penis to become rigid and erect. Impotence is the partial or total impairment of this function.

The primary type of impotence is the inability to get an erection. Secondary impotence is when a man is unable to complete intercourse to the satisfaction of both partners.

Psychological considerations are often causative factors in this condition, such as low self-esteem, strain in the marriage or relationship, depression, job-related stress, and so forth. For instance, if a boss fires a man, he cannot easily enjoy sex. Thus, the inability to get or maintain an erection during sexual activity is often due to some problem with the nerves, but it can also have a physical cause, such as obesity or low testosterone levels.

## Etiological Factors of Impotence

- Imbalance of sex hormones, especially low testosterone
- Structural abnormality of the penis
- Fear of sex
- Fear of pregnancy
- Stress, in relationship, job-related, etc.
- Depression
- Sadness
- Unresolved anxiety
- Major rectal surgery

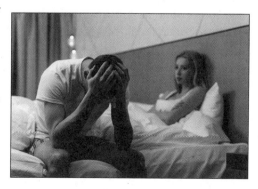

- After a heart attack
- Drug addiction or alcoholism
- Blood pressure medication or diuretic medication
- Obesity
- Diabetes
- High cholesterol, high triglycerides, or high blood pressure; these can all create a slow "heart attack" to the penis.

## Signs and Symptoms of Impotence

- Inability to maintain an erection
- Lack of interest in sex
- Infertility, the inability to father a child

## Diagnosis of Impotence

- Blood test for testosterone levels
- Ultrasound of internal structure of the penis, including the blood vessels
- Cholesterol test
- Triglycerides test
- Blood pressure
- Test the size of erection by measurement

If an erection does not occur during sleep, then it is due to physical rather than emotional factors. These people need more testosterone.

If there are varicose veins of the spermatic cord, surgical repair of the artery and veins can be done. A silicon rod is implanted in the corpus cavernosum. However it creates a permanent erection of the penis, so this is an important psychological consideration.

Seeing a trained sex therapist can be helpful. The person should consume no alcohol or drugs and do daily yogāsana, prānāyāma and meditation.

The man needs a loving, compassionate and cooperative partner, who is patient and helps to stimulate the sexual energy.

Vajikarana herbs and foods help support male sexual health. These include the herbs: Ashvagandhā, balā, vidārī, ātmaguptā, shilājit, vamsha rochan (eye of bamboo), yashthi madhu, gokshura and chyavanprash and foods such as ginseng, pippalī, cardamom, and black whole urad dal [black gram, dal makhani](*Vigna mungo*).

> **AYURVEDIC FORMULAS FOR IMPOTENCE**
>
> The Ayurvedic formula for impotence is equal parts ashvagandhā, balā, vidārī and kushmanda pak. Give 300 mg of this mixture (1/4 teaspoon), three times daily.
>
> Topically, apply a mixture of shatāvarī, balā and ashvagandhā oils to the penis, which can help erectile dysfunction.

Chapter 46

# Enlarged Prostate and Prostatitis

## Ashtila Vruddhi

Fall 2017, Volume 30, Number 1

• • • • • • • • • • • • • • • • • • • • • • • • • • • • • • • • • • • • • • • • •

*Vyadhi pratyanika (antagonistic to the disease) herbs can help with prostate disorders...*

• • • • • • • • • • • • • • • • • • • • • • • • • • • • • • • • • • • • • • • • •

ENLARGEMENT OF THE PROSTATE GLAND and inflammation or infection of the prostate predominantly affects elderly men. There are often chronic, recurring flair ups. Inflammation of the gland is called prostatitis. Although it is not generally a serious disease, prostatitis can be irritating and uncomfortable, because it disrupts urination. It can also cause bladder or kidney damage.

The prostate gland is a walnut-sized gland, located just below the bladder. During old age, the gland can become enlarged, which can constrict the urethra. This condition is known as prostatism, associated with outlet obstruction at the bladder neck and the commonest cause is benign prostatic hyperplasia (BPH). Less than half of all men with BPH have symptoms of the disease.

With BPH, urination requires prolonged effort with repeated attempts to start the flow. There is decreased urine flow, with a dribble towards the end. After urination, there may be urinary retention with a residual amount of urine in the bladder. This amount can be quite high—typically 20 to 30 ml. Some urine is left in the bladder and that is a fertile breeding ground for bacteria to grow. That is why an enlarged prostate can result in bladder infec-

### Benign Prostatic Hyperplasia

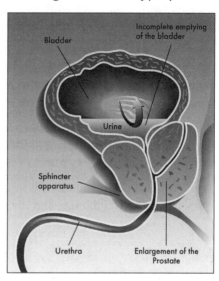

tions or cystitis, or even an ascending kidney infection (nephritis). Prostatitis can cause a total blockage of the urine flow, and the backup of urine may result in kidney damage.

### Causes of Enlarged Prostate or Prostatitis

If we look at the various causes for prostatitis, the most common are:

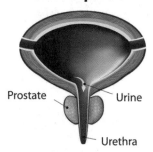

**Normal prostate**

- Genetic predisposition
- Urinary tract infection
- Sexually transmitted disease
- Straining to urinate

### Signs and Symptoms of BPH or Prostatitis

- Reduced urine flow
- Difficulty urinating
- Dribbling of urine at the end of urination
- Increased frequency of urination, especially at night
- Burning urethra
- Fevers and chills

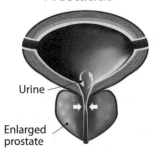

**Prostatitis**

## Assessment of Enlarged Prostate or Prostatitis

Diagnosis is done by physical examination. If you examine the bladder, it looks or feels full. Digital examination of the prostate can be done by putting on gloves. Apply lubricant to the anal orifice. With the patient lying on his left side and ask him to breathe through the mouth, which will relax the anal orifice. Then slowly put your finger up the anus, go to reach toward the top then turn your finger 180 degrees and try to touch the prostate gland.

If you reach the top of the prostate gland and can feel the middle surface, then the gland is normal size. However, if you press the gland and it is tender or painful, that indicates prostatitis. If the top of the gland cannot be reached, that means there is enlargement of the prostate.

If the gland is enlarged but it is firm and smooth, don't worry—it is benign prostatic hyperplasia. Whereas if the mucous lining adheres to the gland and the surface of the gland is nodular and hard, then it indicates a malignancy.

You can massage the prostate gland and collect the residual urine. It may show pus cells in the urine, which indicates bacterial infection. You can send the urine to be tested for various types of bacteria and malignant cells. IVP (intravenous pyelography) can be done to map out the enlargement of the prostate.

Nowadays, the normal way to check for enlarged prostate is through ultrasound, which can show you the size and the shape of the enlargement.

**ANTIBIOTIC TREATMENT TO KILL THE BACTERIA**

Sukshma triphala
Gandha karasayana
Neem
Echinacea
Osha

Use 200 mg of each and give the remedy, ½ teaspoon, three times daily.

**VYĀDHI PRATYANIKA (ANTAGONISTIC TO THE DISEASE) FOR PROSTATE DISORDERS**

Punarnavā 500 mg
Punarnavadi guggulu 300 mg
Goshukrādi guggulu 300 mg
Chandra prabha 200 mg
Shilājit guggulu or Shuddha guggulu 200 mg

Take this mixture three times daily, ½ teaspoon.

Lakshuna shirapaka, garlic boiled with half a cup of milk, twice daily is beneficial.

# Chapter 47

# Female Health Issues

Winter 2005, Volume 18, Number 3 and Spring 2006, Volume 18, Number 4

IN THE ANCIENT Ayurvedic literature, there are many recommendations about ārtava vaha srotas. This is the female reproductive system and it includes the ovaries, fallopian tubes, fundus of the uterus, uterine wall, cervix, cervical canal, and vaginal cavity.

In the process of tissue nutrition, the end product of digested food, called āhāra rasa, nourishes the seven tissues: rasa, rakta, māmsa, meda, asthi, majjā, and shukra or ārtava dhātus. Rasa dhātu is primordially important, as it carries hormones and nutrients, and is responsible for the gaseous exchange of oxygen and carbon dioxide. In the process of tissue nutrition, the immature (asthāyi) rasa becomes mature (sthāyi) and in that transformation, by-products (upadhātus) of rasa dhātu are formed. These include stanya (the lactating tissue) and rajah (menstruation). It takes five days for rasa dhātu to reach maturation, ten days for rakta, fifteen for māmsa, and so on. Hence, it takes ārtava and shukra dhātus up to 35 days to reach maturity.

## The Menstrual Cycle

Menstruation starts at menarche and continues until menopause. Menarche is typically between the ages of nine to 14. In girls with hyperactive pitta, menarche can start at age nine, while in kapha types it usually doesn't begin until age 14, 15, or even 16, because kapha is slow. Menopause is the age of vāta. It may start as early as age 35 in some pitta women, but can occur at age 58 to 60 in kapha types.

Menstruation, a by-product of rasa dhātu, is called rajah. Poetically, Sushruta describes the menstrual process as 'the weeping cry of the vagina for the deceased ovum'. During the 25 to 30 days of the menstrual cycle, the new ovum or egg is formed and enters the fallopian tubes where it eagerly waits to meet with a sperm. However, if the sperm does not show up, the ovum dies. The menstrual flow is a funeral for this deceased ovum.

According to modern science, the endometrial tissue thickens during the menstrual cycle to prepare the uterus for a possible future pregnancy. According to Ayurveda, this thickening of endometrial tissue is due to poshaka kapha,[63] which is a by-product (mala) of rasa. Approximately midway through a monthly cycle of menstruation, ovulation occurs. Ovulation is a process by which the ovary, which is called *antah phala* or 'inner fruit', ripens and releases an egg (ārtava) by means of *ārtava agni,* which relates to estrogen. This egg travels via the fallopian tube toward the uterus.

If fertilized by a sperm, the egg starts to slowly move from the fallopian tube into the uterine cavity, as it is seeks a place for nutrition. Implantation takes place at the fundus. If the fundus is healthy, with many capillaries, implantation occurs and the fetus grows there. However, if the woman is anemic, weak, undernourished, or has tuberculosis, then the fundus is weak as well. Weakness, in combination with apāna vāyu dushti (a disorder of downward vāta), and exacerbated mobility, can lead to implantation in the lower segment of the uterus. This leads to placenta presentation, also called placenta previa, and it is unhealthy, as it can cause hemorrhage prior to or during labor.

If, instead, there is excess kapha, the increased sluggishness can cause the fertilized egg to stay within the fallopian tube, instead of proceeding on its journey to the uterus. If implantation happens there, it gives rise to ectopic gestation. For correct implantation to occur there needs to be poshaka kapha, which relates closely to the role of progesterone in modern science.

If the egg is not fertilized, the thickened endometrial lining tissue starts breaking down. In Ayurveda, it is apāna vāyu that breaks this endometrial wall, due to its dry, hard, and rough qualities. Then those pieces of endometrial wall are passed as part of the menstrual flow.

The menstrual flow contains these broken-down pieces of endometrial wall as well as the unfertilized egg, red blood cells, white blood cells, and mucus. As it is related to rasa dhātu, this monthly cycle is controlled by rasa dhātu agni, ārtava dhātu agni, apāna vāyu, and poshaka kapha.

Modern medicine claims the cycle is controlled by the female hormones secreted by the ovaries and pituitary gland. In Ayurveda, these hormones are nothing other than ārtava agni and they are regulated by prāna vāyu, sādhaka pitta, and tarpaka kapha.

## Dysmenorrhea

Dysmenorrhea, which means painful menstruation, is called *kashthārtava* in Ayurveda. *Prathamik kashthārtava,* meaning primary dysmenorrhea, occurs shortly after the onset of menstruation in young teenagers and in women who have never been pregnant. *Dvitīyak kashthārtava,* which is secondary dysmenorrhea, develops later in life, after the woman has been menstruating for sometime. This can be due to a vāta imbalance leading to narrowing of the blood vessels and cervix, a pitta malfunction leading to endometriosis, or a kapha imbalance leading to a fibroid tumor.

There are two internal causes of vāta dushti (qualitative disturbance of vāta): one is dhātu kshaya (debilitated tissues), which leads to the second, sroto rodha (blockage of the channels). Therefore, dhātu kshaya can bring about a narrowing of the cervix. Generally

---

63. For more information on poshaka kapha, see "Management of Rasa Dhātu Mala," *Ayurveda Today,* Summer 2008, Volume 21, Number 1.

during menstruation, when the uterus contracts, the cervix should dilate. Contraction of the uterus is governed by prāna and dilation of the cervix by apāna vāyu. When this rhythm is disturbed, the cervix remains closed. In this condition, called pinhole os, the woman has severe pain, the blood doesn't flow, and blood clots are held within the uterus. In the passing of these clots, they force a dilatation of the uterus in a type of nature-induced dilatation and curative.

In pitta-type of kashthārtava, rañjaka pitta from the rakta and rasa dhātus goes into the endometrial wall and creates inflammation. This is called endometritis. Due to the hot and sharp qualities of pitta, the mucus lining of the endometrium and cervix become inflamed, causing pitta-type of dysmenorrhea.

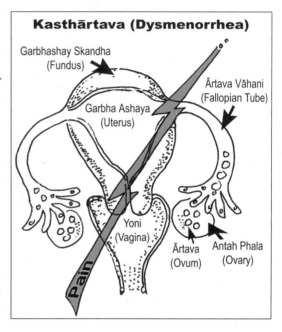

**Kasthārtava (Dysmenorrhea)**

In kapha-type of dysmenorrhea, excess poshaka kapha is produced and it accumulates within the uterine wall, leading to fibrotic changes. These too can lead to dysmenorrhea.

***Etiology (Nidāna).*** In vāta-type dysmenorrhea, a vāta-provoking diet is a common etiological factor. This means the consumption of too many raw vegetables, beans, chickpeas, and so forth. Other causes can be too much traveling, excessive physical activities, especially jogging, jumping, and trampolining as well as unresolved fear and anxiety. Also, prostaglandin, which is present in chocolate, provokes vāta.

There is a path of samprāpti (pathogenesis) for each dosha as it accumulates and then spreads through the system. Here we'll talk about the first four stages of samprāpti as it relates to dysmenorrhea.Vāta undergoes sanchaya (accumulation) and prakopa (provocation) in the colon, then prasara (spread) throughout the body. During this time, there is constipation, gas, and bloating. Then *vāta sthana samshraya* (deposition) happens within the capillaries of the uterus, so there is contraction of the blood vessels and that decreases the blood flow. It is this constriction that causes pain during menstruation in vāta-type of dysmenorrhea.

In pitta-type of dysmenorrhea, the woman's diet is typically pitta-provoking: hot, spicy foods, sour fruits, and citrus fruits. Working in hot conditions, plus emotionally unresolved anger and frustration are also common. These physiological and psychological factors trigger pitta, which undergoes sanchaya and prakopa in the grahani (small intestines), then prasara and sthana samshraya happens through the walls of the blood vessels, causing inflammation of the uterus and endometrium.

In kapha dysmenorrhea, the causes include eating dairy products such as cheese, yogurt, and ice cream, plus eating gluten (mainly from wheat products) as well as insufficient exercise and excessive emotional attachments. Kapha undergoes sanchaya and prakopa in the stomach, then prasara, and in the fourth stage of disease kapha passes through the rasa dhātu of the uterus and enters the endometrium wall. There it produces thickening, possibly causing a fibroid tumor.

***Signs and Symptoms (Lakshana).*** In vāta-type of dysmenorrhea, there is constipation, bloating, lower backache and severe cramps, and the woman also has insomnia, palpitations, fear, and anxiety. There is scanty menstruation, but more clots than normal. Symptoms appear to be more intense during the earlier part of menstruation. Once the woman passes the clots, they cause dilatation of the cervix, and as a result she feels better.

In pitta-type of dysmenorrhea, there are hives, rashes or urticaria, plus mild attacks of urethritis, cystitis and burning urination. In earlier menses, there is acne on the face, nausea, vomiting, diarrhea or loose stools, headache, and irritability. Pitta dysmenorrhea is experienced more during the mid-menses. Once the excessive heat is released through the menses, the woman feels better.

In kapha dysmenorrhea, there is a thick, watery, curd-like, white discharge. There is more mucus and less blood. The uterus looks or feels bulky, and there is a dull, aching pain. There is also increased frequency of urination (polyuria), water retention, and swelling. The woman's bra and rings on her fingers become tight, and she is lethargic and doesn't feel like going to work. She would rather eat candy, cookies, and chocolate and watch TV at home. There is often depression during this period. Lethargy and excessive sleep take over and some women have excess salivation, a runny or stuffy nose, and sinus congestion. This generally occurs during the earlier part of the period, although it may happen throughout the menses.

***Management (Chikitsā).*** For proper management, one must take the family history and personal history. Sometimes, one can take advantage of the support of modern technology, such as an ultrasound, to find out whether there is a uterine fibroid. In some cases, an x-ray may be required.

In Ayurveda, what is important is pulse diagnosis. As well as assessing the prakruti-vikruti paradigm, one would concentrate on the fifth-level dhātu pulse. At this level, dysmenorrhea would show as a weak ārtava pulse, with vāta pushing pitta, pitta pushing kapha, kapha blocking vāta, or pitta in ārtava dhātu.

Management in vāta dysmenorrhea requires abhyanga (oil massage), with nirgundī oil or mahānārāyana oil applied to the lower abdomen and lower back. This should be followed by svedana (sweating), using local fomentation or a hot bath to ease the pain. Internally, the person can begin taking fifteen days prior to the menses, ½ teaspoon of an herbal combination of:

| | |
|---|---|
| Dashamūla | 500 mg |
| Ashvagandhā | 400 mg |
| Mustā | 300 mg |
| Tagara | 200 mg |
| Yogarāja Guggulu | 200 mg |

This should be taken TID with warm water, before meals. This remedy pacifies vāta dosha and relieves pain. After cessation of menses, one should administer a dashamūla tea basti (enema) containing ½ cup of sesame oil. This is followed by a vāta-pacifying diet. For vāta dysmenorrhea, the best yoga poses are camel, cobra, and cow pose, while best types of prāṇāyāma are nāḍī shodana and anuloma viloma.

Management in pitta dysmenorrhea requires abhyanga with coconut oil or sunflower oil. No svedana is generally needed, because pitta is already hot by nature. However, a baking soda bath is effective during painful periods. To do this, put one-third of a cup of baking soda (not baking powder) into the bathtub and fill with warm water.

Internally, beginning fifteen days prior to the menses, the person can take ½ teaspoon of an herbal combination of:

| | |
|---|---|
| Shatāvarī | 500 mg |
| Gudūchī | 300 mg |
| Kāma Dudhā | 200 mg |
| Ashoka | 300 mg |

This should be taken TID with aloe vera gel, before meals. After the cessation of menstrual bleeding, virechana (purgation) can be performed with one teaspoon of bhumi āmalakī at bedtime. For pitta dysmenorrhea the best yogāsanas are boat, bow, and bridge poses, and the best prāṇāyāma for pitta is shītalī.

Management for kapha type of dysmenorrhea requires snehana with visha garbha tailam or a kapha-pacifying oil medicated with heating herbs, such as trikatu or chitrak. Chitrakadi tailam is a good example. This should be followed by svedana, either using dry heat from the topical application of ginger paste to the lower belly, or wet svedana by means of a ginger bath. This means adding ginger powder to a bathtub of hot water. Internally, fifteen days prior to the menses, ½ teaspoon of an herbal combination of:

| | |
|---|---|
| Punarnavā | 500 mg |
| Kutki | 200 mg |
| Shilājit | 200 mg |
| Trikatu | 200 mg |

This should be taken TID before meals with honey. After the cessation of menses, a kapha-pacifying diet and exercise routine should be followed. For kapha, the best āsanas are lotus, locust, lion, palm tree, and spinal twists, and the best prāṇāyāma are bhastrikā and kapāla bhāti.

## Premenstrual Syndrome

Premenstrual syndrome or PMS is a complex set of physical and emotional symptoms that is experienced a week or so before the menstrual cycle begins. It appears five to fourteen days before the menstrual cycle and usually disappears after menstruation. In the past, PMS was thought to be caused by emotional instability or hysteria. The word *hysterus* is Greek and it means uterus. Uterine dysfunction is called hysteria. However, there is a definite cause and reason for PMS and it is not only an emotional disorder.

| Signs and Symptoms of PMS |
|---|
| **Vāta** |
| Sadness |
| Hopelessness |
| Self-deprecation |
| Tenseness |
| Anxiety |
| Feeling 'on edge' |
| Mood swings |
| Fear |
| Loneliness |
| Insomnia |
| Overwhelm |
| Lower backache |
| **Pitta** |
| Irritability |
| Anger |
| Interpersonal conflict |
| Judgment |
| Criticism |
| Lack of patience |
| Breast tenderness |
| Swelling |
| Suicidal thoughts |
| Cystitis |
| Acne |
| Hot flashes |
| **Kapha** |
| Depression |
| Decreased interest in usual activities |
| Withdrawal from social relationships |
| Difficulty concentrating |
| Fatigue |
| Lethargy |
| Poor appetite |
| Bloating |
| Weight gain |
| Leukorrhea |
| Food cravings |

*Manifestation.* Like dysmenorrhea, PMS can be a mono-doshic, dual-doshic, or triple-doshic disorder. The etiological factors are also similar to those of dysmenorrhea.

In vāta-type PMS, systemic vāta undergoes sanchaya, prakopa, and prasara and then the sthana samshraya happens in the ārtava vāta srotas, leading to fluctuations of the hormones. In pitta PMS, the pitta accumulates and is then provoked and spreads. In kapha PMS, increased kapha spreads through the body and fluid retention is the result.

*Signs and Symptoms (Lakshana).* In vāta-type of PMS, there is nervousness, anxiety, tachycardia, insomnia, debility, and lower backache. In pitta-type of PMS, there can be hives, rashes, urticaria, acne, cystitis, irritability, and migraine headache. The nipples become sensitive to the touch and the breasts become tender. There may be repeated attacks of cystitis or urethritis, with burning sensations while passing urine. In kapha-type of PMS, there is fluid retention, bloating, enlarged breasts, and ankle swelling. The woman may put on a couple of pounds of excess weight, have white discharge, and a bloated, puffy face.

*Management (Chikitsā).* Before approaching management, one should take the client's history: her personal history and family history. One must also find out the symptomatology and read the pulse, especially the prakruti, vikruti, and ārtava dhātu pulses.

Whenever we are dealing with PMS, it is rare to have a mono-doshic disorder, as this syndrome is almost always a combination of two or three doshas.

When there is anxiety, tachycardia, palpitations, and headaches, the woman should avoid methylxanthine, a group of naturally occurring agents in caffeine. This means avoid coffee, chocolate, tea, and colas.

For headaches, herbs such as tagara and jatamāmsi can be taken in equal proportion: ½ teaspoon of the mixture TID. Also for headaches, nasya with vacha oil is highly recommended.

When a woman has anxiety, tachycardia, or insomnia, tranquilizing herbs such as brahmī, jatamāmsi, and shankha pushpī can be used or she can try my formula, Tranquility Tea©.

For edema, reduce salt intake and avoid pickles, cucumber, watermelon, ice cream, candy, cookies and chocolate. Some diuretic herbs, such as punarnavā and gokshura, can be helpful in the quantity of ½ teaspoon TID.

To create emotional balance, one can do alternate nostril breathing, called anuloma viloma prānāyāma, and also have an oil massage and take a hot bath. Marma chikitsā is also helpful and the best marmas for PMS are Nābhi, Bhaga, Sakthi Ūrvī, Jānu, Gulpha, and Trik. Nutmeg essential oil can be applied to these energy points. (see illustrations page 459)

If a woman has a hormonal imbalance, Ayurveda suggests the use of food precursors of estrogen, such as shatāvarī, kumārī, ashvagandhā, vidārī, and soy, or precursors of progesterone, including nirgundī, kapikacchū, and balā. Also, primrose oil in a 500 mg capsule daily can help in maintaining hormonal balance.

Uterine tonics to strengthen and tonify the uterus are shatāvarī ghrita (or shatāvarī ghee), yashthi madhu ghrita (licorice ghee), and vidariadi ghrita (vidārī ghee). Note that shatāvarī should not be given if there is pathology involving āma. Ideally, to maintain balance, one would use dashamūla ghee for vāta, shatāvarī ghee for pitta, and tikta ghee for kapha.

For prevention of PMS, daily yogāsana and prānāyāma are beneficial as well as abhyanga (oil massage) and svedana (steam therapy), plus weekly *uttara basti* (see Uttara Basti on page 378) to pacify vāta in the lower uterine passage. For abhyanga, cottonseed oil can be applied topically along with lotus oil.

> **SHATAVARI MEDICATED GHEE**
>
> Shatāvarī, powdered
> Water, filtered
> Ghee
> Take one part of shatāvarī to 16 parts of water, stir together in a stainless steel cooking vessel.
>
> Bring this to a boil then turn the heat down until the concoction is simmering. Cook at a simmer until the mixture is reduced to ¼ the original amount. Cool and strain.
>
> Then add ghee that is equal in volume to the volume of the concoction. Cook this mixture over medium heat until all the water evaporates. It is very important that the water is completely eliminated as otherwise the ghee will spoil.
>
> Pour into a glass container with a tight fitting lid. This will keep indefinitely. You can use the same principles of this recipe to make other medicated ghees.

## General Rasāyana and Foods to Favor

Rasāyana (rejuvenation therapies) for dysmenorrhea and PMS include shatāvarī and kumārī (aloe vera). Medicated wines, such as ashok arishta and kumārī arishta, can be taken in the dosage of four teaspoons with an equal amount of water after lunch and dinner.

The best foods to favor in dysmenorrhea and PMS are broths, urud dhal soup, winter squash, zucchini, and pumpkin for vāta. Mung dal soup, red lentil soup, grapes, shatāvarī milk, and coconut milk are good for pitta. Kapha should favor light and easily digested foods.

Avoiding grief and sadness is the rasāyana for vāta, avoiding judgment and argument is that for pitta, while letting go of attachment as well as not sleeping during the daytime is the rasāyana for kapha.

### Part Two

We have discussed the menstrual cycle, managing imbalances, and the role of diet as well as PMS, its symptoms and management. In this next section, we cover disorders of menstrual flow and maintaining vaginal health.

# Menorrhagia

Menorrhagia is a disorder characterized by excessive bleeding at the time of a menstrual period, either in the number of days or the amount of blood passed or both. In Ayurveda, this condition is called *asrugdhārā* or *adhoga rakta pitta*. This pitta disorder is quite common during the pitta time of life, mainly between the ages of thirty to forty. It can lead to iron deficiency anemia.

For a woman with pitta prakruti and/or pitta vikruti, one should look at her diet as well as her lifestyle activities. Physical activities like jogging, jumping on a trampoline, heavy weight lifting, or hiking can provoke vāta dosha and this can lead to menorrhagia.

*Etiology (Nidāna).* The samprāpti (pathogenesis) of menorrhagia varies according to the condition. There is an assortment of ways that pitta becomes aggravated and excessive bleeding is one of the signs of high pitta. In the tissue nutrition of rasa dhātu, its upadhātus (by-products) are stanya (lactating tissue) and rajah (menstruation). When vāta dosha is provoked, vyāna vāyu (systemic vāta dosha) will push rañjaka pitta into the rasa and rakta dhātus (blood and plasma tissues). In the case of excessive physical activities, vāta is pushing pitta in the *rajo vaha srotas* (menstruation channel). Surplus pitta in this channel will show up as increased bleeding during menstruation.

Vāta pushing pitta in the ārtava vaha srotas may be also responsible for the disturbance of hormones controlling the overall menstrual cycle. The vāta symptoms of this are lower back ache, lower abdominal pain, distention, palpitation, anxiety, and fear with slight insomnia. The pitta symptoms would manifest as burning sensation in the urethra, cystitis of unknown origin, nipples becoming sensitive to touch, tender breasts with cravings for sweets, irritability, and a judgmental and critical attitude for no apparent reason. In the case of a fibroid tumor, especially the intramural type with increased vascularity, this is also vāta pushing pitta in the blood vessels and it can rupture the capillaries, creating heavy menstrual flow.

As vāta becomes provoked, apāna vāyu in the pelvic cavity also pulls rañjaka pitta into the pelvic area, causing further inflammation of the pelvic organs. There is no inflammation without the ushna (hot) and tīkshna (sharp) qualities of pitta and these are contributing factors in menorrhagia.

Another consideration in prolonged menstrual flow is the strength of agni. When dhātu agni is low (manda or slow agni), there is undue production of raw tissue. This unprocessed tissue from rasa dhātu is eliminated as raw rajah (menstruation), producing excessive menstrual bleeding. Low dhātu agni is attributed to hypothyroidism.

The assessment and diagnosis of abnormal menstrual flow is important and should be continued until resolved. Pap smear tests are needed in order to detect serious underlying causes, such as cervical erosion and cervical dysplasia. For some individuals a biopsy of cervix and uterine membrane tissue is done in order to find possible abnormality and to rule out adhoga rakta pitta, a bleeding disorder. A blood profile is also recommended, to find if there is any sign of blood dyscrasia, hemophilia, polycythemia, and/or anemia. Even leukemia can be the cause of severe bleeding.

*General Management (Chikitsā).* For management of menorrhagia, it is wise to build the health of the client as the loss of blood can be depleting. First, reduce physical activity and get rest. Second, administer sufficient iron to improve the quality of the blood. For iron supplementation in India, we give loha bhasma and abhrak bhasma. In the west, we use foods such as currants, raisins, beet juice, and carrot juice; and we can give kumārī āsava (an herbal fermented wine) and aloe vera. Third, for balancing the hormones, ingest the food precursors of estrogen such as one of the following for a month.

| | |
|---|---|
| Shatāvarī | 500 mg, TID |
| Kumārī Āsava (an herbalized wine) | 4 tablespoons with an equal amount of water, after lunch and dinner |
| Primrose oil capsules | 500 mg at bedtime |

The typical formula for asrugdhārā (menorrhagia) is shatāvarī 500 mg, as dosha pratyanika, then gulvel sattva 300 mg, as an anti-inflammatory, ashoka 300 mg as a hemostatic, and vāsaka 300 mg also as a hemostatic. This formula is given TID, ½ teaspoon with pomegranate, cranberry, or aloe vera juice.

Bhumi āmalakī, is a mild laxative, hemostatic and anti-inflammatory, and a good source of iron. It should be taken in the quantity of one teaspoon at bedtime. Whenever there is a pelvic floor, inflammatory disorder causing profuse bleeding, bhumi āmalakī is the herb of choice. Other very famous hemostatic herbs in Ayurvedic literature are ushīra/khus, dūrvā grass/conch grass, lodhra, ashoka, and vāsaka. Hemostatic minerals are laksha, and pravāl pañchāmrit and kāma dudhā.

Other traditional Ayurvedic compounds used for menorrhagia are shatāvarī ghee, dūrvā ghee, pradarāntak vati and lodhra āsava. In some instances ghee should not be given. For example, if there is āma (toxins) present, then there should be dīpana (kindling of agni) and pañchana (digestion) first.

# Amenorrhea

Amenorrhea is an absence of or abnormal stoppage of the menstrual flow and is called nasthartava or rajah kshaya in Ayurveda. It can be primary (prathamik) or secondary (dvitayak). Prathamik nasthartava, or primary amenorrhea, is lack of menarche or failure to begin the menses by the age of 16. This condition can continue indefinitely. Dvitayak nasthartava, or secondary amenorrhea, is the absence of two, three or more periods in a row in a woman who has been menstruating for some time. Secondary amenorrhea may be a temporary phase.

It is completely normal for menses to be absent during pregnancy, the period of lactation, and after menopause.

*Etiology (Nidāna).* The samprāpti of amenorrhea creates endocrine gland disorders and hyperthyroidism. When there is hyperthyroidism due to an excess of dhātu agni, the dhātus become depleted, leading to nasthartava. This is usually caused by increased vāta and kapha doshas. In this situation, kapha is blocking vāta or vāta is pushing kapha in ārtava dhātu (female reproductive tissue) as well as in majjā dhātu (bone marrow and nerve tissue).

The occurrence of extreme kapha disorders can also cause primary amenorrhea. This elevated kapha would manifest as hypothyroidism or myxedema, or as a genetic abnormality such as damage to or missing ovaries, the absence of a uterus or vagina, an excessively thick hymen or un-open hymen requiring surgery. Other etiological factors include congenital diabetes, malnutrition, obesity, deep-seated emotional anxiety, extreme stress, or anorexia.

Some things responsible for secondary amenorrhea are activities such as strenuous exercise, aggressive sports, and taking part in marathons, since intense physical training provokes vāta. Also, poor nutrition, fasting, drastic weight loss, jet lag, and traveling can cause dvitayak nasthartava. It may seem surprising but intense spiritual practices—yoga, meditation, and prānāyāma where the goal is enlightenment—can cause secondary amenorrhea as well. These practices cause the energy of the body move up to the higher chakras thereby diminishing the downward movement necessary for menstruation.

Other causative factors for secondary amenorrhea are taking drugs such as corticosteroids and birth control pills, major surgery, severe shock, stress, and loss of body fat.

*Signs and Symptoms (Lakshana).* Samprāpti differs according to the etiology but common signs and symptoms of primary amenorrhea are general abnormal physical maturation. This includes the young girl failing to develop breasts and an absence of secondary sexual characteristics, i.e., pubic and auxiliary hair. The girl may also exhibit minimal sexual maturity such as at the age of 16 she acts like a little girl or infant and has stunted growth. In secondary amenorrhea there are no symptoms at all other than anemia and weight loss. However, this can be detected by pulse analysis. The 5th level pulse, that is the dhātu pulse, will show either a strong vāta or kapha spike at the ārtava dhātu site.

For assessment and accurate diagnosis, a blood test for genetic hormonal disorder should be done. An x-ray or ultrasound study should be performed to check for the development of the uterus. A complete blood profile for anemia and, if found, discovering the cause of the anemia. One should also check if there is tuberculosis, severe anemia or blood dyscrasia.

*Management (Chikitsā).* The treatment for primary amenorrhea is a hormonal therapy program including including building therapies such as *brahmana chikitsā* and *tarpana chikitsā.*[64] These are complex programs that should be done with the guidance of an Ayurvedic physician.

Panchakarma, the Ayurvedic cleansing program, is also helpful. For the panchakarma procedure of snehana (oil applied by a specific massage), the best oil to use would be a

---

64. Refer also to *Textbook of Ayurveda,* Volume 3 for more on these therapies.

balā tailam (an herbalized oil prepared by a specific sequence of techniques), a vāta-pacifying tailam or almond oil. The svedana (sudation) would be encouraged with nirgundī. Herbs such as shatāvarī, ashvagandhā, balā, vidārī, and ātma guptā would be used to promote *bālya jīvinīya* (strength, life-giving).

For an intact hymen that needs to be opened, a surgical procedure is required. Unfortunately there is nothing that can be done in cases of infantile uterus, the absence of an ovary, or the presence of two small uteri.

If the amenorrhea is due to poor nutrition, then one should undergo a blood nutritive program. If it is from drastic weight loss, then one would help balance meda dhātu (adipose tissue) with meda rasāyana (rejuvenation) herbal combinations like shatāvarī ghee or balā ghee. Take 1 teaspoon TID before meals. When the cause is jetlag-induced amenorrhea, one should have an oil massage and take 1 teaspoon each of balā and trikatu or balā and ginger, mixed together in milk. If the origin is from one's spiritual practices, then reduce or stop these practices entirely. If the patient is taking steroids then they should consider discontinuing the steroidal therapy. Of course they would discuss alternatives with their primary care provider. If amenorrhea is due to stress then one should do less, relax, rub bhringarāja or brahmī oil on the scalp and the soles of the feet, and try So'Hum meditation. You can supplement this with herbs. Take ½ teaspoon TID of a mixture of ashvagandhā 500 mg, jatamāmsi 300 mg, and shankha pushpī 200 mg

If the amenorrhea is a result of major surgery, then one should have rasāyana (rejuvenation) therapy with the herbs shatāvarī 500 mg, balā 300 mg, and vidārī 200 mg. Take ½ teaspoon of this mixture TID. For hormonal imbalance, one can use primrose oil or phytoestrogens like aloe vera, soy, and shatāvarī ghee. For emotional imbalance the ideal herbs are brahmī 200 mg, jatamāmsi 200 mg, and sarasvatī (herbal compound) 200 mg, ½ teaspoon TID. You can also use 10 drops of Deep Love® tincture taken before meals.

### Prevention

Prevention is always better than a cure. So, to prevent amenorrhea and the possibility of amenorrhea, one should seek good nutrition through diet. Be sure to get plenty of iron in the diet and consume food items that are good sources of iron such as papaya, pomegranate, mango, pumpkin, pineapple, currants, raisons, soaked almonds, garlic milk, shatāvarī milk, or shatāvarī kalka with milk at bedtime. Shatāvarī kalka is a compound of shatāvarī roasted with ghee and to which saffron, cardamom, and sugar are added.

For someone who is prone to problems with amenorrhea, maintaining proper body weight by following a healthy, vāta-pacifying diet is important. These women should also avoid excessive strenuous exercise and sports and instead rest, read, and relax!

# Vaginitis

Vaginitis in Ayurveda is called is called *yoni paka*. *Yoni* means vagina and paka means digestion or inflammation. It is an inflammation of the vagina usually accompanied by burning and itching of the external genital organ.

Flare ups are more likely occur in the summer, due to heat and moisture. Common causes are:

- Increased systemic pitta.
- An imbalance in the vagina caused by micro-organisms such as fungus (Candida albicans), bacteria (Gardnerella vaginalis), and protozoa (Trichomonas vaginalis) and by pinworms, roundworms, and threadworms.
- Birth control pills.
- Antibiotics, like tetracycline or erythromycin, which may kill certain flora allowing other to flourish.
- A hot, moist environment or climate.
- Wearing tight pants and synthetic underwear.
- Putting on a wet bathing suit, which is a breeding ground for infectious organisms.
- Sexual intercourse with an infected individual.

Causes of noninfectious vaginitis or vaginitis due to direct irritation are chemical irritation from douches, sprays, bubble bath, talcum powders, poor feminine hygiene, and using scented, colored toilet paper, which will have more chemicals and hence, be more irritating. Vaginitis may also occur during pregnancy, diabetes, and gonorrhea.

***Signs and Symptoms; Management.*** Signs and symptoms vary according to etiological factors. Diagnosis can be complex. It is done by collecting a specimen from the woman and then determining the microorganism involved by microscopic examination of the sample. Once you have a diagnosis, your doctor is likely to prescribe medicines such as metronidazole. However, these can be toxic to the liver. If you would like to try a more natural approach, the following are some suggestions. You can take these herbal formulas for one to two months, along with the medicine prescribed by your physician.

If there is a fungal infection, try licorice tea uttara basti. (see instructions page 378) For bacterial infection, antibacterial herbs like goldenseal, echinacea, haridrā, pushkaramūla, yavānī, and mahāsudarshan and are very effective. Try them alone in tea form or in a base of ghee.

If the woman has an infected sexual partner, she and her partner should be treated for the condition and they should use condoms until the condition has cleared up. Helpful are also chandana āsava, kumārī āsava, and shatāvarī ghee. The ghee can be taken before meals at a dose of one teaspoon. For the herbal wines, take 4 tablespoons mixed with an equal amount of water after lunch and dinner.

In the case of candidal vaginitis, there is more itching, pain during intercourse, and a thick, white discharge resembling cottage cheese with a yeast-like odor. This is quite common during pregnancy and diabetes. The treatment for this is shatāvarī 500 mg, gudūchī 300 mg, shardunikā 200 mg, neem 200 mg, and vidanga 200 mg. This mixture is taken ½ teaspoon TID using aloe vera gel as the anupāna, carrying medium. Also one should do a licorice tea uttara basti (medicated douche) by using one pint of water, two tablespoons of licorice, and one teaspoon of neem, boiled together for three minutes; once cooled, it should be strained before use. This douche should be done at least every other night, until the symptoms disappear.

In the instance of Gardnerella vaginalis vaginitis (formerly called non-specific vaginitis or hemophilus vaginalis), there is itching, burning, with a creamy white, grayish, foul-smelling discharge. It is more common in the summer season. In this case one should do a triphalā tea uttara basti by taking two tablespoons of triphalā and boiling it in pint of water. Once cooled, it should be strained before use. Also take ½ teaspoon of the following formula with pomegranate juice.

| | |
|---|---|
| Ashoka | 300 mg |
| Manjishthā | 200 mg |
| Katukā | 200 mg |
| Shilājit | 100 mg |

If the client has Trichomonas vaginalis vaginitis, there is more itching and burning accompanied by a greenish, whitish discharge having a foul odor. This condition usually starts after menstruation. The uttara basti in this case combines two tablespoons each of ashoka and yashthi madhu, boiled together in a pint of water. Cool and strain before use. Take ½ teaspoon of the mixture below TID with gheemadhu, honey and ghee.

| | |
|---|---|
| Shatāvarī | 500 mg |
| Ashoka | 200 mg |
| Manjishthā | 200 mg |
| Kāma Dudhā | 200 mg |

In cases of non-infectious vaginitis, there is more dryness of the vaginal mucus membrane and there are red, inflamed patches with irritation but no discharge. This is high pitta in ārtava dhātu. For non-infectious vaginitis where the cause is contact with an external irritant, one should avoid the cause and maintain strict feminine hygiene. To soothe and heal the membranes, coat a tampon with shatāvarī ghee and insert in the vaginal canal. To help the symptoms, take ½ teaspoon of the following mixture TID with aloe vera gel. Be sure to take each dose before food so it will act on the vagina.

| | |
|---|---|
| Shatāvarī | 500 mg |
| Gulvel Sattva | 200 mg |
| Kāma Dudhā | 200 mg |
| Motibhasma | 200 mg |

The female reproductive system, ārtava vaha srotas is profoundly important in the life of every woman. In some individuals, ārtava vaha srotas is extremely sensitive to changes in environment, lifestyle, and diet. To help your awareness of your cycle and symptoms, keep a calendar of the dates of onset of menstruation and the cessation of menstruation (the moon cycle) along with a detailed record of the signs and symptoms. In cases of amenorrhea too much physical activity could be responsible, so keeping a balanced yoga, meditation, and exercise practice is important to help maintain healthy biorhythms of the menses. Emotional factors also play an important role in the rhythm of menses. As much as possible one should keep an easy schedule, try not to have sex during menses, and avoid hot, spicy food and alcoholic beverages that can trigger pitta. Any change in the menstrual cycle is a warning sign that the reproductive system may be experiencing detrimental change.

## UTTARA BASTI

The nine gates of the body (seven openings in the head and two below) are constantly open to outer environmental changes. These are also the main gates of prāna, tejas and ojas into majjā dhātu (in this case, primarily nerve tissue). Through these openings, the external qualities of rough, dry, hot, cold, and others enter directly through majjā dhātu into the mental faculty. These attributes can affect the mind and the functioning of related srotāmsi (channels).

The ancient Ayurvedic literature speaks a great deal about obtaining female health by means of uttara basti (a form of medicated douche). This treatment works on the pelvic space, lumbo-sacral plexus, and mūlādhāra chakra. It has a wide range of actions on the bladder, uterus, ovaries, and sigmoid colon. In uttara basti, herbal medicated teas are injected into the vagina, working directly on the vaginal mucus membrane, cervix, uterus, fallopian tubes, ovaries, and endometrial tissue. Hence, in Ayurveda, dryness of the vagina, constriction of the cervix, inflammation of the endometrium, fibroid tumors, and several other PMS syndromes can often be effectively managed through the administration of specific herbal teas via uttara basti.

In general, the preferred substance used for uttara basti in vāta predominance is dashamūla tea. For pitta, gudūchī tea is the best uttara basti, while for kapha one can use yashthi madhu (licorice) basti. However, in cases of vaginitis and cervicitis, shatāvarī tea with ghee would be used as an uttara basti. In dryness of the cervix and vaginal wall and dysmenorrhea, use a dashamūla tea uttara basti with added nirgundī oil. In fungal or yeast infections, a shardunikā and neem tea uttara basti is used. When there is kapha dusthi with leucorrhea and fibroids, a punarnavā and yashthi madhu tea uttara basti is recommended. It is also said that if a woman takes a simple triphalā tea uttara basti with plain ghee once a week on a Saturday, good female health will be maintained.

In cases of PMS, uttara basti is done every day for one or two weeks, until the person is symptom free. Uttara basti should not be done during menstruation, the bleeding phase of rakta pitta conditions, vaginal prolapse, pregnancy, or when malignant lesions are present, especially during chemotherapy or active cancer.

To make an uttara basti tea, two tablespoons of the herb or herbs are added to one pint of water and boiled for two minutes. Once this has cooled down, half a cup of any recommended medicated oil or ghee can be added.

Chapter 48

# Endometriosis
## Kapha Āvrita Rakta

Summer 2013, Volume 26, Number 1

THE DEFINITION OF DISEASE in Ayurveda is *dosha dūshya sammurcchana*. This means that the doshas from the gastrointestinal (GI) tract enter rasa and rakta dhātus (the bloodstream) and circulate throughout the body. Then, when they find a khavaigunya (defective space), they deposit in the weakened dhātu (tissue) and create a pathological lesion.

Endometriosis occurs in a part of endometrium[65] that is weakened by lifestyle or genetic defect. Vāta or pitta dosha push kapha in ārtava vaha srotas (the female reproductive system), and that can cause thickening of the wall of the endometrium. Endometriosis arises when the endometrial cells lining the uterus thicken and detach from the wall of the uterus. The endometrial tissue sometimes starts to grow outside of the uterus, in other areas of the body such as the pelvic or abdominal cavity. This can lead to pain, irregular bleeding, and infertility. Endometriosis is non-malignant disorder. It generally happens in the pitta stage of life, from about age 25 into the 40s. That is also the typical childbearing age in the West.

The endometrium is the mucous membrane that lines the wall of the uterus. It undergoes changes during the menstrual cycle and in pregnancy. The endometrium consists of two highly vascular layers of areolar connective tissue. The bacillary layer is adjacent to the myometrium and the functional layer is adjacent to the uterine cavity. In endometriosis, each of these layers undergoes growth and pierces the wall of the uterus. It can spread outside the uterine cavity and grows on the surface of the small intestine, colon, bladder, and vagina. It can even grow on the pericardium and pleura. It looks like a surgical scar.

## Nidana, Etiological Factors

Between 1% and 7% of women in the United States are prone to this condition. It is a relatively common disorder amongst women of Asian and European descent. Women who are tall and thin, with a low body mass, have a higher risk. Genetic predisposition and hereditary factors play an important role. Delayed pregnancy is another factor.

---

65. The glandular mucous membrane that lines the uterus.

During each menstrual cycle, the endometrium naturally becomes thick and swollen in the preparation for a possible future pregnancy. Then, if no conception occurs, a portion of the endometrium tissue breaks down and passes out of the uterus as a part of the menstrual flow.

In endometriosis, some of the cells are not expelled and remain in the uterus. The endometrial tissue then forms on top of these displaced cells. These displaced pieces of endometrial tissue continue to swell and bleed each month. The blood has no outlet, because it is enclosed within the endometrium.

The body responds to the presence of this accumulated blood by surrounding it with scar tissue. This builds up month after month, until blood-filled pockets are formed within the uterine wall. These pockets disturb apāna vāyu, which becomes retrograde, flowing upwards instead of in its natural downward and outward direction. The cervix and vagina may be blocked by blood, scar tissue, or endometrial tissue, so menstruation cannot flow out normally. Thus, the menstrual blood may back up through the fallopian tube and into the ovaries, and sometimes even up into the abdominal cavity.

Endometriosis starts off confined in the uterus, so how does it spread to other organs? One reason is that the surgeon can transplant the endometrium wall into the peritoneal or abdominal organs during abdominal surgery. That may lead to the displacement of some tissue from the uterus onto the bladder, intestines, or other abdominal organs.

When a new endometrial lining is developed, it mixes with a portion of the displaced endometrial tissue from the previous cycle, and this continues to swell and bleed. This persistent growth of the endometrium starts to spread through the wall of the uterus. This condition is called *kapha āvrita rakta* (kapha covering rakta). The endometrium starts to metastasize (spread) into the fallopian tubes, ovaries, and neighboring pelvic organs. It is a non-malignant growth.

## Samprapti, the Disease Process

The samprāpti begins in rasa dhātu, due to increased systemic kapha in rasa vaha srotas. The upadhātu (superior by-product of the dhātu) of rasa are stanya (lactation) and rajah (menstruation), and its mala (inferior by-product of the dhātu) is poshaka kapha. The functions of rajah and poshaka kapha are the thickening and swelling of the endometrium to prepare a bed for a possible pregnancy. If pregnancy does not occur, a portion of the endometrial tissue breaks down and passes out of the uterus with menstruation.

When dhātu agni is low, there is undue production of raw tissue. When dhātu agni is high, the tissue gets roasted and toasted and emaciation can result. Endometriosis is a classical picture of low rasa dhātu agni, which causes a buildup of unprocessed rasa dhātu and its by-product (poshaka kapha), as well as unprocessed stanya and rajah. This unprocessed rasa dhātu is responsible for abnormal development of the endometrial wall. The endometrial growth migrates due to disturbed pīlu pāka and pithara pāka (cellular digestion and assimilation).

Hormonal changes throughout the menstrual cycle are an important cause of endometriosis. Endometrial cells migrate into the newly formed endometrial wall, and this affects cellular agni.

One school of thought says that endometriosis is caused by an auto-immunological dysfunction. In Ayurvedic terms, this is raw ojas suppressing tejas. The immune system does not recognize its own endometrial cells, so it attacks the body's own cells. Any woman who has an autoimmune disease can have a higher risk of developing endometriosis. Therefore, the woman should boost her immune system with a healthy diet and good nutrition, including plenty of kapha-reducing fruits and fresh vegetables.

There are two main categories of endometriosis. The first type is vāta pushing kapha. This creates pain in the pelvic area, lower abdomen, rectal area, vagina, and lower back. The pain may occur during the last phase menstrual cycle, during intercourse, ovulation, and defecation, or even all the time. The woman gets fear, anxiety, and insomnia, and there is often constipation.

The second type of endometriosis is due to pitta pushing kapha. Common symptoms include abnormal bleeding, heavy menstrual flow or spotting, bleeding between periods, bleeding after sexual intercourse, and blood in the urine and stools. The breasts become swollen, painful, and tender, and the nipples are sensitive to the touch. There may be diarrhea.

Pitta is hot and sharp, so when pitta dosha is involved, the endometrium pierces the endometrial wall and develops in the peritoneal lining of the pelvic organs. Whenever the endometrium spreads quickly or further away from the uterus, it is due to pitta pushing kapha. Whereas when the disease spreads more slowly or is more localized, it is due to vāta pushing kapha.

| MAIN SIGNS & SYMPTOMS OF ENDOMETRIOSIS |
| --- |
| Pain |
| Adnexal mass (bulky lump) |
| Infertility |
| Alteration of menstrual cycle |
| Dysmenorrhea |
| Dysuria |
| Cyclical pelvic pain |
| Painful, enlarged swollen breasts, with lactation |
| Premenstrual pain during sexual intercourse, lower backache, painful urination, lower abdominal pain, vaginal pain |

## Signs and Symptoms

No single symptom is diagnostic. A patient of endometriosis often complains of dysmenorrhea, pelvic pain, premenstrual pain during sexual intercourse, lower backache, infertility, painful urination, lower abdominal pain or discomfort, pain in the lower urinary tract, and/or vaginal pain. The symptoms of pain typically worsen five to seven days before menses, and reach a peak two days prior to menstruation. Many times the woman also has heavy, irregular bleeding or bleeding through the urethra or rectum. Because stanya (lactation) is an upadhātu of rasa dhātu, there may be painful, enlarged swollen breasts, with lactation.

In endometriosis, the uterus looks bulky; this indicates an adnexal mass.[66] The woman can experience infertility because the sperm have to travel over larger than normal folds of the uterine wall, and they usually get exhausted and die in that journey.

A chocolate cyst is an ovarian cyst that contains pockets of stagnant blood, surrounded by endometrial scar tissue. The appearance is these is chocolate-colored—hence their name. Retrograde apāna vāyu pushes the rakta (blood) of the menstrual flow up into the fallopian tube and abdominal cavity. The blood that backs up into the ovaries is surrounded by endometrial tissue.

Some patients of endometriosis are completely asymptomatic. This is because there is no correlation between the degree of pain and the progress of the endometrial growth. Some young women may not notice anything if the growth hasn't pierced the endometrial wall.

Diagnosis is done by taking a thorough medical history and a full medical examination, including a pelvic exam. Ask about the woman's menstrual history, including first menstrual period, last menstrual period, her menstrual cycle, and the rhythm of her menstruation. An ultrasound can show a thickened endometrial wall and growth outside the uterus. A laparoscopy will give more details of the area of any endometrial spread. Definite diagnosis can be established by direct visual observation of an ectopic lesion by endoscopy. An endoscope allows one to see the growth on the walls of the uterus.

## Chikitsā, Management of Endometriosis

These endometrial growths of raw tissue migrate due to low pīlu and pithara agni. One needs to do dīpana (kindling of agni, the digestive fire) with 200 mg each of chitrak and trikatu before food, and *āma pāchana* (burning of toxins) with 200 mg of chitrak after food. Lekhana (scraping of fat) is another treatment and it can be done with kutki, shilājit and flaxseeds. These dīpana, pāchana, and lekhana treatments will help to shrink the endometrial tissue. In order to halt the condition, reduce the amount of pain, and re-establish a normal menstrual cycle, one has to pay close attention to ārtava vaha srotas.

To kindle pīlu and pithara agni and inhibit future abnormal endometrial growth:

| | |
|---|---|
| Punarnavā | 500 mg |
| Ashoka | 300 mg |
| Chitrak | 200 mg |
| Trikatu | 200 mg |
| Shilājit | 200 mg |

Half teaspoon, three times daily with warm water.

Punarnavā helps to develop a normal, healthy endometrium. Ashoka inhibits the release of certain hormones by the pituitary gland. It is agonist therapy[67] and will help treat chocolate cysts by its astringent properties. Shilājit is a lekhana treatment, which scrapes excess raw endometrial tissue. Chitrak and trikatu do dīpana and pāchana.

---

66. A lump in tissue of the adnexa of uterus, usually in the ovary or fallopian tube.
67. A substance that acts like another substance and therefore stimulates an action.

A warm flax seed oil compress placed on the lower abdomen over the uterus will do further lekhana of localized endometrial tissue. Use a handkerchief dipped into warm oil.[68]

To further shrink the tissue, give a vacha oil nasya. Vacha has a lekhana action.

Give triphala every evening at bedtime, to maintain a normal flow of vāta dosha.

## Modern Treatments

A woman's fertility plays an important part in endometriosis. These days, birth control pills are used to suppress hormonal balance. Modern medicine also uses drugs to induce menopause, and these will stop the menstrual cycle. Sometimes a nasal spray is given to stop the brain from creating hormones that cause ovulation and menstruation. This is called drug-induced menopause.

These drugs and sprays will slowly shrink the endometrial tissue and any endometriosis can disappear. If it doesn't shrink completely, a hysterectomy with oophorectomy[69] will remove any remaining scar tissue. For a woman in her 40s or 50s with severe endometriosis, these medical treatments can help. Laser surgery is sometimes also incorporated into the treatment protocol. Surgical intervention helps to remove any scar tissue. Pregnancy and breastfeeding can end the symptoms of endometriosis for the same reason—there is cessation of the menstrual cycle.

## Self-Care

Exercise is an important aspect of treatment. Daily walking for two or three miles, or a short period of vigorous exercise, will help to relieve pain. Women who do regular exercise also have less likelihood of developing endometriosis, because it helps to keep kapha dosha in balance.

Kapha-reducing fruits and fresh vegetables are an important part of dietary treatment. Examples include apricots, plums, peaches, pears, apples, cantaloupe, strawberries, oranges, grapefruit juice, broccoli, Brussels sprouts, and red bell pepper. Omega 3 fatty acids can also be beneficial. Rich sources include certain types of fish, walnuts, flaxseeds, and flaxseed oil.

A woman with endometriosis should keep a calendar of her symptoms. List when any pain starts, when it goes away, what other symptoms are happening, and when these occur. Endometriosis is a great imitator, with symptoms that may mimic irritable bowel syndrome, urinary tract infections, tubule pregnancy, and other medical disorders. Hence, it is good to see your doctor to rule out other diseases. Keeping a calendar will help the doctor to determine if you have any of these other ailments.

Lower abdominal pain is another symptom of endometriosis. Anything that stimulates vāta dosha and increases peristaltic movement should be avoided. This includes coffee, black tea, chocolate, cola drinks, and smoking cigarettes, which can all cause lower

---

68. No more than 110° F.
69. The surgical removal of the ovaries.

abdominal pain. Application of a warm castor oil compress to the lower abdomen will help with these symptoms.

## The Ayurvedic Approach

The Ayurvedic approach to endometriosis is to understand which dosha is pushing kapha into the endometrium—whether it is vāta pushing kapha or pitta pushing kapha.

The Ayurvedic protocol to manage endometriosis is comprehensive. First, give dīpana to kindle the agni (digestive fire), including pīlu agni and pithara agni at the cellular level. Trikatu (ginger, black pepper and long pepper) is useful in this regards. Then give pāchana to burn the āma. Chitrak is particularly effective at eliminating āma from cells in the deep tissue.

Many women with this condition also need lekhana chikitsā to eliminate excess fat and to remove any abnormal endometrial tissue. Kutki and tambra *bhasma* (copper ash) are commonly used as lekhana. Loha bhasma (iron ash) is also given as a hematinic[70] tonic.

Herbal formulas to treat the causative doshas and the disease as well as to heal the reproductive tissue are of benefit. (see "Herbal Management for Endometriosis" on page 385)

Lepana[71] is another treatment that can be used for endometriosis. One can give gentle *lepa* using an astringent herb, such as punarnavā, manjistha, red sandalwood, turmeric, or alum. These astringent herbal lepana can be placed on the lower abdomen to try to minimize the spread of endometrial growth. Lepana can also help to reduce the thickening of the endometrium wall.

## Marma Chikitsā for Endometriosis

Nābhi 3      Nābhi 4
Bhaga        Vankshana
Trik         Kati
Gulpha (lateral)

| AIMS OF TREATMENT |
| --- |
| To halt the condition |
| Pain reduction |
| Restore normal menstrual cycle |
| Restore fertility in younger women |

Use nutmeg essential oil diluted in sesame oil and apply to each of these marma points. This marma chikitsā will help to minimize pain, normalize any retrograde apāna, and minimize displacement of the endometrium. (see illustrations on page 459)

*Basti basti* (bladder basti) with flaxseed oil is another treatment that can be used for endometriosis. This is applied topically to the area of the abdomen above the bladder, in the same way as a *kati basti*. Oil is poured into a doughnut-like structure made with whole-wheat dough. Allow the oil basti to sit there for 40 minutes. The oil should be room temperature and no more than 110° F. The oil molecules penetrate through the skin and superficial fascia, down to the nerve endings. There, the oil stimulates the release of certain neuropeptides. These same neuropeptides released from the central nervous system

---

70. A medicine that increases the hemoglobin content of the blood.
71. Ointments or pastes applied to the skin.

also maintain psycho-neuro-immune balance. They help to relieve localized pain and inhibit endometrial growth.

*Nasya chikitsā* using vacha oil nasya will also help to minimize hormonal disturbance.

There are certain *yogāsanas* that will stretch the lower abdomen. *Dhanurāsana* (bow pose), *ustrāsana* (camel pose), *mandhukāsana* (frog pose), *shalabhāsana* (locust pose), *matsyendrāsana* (spinal twist), and *gomukhāsana* (cow pose) are all particularly beneficial. (see page 450)

Prānāyāma is also helpful. Analoma viloma, bhastrikā, kapāla bhāti, and ujjāyi prānāyāma can help to manage the symptoms of endometriosis.

Following this protocol for 3 to 6 months will usually show remarkable changes. If it doesn't help for some reason, the woman can always follow the medical path of surgical removal of the scar tissue and a hysterectomy. Nowadays they use a medical laser to destroy the endometrium.

Ayurvedic treatment is safe and without any significant side effects. However, endometriosis is stubborn, because it is a long-lingering kapha disorder within the wall of the endometrium, so one should treat this problem skillfully. You need a basic understanding of the prakruti-vikruti paradigm and keen observation of the signs and symptoms, to determine whether it is due to vāta pushing kapha or pitta pushing kapha.

Ayurveda has good treatments for endometriosis. One should follow these protocols according to the different causes of the disease. If one does that, one will get good results in the management of endometriosis.

# Herbal Management for Endometriosis

**ENDOMETRIOSIS TYPE 1**

Vāta pushing kapha in the endometrium creates less bleeding but evidences more metastasizing (spread).

An effective herbal protocol is:

| | |
|---|---|
| Punarnavā | 500 mg |
| Ashoka | 300 mg |
| Chitrak | 200 mg |
| Trikatu | 200 mg |
| Shilājit | 200 mg |
| Kāñcanāra | 200 mg (for bulky uterus and adnexal growth) |

Give this mixture three times daily.

Additionally, give 1 pill of triphala guggulu or yogarāja guggulu along with the formula above.

**ENDOMETRIOSIS TYPE 2**

Pitta pushing kapha in the endometrium creates more bleeding and includes the possibility of chocolate cyst(s) in the ovaries.

An effective herbal protocol is:

| | |
|---|---|
| Gulvel sattva | 400 mg |
| Manjistha | 300 mg |
| Ashoka | 200 mg |
| Neem | 200 mg |
| Mustā | 200 mg |

Give this mixture three times daily.

Additionally, give 1 pill of kaishore guggulu or amrita guggulu along with the formula above.

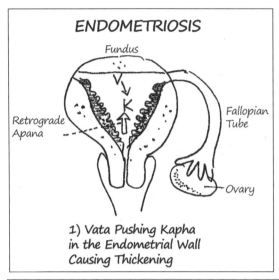

## ENDOMETRIOSIS

Fundus

Retrograde Apana

Fallopian Tube

Ovary

1) Vata Pushing Kapha in the Endometrial Wall Causing Thickening

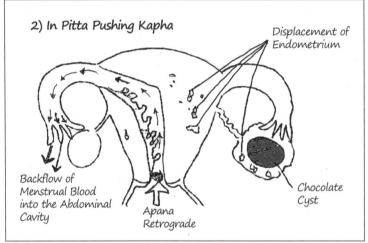

2) In Pitta Pushing Kapha

Displacement of Endometrium

Backflow of Menstrual Blood into the Abdominal Cavity

Apana Retrograde

Chocolate Cyst

# Chapter 49

# Irritable Bowel Syndrome
## Pakvāshāya Kūpita Dosha

Winter 2008, Volume 21, No 3 and Winter 2013, Volume 26, Number 3, Integrated

ACCORDING TO AYURVEDIC LITERATURE, the *koshta* (gastrointestinal tract) is a *mahā srotas* (major channel). The first line of this sūtra states that the gastrointestinal (GI) tract is a large passage. It includes the āmāshaya (stomach), *grahani* (small intestine), and *pakvāshāya* (colon). This whole space is called the koshta and is the home of all three doshas. The stomach is the seat of gastric mucous secretions and kapha dosha, the small intestine is the seat of agni and pitta dosha, and the colon is the seat of vāta dosha.

> *Anta koshta mahā srotas, āma pakvāshāyāshrāyam,*
> *muhuh badam, muhuh dravam*
>
> The gastrointestinal tract is a large passage, (it has) periods of loose stools and those of hard constipation
>
> **MADHAVA NIDANA, CHAPTER 4**

According to Ayurvedic samprāpti (pathogenesis), the disease process has six stages. The first two stages happen in the dosha's own site. Hence, the first two stages of vāta disorders will take place in the large intestine, while the first stages of pitta disorders take place in the small intestine, and the early stages of kapha disorders occur in the stomach.

Irritable bowel syndrome (*pakvāshāya kupita vāta*) is the continuous inflammation of the intestinal mucous lining, anus, rectum and distal part of colon. In some seriously ill patients, the entire large intestine is affected. This disorder usually becomes apparent during the second and third decades of life.

According to Ayurveda, irritable bowel syndrome (IBS) is a collection of symptoms or syndrome that is a dual-dosha samprāpti. It is due to vāta pushing pitta or pitta pushing kapha in the colon. The moment the third dosha gets involved, it can lead to colon cancer. If that happens, it will usually occur about 20 to 30 years after the onset of IBS.

## Etiology
When we look into vāta-provoking etiology, one important causative factor is eating a vāta-increasing diet, such as black beans, pinto beans, adzuki beans, or raw vegetables.

387

Eating too little or too much, irregular eating, eating at the wrong time, and eating while driving or traveling also aggravate vāta dosha. Food that is bitter, pungent, or astringent is particularly vāta-provoking. These dietary factors, along with various lifestyle factors, may be the cause of vāta aggravation.

If all the stages of a vāta disorder happen within the colon, that condition is called *pakvāshāya kūpita vāta,* which means vāta is aggravated in the large intestine. Irritable bowel syndrome (IBS) is described in Ayurvedic literature under this heading, as the symptoms given are very similar to modern symptomatology.

IBS is sometimes called spastic colon or mucous colitis. It is not a disease, but a collection of signs and symptoms caused by irritability and irregularity in the small and large intestines. The condition is marked by abdominal pain that is relieved by the passing of stools or gas. There is a disturbance of evacuation—causing either constipation, diarrhea, or alternating episodes of diarrhea and constipation. The phrase in the sūtra, *muhuh badam muhuh dravam,* means there are periods of loose stools and times when there is hard constipation.

Muscle contractions of the small intestine are called intestinal peristalsis, and they are governed by samāna vāyu. The brief forcible peristaltic movement of the colon is called mass peristalsis. In IBS, there is irregularity in the mobility of both the small and large intestines because of increased *chala* (mobile) and *vishama* (irregular) qualities.

### Table 11: Main Causes of IBS

Typically, IBS begins with pāchaka pitta undergoing sanchaya and prakopa in the small intestine, at the same time as apāna vāyu is undergoing sanchaya and prakopa in the large intestine. Then, during the prasara stage, either vāta pushes pitta or pitta pushes kapha in the colon.

Symptoms are caused by intestinal irritability and irregularity in the bowel movements, with the symptoms occurring in both the small and large intestines.

Some specific pathogens are a second causative factor associated with IBS. Amoebic dysentery and amoebic colitis are examples of illnesses that can result in IBS symptoms.

Antibiotic-associated diarrhea is a third etiological factor. Prolonged antibiotic therapy can disturb the normal bowel flora, leading to either IBS or colitis.

A fourth factor that can lead to IBS is a chronic debilitating illness caused by exotoxins or environmental pollutants such as heavy metals.

Number five in this list is pseudo-membranous colitis. Exotoxins or prolonged exposure to radiation can damage the colon mucous membrane and produce inflammation and IBS symptoms.

Sixthly, there are commonly dietetic factors involved. Excessive consumption of coffee, chocolate, raw fruits or raw vegetables can lead to irritable bowel, as well as consumption of hormones or toxins in the diet. Lactose intolerance is also associated with IBS, due to an inability of the body to digest lactose milk sugar, and so is wheat intolerance.

Seventh, an overuse of laxatives is a causative factor. In fact, many drugs can be involved in the formation of irritable bowel syndrome.

Finally, genetic predisposition is an important etiological factor that should always be kept in mind.

Irritable bowel syndrome is influenced by emotion. Fear, nervousness, anxiety, guilt, depression, and anger can all cause an aggravation of the condition. If we look at these emotions, we can understand why. Fear causes emptiness, while insecurity and nervous-

bile, so those emotions aggravate the condition. Anxiety creates agitation and uces withdrawal. These emotions disturb vāta dosha, while anger may disturb ce, nervousness, anxiety, fear and insecurity can trigger symptoms in a person prakruti or vikruti. On the other hand, anger, hate, and envy may bring on or symptoms in someone with pitta prakruti or vikruti.

often occurs in people who have experienced physical abuse or sexual abuse in dhood. Physical abuse can create fear and anxiety, which often builds up vāta in Sexual abuse may cause trauma in the rectum. Both result in khavaigunya pace) in the large intestine and may bring about irritable bowel syndrome. have found a relationship between IBS and anxiety, psychological stress, and personality disorder. This can result in either an increased or decreased rate of bowel mobility.

Certain foods are particularly aggravating to the condition. Examples are coffee, raw vegetables and some raw fruit. Hormones and certain drugs can aggravate IBS. Overuse of laxatives, including strong natural laxatives such as senna, castor oil, cascara sagrada or jamalgota, can create more irritation.

## Signs and Symptoms

IBS is a syndrome, which means the presence of several clinically recognizable signs, symptoms or other characteristics that usually occur together. Predominant symptoms can include alternating diarrhea and constipation, accompanied by abdominal cramps and straining during elimination. The stools may be loose, or they may be compacted. At times, the patient can pass mucous with the stools, produced by irritation of the bowel lining. There is often gas, bloating, occipital headache, and fatigue, which are vāta symptoms. Pitta symptoms include diarrhea, nausea, temporal headache and burning of the anal canal.This syndrome is commonly found in women aged between 20 and 40 years. The most common symptom is abdominal pain, occurring in attacks. The pain refers to the left or right iliac region, or to the hypogastrium, which is the suprapubic area. This pain is generally relieved by defecation, and may be provoked by food.

In vāta type of IBS, there is colicky pain, and usually constipation with hard, pellet-like stools. In the *vāta-pitta* type of IBS, there is a more sharp pain and bouts of diarrhea. Most people with IBS suffer from a vicious cycle of alternate diarrhea and constipation.

If we look at the symptomatology of IBS, there is constipation due to an accumulation of gas and the dry attribute of vāta, diarrhea because of the spreading quality of pitta, abdominal cramps due to mobile and cold attributes of vāta, and straining during defecation because of the astringent quality of vāta

**Areas of Pain in IBS**

| | | |
|---|---|---|
| Right Hypochondrium | Epigastric Region | Left Hypochondrium |
| Right Lumbar | Umbilical Region | Left Lumbar |
| Right Iliac Region | Hypogastrium | Left Iliac Region |

and the sticky attribute of kapha. The patient often has loose stools, with or without mucous, because vāta pushing pitta in the colon creates loose stools and vāta pushing kapha in the colon creates mucous. Other common symptoms include irritation, inflammation, bloating, nausea, and fatigue.

In the first two samprāpti stages of IBS (sanchaya and prakopa), accumulated vāta produces constipation, gas and bloating. When vāta moves into the third stage (prasara), it produces diarrhea, abdominal cramps, and straining during elimination. If there is also increased pitta, there will be loose stools with irritation, nausea, and fatigue.

In irritable bowel syndrome, agni (digestive fire) is usually vishama (irregular). Vishama agni and tīkshna (sharp) agni can both create this condition, because in tīkshna agni there is an inability to digest lactose (milk sugar), which creates lactose intolerance. If a person with lactose intolerance drinks a glass of milk, he or she will get diarrhea and purging.

## Categories of IBS

There are three main types of IBS. The first category is spastic colon, in which there are cramps and dull aching pain in the lower abdomen. This type is due to increased vāta. It is associated with constipation. Individuals with this type of IBS have a decreased rate of bowel mobility. There is discomfort at mealtimes and the pain often begins immediately after eating. People with this condition often have to run to the toilet while eating food. Symptoms usually disappear after a bowel movement, but they can then lose their appetite. It is marked by cramps, bloating and dull, aching pain in the lower abdomen.

The second category of IBS is characterized by loose stools with watery diarrhea or mucous colitis. This type is due to both increased vāta and the involvement of pitta. There is often sharp, burning pain, and an urgent need for a bowel movement, especially on awakening or immediately following a meal. The moment the person gets up, they run to the toilet. This often happens during or right after a meal. This kind of IBS is due to vāta pushing pitta.

The third category is mucoid IBS or nervous colon. It is due to increased vāta with kapha involvement, and there is generally vague pain or discomfort. People with this type of IBS have a full colon and an urge to go to the toilet, but are unable to eliminate the feces, which are sticky due to the involvement of both vāta and kapha. Vāta is pushing kapha – dryness of vāta makes the kapha mucous sticky.

Many diseases are similar to IBS, such as sprue syndrome, amoebic dysentery and bacillary dysentery. So, when a person comes to you with IBS symptoms, one has to rule out all those other diseases that have similar signs and symptoms. A stool examination is helpful in that regard, and possibly a barium enema to assess the colon. In certain cases, a doctor needs to examine the lower colon using a proctosigmoidoscope, to rule out ulcerative colitis and other diseases.

Grahani is the name given in Ayurveda to tropical sprue syndrome, which is also known as malabsorption syndrome. In grahani, there is alternating diarrhea and constipation, with periumbilical pain. While in IBS there is also alternating diarrhea and constipation, the pain is generally on the right or left flank and there is no malabsorption. This is because the khavaigunya (lesion) is in the colon in the case of IBS, while in grahani the khavaigunya is in the small intestine.

Another condition in the large intestine is ulcerative colitis, or inflammatory bowel disease, which is a pitta disorder. In ulcerative colitis, a sigmoidoscopy shows multiple patches of ulceration, whereas in IBS there are only patches of inflammation but no ulceration. It is interesting to note that pitta type of IBS can result in ulcerative colitis.

## Diagnosis of IBS

Whenever one sees a person with IBS, one should do a thorough examination to find out the subject's weight and their color and complexion. Look at the tongue, then feel the pulse and find out the person's prakruti and vikruti. Give special emphasis to the colon pulse, which is felt on the person's right wrist under the practitioner's index finger.

If the colon pulse is feeble, then see whether there is a vāta spike, or vāta pushing pitta, or vāta pushing kapha. If there is only a vāta spike, that indicates spastic colon. If it is vāta pushing pitta, it points to IBS with diarrhea and urgency of bowel movement. If there is vāta pushing kapha, it indicates IBS with mucous.

Examine the abdomen. Generally, pain and soreness in the sigmoid colon and descending colon falls under vāta type of IBS. Pain, flatulence, and distension in the ascending colon (right side) indicate vāta-pitta type of IBS. Usually in IBS there is no involvement of parasites. However, if there is amoebic infection, pain is more common in the ascending colon. If there is bacillary dysentery, it normally affects the descending colon.

**Colon**

Ascending / Descending / Sigmoid

Ascending
Vāta-pitta type of IBS indicated by pain, flatulence, and distension.

Descending/Sigmoid
Vāta type of IBS typified by pain and soreness.

Diagnosis can also be done with a stool examination. Look for blood, mucous, and micro-organisms in the stools. Sometimes one has to do a barium enema with an x-ray plate, or a proctosigmoidoscopy to rule out ulcerative colitis. We can tell the patient to go to a gastroenterologist and get these examinations. Fortunately, most people have already done these tests before coming to the Ayurvedic practitioner for help.

There is a definite link between irritable bowel syndrome and a history of anxiety, psychological stress, or personality disorder. Psychologically, irritation of the bowel occurs more often in people who have a history of physical or sexual abuse during childhood. Sexual abuse in childhood can aggravate apāna vāyu and create khavaigunya (weakness) in the colon.

## Management of IBS

Management is generally symptomatic, because IBS is a complex syndrome.

For vāta (and kapha) type of IBS, one can use:

Jati phaladi guti        200 mg

Kutaja vati          200 mg (or kutaja churna)
Bhallataka guti      200 mg
These three tablets are given three times a day.

Other remedies for vāta IBS include:

+ Roasted cumin, fennel, vidanga and nutmeg powder (1 part cumin, 1 part fennel, ¼ part vidanga, pinch of nutmeg) with a teaspoon of ghee.
+ Tagara 200 mg is a tranquilizer that helps with anxiety or insomnia.
+ Vidārī 300 mg is a mild analgesic and sedative that is good for vāta IBS symptoms.
+ Ashvagandhā 500 mg is a mild analgesic, sedative and muscle relaxant that is also good for vāta IBS symptoms.
+ Lashunadi vati 200 mg is a common remedy for gas and bloating.
+ Shankha vati 200 mg is useful for abdominal cramps.
+ Chitrakadi vati 200 mg can be given for nausea, low appetite and poor digestion.

An anti-inflammatory herbal formula that helps with pitta-type IBS is:

Shatāvarī       500 mg
Gudūchi         300 mg
Kama dudhā      200 mg
This mixture is given three times daily.

Another good formula for pitta-type of IBS is:

Shatāvarī           500 mg
Kama dudhā          200 mg
Praval pañchāmrit   200 mg
Bilva               200 mg
Take half a teaspoon three times daily, with pomegranate juice (or cranberry juice if pomegranate juice is not available).

Other pitta-pacifying remedies that can help include:

+ Maha tikta ghrita (or tikta ghrita)
+ Bilva avaleha (or bilva churna)
+ Cumin, coriander and fennel tea (equal parts of the whole seeds boiled in water)
+ A specific remedy for all types of IBS is kutaja arishta.

**Cramps and abdominal pain are common IBS symptoms.** To deal with abdominal pain, we can use one or more of the following herbal analgesic remedies:

Hingvastak churna   200 mg
or Ajvain           200 mg
or Garlic powder    200 mg
or Āma pachak vati  1 tablet
or Shankha vati     1 tablet
or Shulahara vati   1 tablet

According to Ayurveda, pain is due to āma. The following herbal formula helps to manage spasmodic pain. These herbs do dīpana to kindle agni, pāchana to burn āma, anulomana to maintain normal peristalsis, and shamana to palliate any pain.

| | |
|---|---|
| Dashamūla | 500 mg |
| Ajvain | 200 mg |
| Garlic powder | 200 mg |
| Chitrak | 200 mg |
| Shakha bhasma | 200 mg |

This is given after each meal. It acts like an anti-cholinergic medicine, so it helps to relieve any spasms.

One can also use a warm castor oil compress over the site of the pain. Application of heat is a beneficial treatment for any IBS caused by vāta.

If the IBS patient gets diarrhea, one can give:

| | |
|---|---|
| Kutaja | 200 mg |
| Sanjīvanī | 200 mg |
| Bilva | 200 mg |

This is given after each meal.

A second line of treatment is used to manage depression and emotional factors. If the person has depression, the following tranquilizing and antidepressant herbs can be useful:

| | |
|---|---|
| Sarasvatī | 300 mg |
| Brahmi | 300 mg |
| Jatamāmsi | 300 mg (if available, or increase Shankha pushpī to 300 mg) |
| Shankha pushpī | 200 mg |

This mixture may be taken three times daily after every meal.

We are not allowed to use the herb vacha internally in the USA, but vacha can be used externally. It is made into a paste by mixing it with water, and then applied to the abdomen. This can be effective for dealing with the depression in IBS.

Anxiety is a common symptom, due to vāta dushti. Tranquility Tea® is effective at calming a person's mind. Give 1 teaspoon of the tea, steeped in a cup of hot water for 10 minutes. It can be drunk after breakfast, lunch, and dinner.

The following herbal protocol will help with the anxiety:

| | |
|---|---|
| Ashvagandhā | 500 mg |
| Tagara | 200 mg |
| Jātīphalā | 100 mg |

This can also be given after each meal.

Also rub bhringarāja oil on the soles of the feet and the scalp, before bedtime.

*Nābhi basti,* with warm sesame oil, is another good treatment for anxiety. (see instructions on page 449)

Exercise is an important part of the therapy for a person with IBS. A patient of IBS should have a daily walk. Walk for 2 miles, because long walks will improve the tone, power, coordination of pelvic organs and abdominal muscles. Bike rides, swimming and underwater exercise can all help the person to relax, thereby promoting better bowel movements.

Yogāsana are beneficial for IBS. The following āsanas (poses) are particularly beneficial:

- uttāna pādāsana (leg lifting)
- pāwanamuktāsana (chest-knee pose)
- halāsana (plough pose)
- shalabhāsana (locust pose)
- ūrdhva padmāsana (shoulder stand with lotus pose) (see poses page 450)

Also *tadagi mudra,*[72] which means lying on the back exhaling while drawing in the abdomen.

Beneficial prānāyāma are anuloma-viloma, kapāla bhāti, ujjāyi and utgīta prānāyāma. This yoga and prānāyāma protocol should be done under the guidance of an experienced yoga teacher.

Specific yogāsana and prānāyāma, according to the person's prakruti and particularly their vikruti, include:

- Vāta vikruti: camel and cow āsanas; alternate nostril breathing and ujjāyi prānāyāma
- Pitta vikruti: boat, bow and bridge āsanas; shītalī and shītkāri prānāyāma
- Kapha vikruti: locust, lotus and lion āsanas; gentle bhastrik and kapāla bhāti prānāyāma
- So'ham meditation[73] is good for all body types.

## Diet

If there is no organic disease found, the Ayurveda practitioner has to recommend a suitable diet and lifestyle, and help the patient with any emotional factors. The first principle is to avoid the cause. That often includes reducing the amount of raw food that is eaten, as well as any alcohol and cigarettes.

IBS patients get gas, so they should avoid cabbage, kidney beans, black beans, pinto beans, adzuki beans, chickpeas, and other beans that are difficult to digest.

Someone with IBS should also avoid milk, because IBS often goes with lactose intolerance, which is an inability to digest milk sugar. Instead of milk, take whey (called *morat* in Sanskrit). Take one gallon (4 liters) of milk, boil it and squeeze the juice from half a dozen limes into it. If limes are unavailable, use lemons. This will curdle, so leave it for at least an hour. Then filter this milk through cheesecloth. The thick part is fresh paneer cheese, which is light to digest and okay for people with IBS to eat. The liquid portion is

---

72. Tadagi Mudra is also known as Uddiyana Bandha.
73. Visit https://www.ayurveda.com/resources/articles/soham-meditation for instructions.

whey (morat). Whey is anti-inflammatory, a good source of protein, and beneficial for IBS.

IBS can easily cause constipation, so soluble fiber is helpful. This is found in many vegetables and fruits, along with oat bran and soaked psyllium husks. Soaked raisins are also okay. Alternatively, one can give triphala to deal with the constipation. Be aware that sources of insoluble fiber, such as wheat bran, can irritate the colon. Therefore, if you want to take wheat bran, soak it overnight and then eat it the next day.

Fresh juices are beneficial, but don't drink canned or bottled juices because most of those contain some type of preservative, which are irritating substances that will aggravate the IBS. Fresh juice made from apples, pears, plums, grapes or certain vegetables can be helpful for people with IBS. Therefore, a juicer can be a useful addition to your kitchen.

Don't be too sweet on sweet—in other words, minimize the amount of sugar in the diet, because excessive sugar often produces gas and indigestion. Only munch when you are mellow—this means don't eat emotionally. Eat slowly, in a relaxed manner, with mindfulness.

Helpful foods for most people with irritable bowel syndrome include basmati rice, mung dal and kitchari. Banana, pomegranate, and cranberry are the best fruits for IBS patients. Ghee is also good for most people with IBS, because there is no lactose in the clarified butter.

In general, people with IBS should eat a diet that pacifies the doshas and see an experienced Ayurvedic practitioner who can give them appropriate lifestyle and herbal remedies.

Someone with IBS should follow a yogic or spiritual discipline. They should do yoga or some relaxation technique. Although Ayurveda is not a quick fix, the use of Ayurvedic herbal protocol, diet, lifestyle, yoga, and prānāyāma will truly unfold radical healing for a person with irritable bowel syndrome.

Even though IBS is not a serious disease, it can continue to be a problem despite having treatment. Therefore, regular medical checkups should be scheduled to be on the safe side. This is especially true for people over the age of 40.

# Chapter 50

# The Art of Parenting Hyperactive Children
## Chanchalatā

Fall 2009, Volume 22, Number 2

THERE ARE INNUMERABLE srotāmsi in the human body, but we use thirteen main channels in Ayurveda. These include the seven *dhātu-srotamsi* and majjā vaha srotas (the nerve channel) is one of those important channels. Even though the mind functions throughout the body, the mental functions are intimately connected to majjā dhātu (nerve tissue and bone marrow) and thus to majjā vaha srotas. Hence, any nervous disorder is bound to affect the mind.

Attention Deficit Hyperactivity Disorder (ADHD) is known in Ayurveda as *chanchalatā*. It is a nervous disorder that usually affects children. Though ADHD is a relatively new term in Western medicine, this disorder has been known to Ayurveda for many centuries and can be understood by ancient Ayurvedic principles.

In chanchalatā (ADHD), high systemic vāta undergoes accumulation (sanchaya), then provocation (prakopa), and then spreads into majjā dhātu, affecting majjā vaha srotas and mano vaha srotas (the mind channel) simultaneously. The qualities of vāta that are most aggravated determine the types of symptoms that occur.

Due to increased mobile (chala) quality, the child is hyperactive. Increased mobile and light qualities of vāta make the affected child consistently impulsive and create an extremely short attention span. Owing to an imbalance of erratic (vishama) attribute, he or she cannot concentrate well or stay focused on a task. Vāta's cold, dry and rough attributes may be responsible for immature behavior, just as a cold, dry, refrigerated fruit will never ripen and become fully mature. The clear and empty attributes mean that these children live in their own world and don't respond to other people in a normal way. Vāta is also subtle, so when it is aggravated, there is an increase of subtle thoughts, feelings and emotions. According to modern classifications, there are different types of ADHD: hyperactive impulsive, hyperactive inattentive and hyperactive combined. From an Ayurvedic perspective the hyperactive impulsive has excess vāta qualities, the hyperactive inattentive has both kapha and tamasic qualities and the hyperactive combined has more pitta qualities and is due to the fluctuations of *drava guna* (the liquid quality).

ADHD may physically damage the body and it can trigger long-lasting social, emotional and educational problems. Teachers may complain about the child. The child is often not able to sit still and concentrate for long periods of time, which can lead to trouble in schooling, as the child appears immature, uncoordinated and boisterous. He or she usually has trouble getting along with other classmates, and with teachers and parents, and invariably suffers from a poor self-image. This is a book picture of disturbed vāta dosha.

The behavioral patterns depend upon the severity of the vāta disorder. If there is a lower intensity of vāta aggravation, the child probably won't be a disturbance in the classroom, nor show all the above signs. However, he or she may still have difficulty in paying attention and will appear unusually active.

> There are two systems of the brain that respond to situations. One results in prompt action, and in Ayurveda this is known as prāna vāta. The other encourages hesitation (tarpaka kapha) and consideration (sādhaka pitta). If prompt action is stimulated, hesitation is diminished, and that can be the mechanism that causes impulsive behavior.
>
> For instance, a hyperactive child may see a flower in a pot on a table above and will jump to catch it, no matter how high, without considering the consequences of grabbing the flower. For a normal child, the prompt action is controlled by consideration and hesitation. The neurotransmitters that control the hesitation response are malfunctioning in the case of a child with ADHD. One factor may be vaccination shots, which can be hugely stressful to the immunological system. Mercury was previously used as a preservative, and one school of thought says that this mercury resulted in toxins affecting the brain. Consuming food preservatives, canned food, or frozen food may also be an important factor in disturbing the functional integrity between prāna vāta, sādhaka pitta and tarpaka kapha.

## Causes (Nidāna)

- Vāta-provoking diet or malnourishment during pregnancy, especially stimulants such as caffeine, tobacco, sugar and chocolate, can disturb the central nervous system of the fetus, which may cause central nervous system malfunctioning. Watching movies excessively or visiting busy locations such as shopping malls may also disturb vāta dosha in the fetus.
- Mother drinking alcohol or taking drugs during pregnancy
- Food additives – chemical colors and preservatives that are added to food that the child eats, or those eaten by the mother when she is pregnant or breastfeeding
- Exposure of pregnant mother to radiation, such as repeated X-rays or radiation therapy
- Chemical toxicity, such as exposure to dyes, formaldehyde and so forth
- Damage during pregnancy, e.g., induced delivery, obstructed labor, premature rupture of amniotic fluid bag, forceps delivery, administration of drugs during delivery
- Premature delivery – this gives rise to congenital vāta disorders that may affect majjā dhātu, rendering the child hyperactive
- Complications of child birth that can cause neurological defects, e.g., CPD (cephalopelvic disproportion), face presentation, hand presentation, cord presentation or hip presentation
- Gender – boys are more prone to ADHD than girls

- Hereditary traits – genetic predisposition to ADHD; pitta- or vāta-predominant individuals are more likely to get ADHD—specifically those with $V_3 P_3$, $V_3 P_2$, or $V_2 P_3$
- Deficiency of tarpaka kapha; malfunctioning neurotransmitters that control the hesitation response

## Signs and Symptoms (Lakshana)

A child affected by ADHD can display the following signs and symptoms:

- Overactive
- Fidgety
- Restlessness
- Overly talkative
- Boisterous
- Overly excited
- Impulsive
- Poor coordination
- Short attention span (especially noticeable at school)
- Creates disturbances in the classroom
- Skips words when reading
- Laughs loudly
- Prefers to play with younger children

## Diagnosis (Roga Nidāna)

There is no specific laboratory test to diagnose ADHD. Diagnosis is done by consideration of the signs and symptoms that the child presents. Vāta vikruti children are hyperactive in behavior, so ADHD can seem like a rather vaguely defined term for these children. The quantity, intensity, and duration of symptoms should be carefully observed before diagnosing ADHD. Only then should one say that a particular child has attention deficit and hyperactive disorder.

Many times, ADHD is wrongly diagnosed and the child is put on medication that really affects the growth of that 'flower.' Don't label a child by the word 'hyperactive' simply because the parents or teachers may have a low level of tolerance for the child's activity level. They may not tolerate the normal intense activity of a child with vāta prakruti or vāta vikruti. That in itself does not mean that the child has ADHD.

**AUTISM**

ADHD is a disorder of increased vāta, whereas autism is caused by kapha blocking vāta. In that disorder, tarpaka kapha blocks prāna vāyu and causes mental introversion. The person's attention is focused mainly on himself or herself. There is withdrawal from communication with other people and repetitive, childish behavior. This means that the child is self-absorbed and there is inaccessibility, aloneness, an inability to relate, and highly repetitive play. There can be strong resistance if this play is interrupted. The child also has language disturbances, as he or she is too introverted to learn what others are trying to communicate. Autism is more passive and introverted, whereas ADHD is more active and extroverted.

## Treatment (Chikitsā)

In the standard medical treatment protocol, several stimulant medications may be given to treat ADHD since these stimulants affect the hesitation response thereby having a calming effect. This is an example of *tadarthakāri* (protagonistic) *chikitsā*. Methylphenidate and amphetamines are two common drugs of choice. After taking the drug, the child ends up being exhausted and does not have much energy left to act hyperactively. The drug makes the child's nervous system exhausted and the child appears calm. However, the child is made quiet, rather than being quiet.

These stimulant drugs have some hazardous side effects, such as stomachaches, muscle cramps, runny nose, colds, congestion, and stunted growth. In extreme cases, it is okay to use these drugs for a short period of time. However, it is better to bring the child back into balance by nature's way, through Ayurveda.

The Ayurvedic protocol for hyperactive children is to calm down vāta dosha. First, do oil massage (abhyanga) with a mixture of balā, dashamūla, and mahānārāyana oils. This can be followed by sweating therapy with nirgundī svedana, because nirgundī helps to relax the muscles. Anuvāsana basti is then given, with plain sesame oil. Also, rub bhringarāja oil onto the soles of the feet and scalp at bedtime.

Internally, give an herbal formula made of some or all of the following herbs:

| | |
|---|---|
| Dashamūla | 500 mg |
| Ashvagandhā | 400 mg |
| Vidārī | 300 mg |
| Yogarāja guggulu | 300 mg |
| Jatamāmsi | 200 mg (or Mustā 200 mg if jatamāmsi is unavailable) |
| Shankha Pushpī | 200 mg |
| Licorice | 200 mg |
| Tagara | 200 mg |

Children can be given ¼ teaspoon of this mixture three times daily (TID), and it is best taken with a teaspoon of honey and a teaspoon of ghee, all mixed together. One can also keep the doshas flowing well (anuloma) by using ¼ teaspoon of nishottara or triphalā before bedtime.

The child should be put on a vāta pacifying diet. Good foods are basmati rice and mung dal kitchari, with mustard seeds, cumin, and cilantro. Soaked almonds or almond milk are good, as are walnuts and cashews. A quarter teaspoon each of holy basil (tulsi) and turmeric can be boiled in a cup of milk and given to the child to drink at bedtime.

Brahmī-almond-date-cashew milk is a rich nervine tonic that can really help a child with ADHD. To make this, boil a cup of milk with a few dates, almonds, and cashews, and ½ teaspoon each of date sugar and brahmī (gotu kola) powder.

One special Ayurvedic treatment is to rub some pure gold on a rough stone, along with the fresh juice of brahmī, anantā mūla, and vacha and a teaspoon of honey. Give this mixture regularly for a month or two and it will really calm down a hyperactive child.

Ayurveda also recommends a number of rejuvenative therapies (rasāyana) for ADHD. Jatamāmsi, sarasvatī, and brahmī are three herbs that help to improve the attention span.

One can give a child with ADHD 200 mg of each of these herbs TID. Shankha pushpī syrup is another beneficial remedy, and it enhances the ability to focus. Brahmī prash, brahmī ghee, and sarāvat arishta are good nervine tonics that enhance the attention span. One teaspoon of sarasvatī ghee can be given twice a day to calm the child down.

Suvarna vacha (calamus root in gold water) is another specific rejuvenative remedy for ADHD children. One can also boil a quarter ounce of pure gold in two cups of water, until the liquid evaporates down to one cup. Then remove the gold and give five to ten drops of this 'gold water' to the child, twice a day.

## Conclusion

Children with ADHD need tender, loving care. Don't order around a child with ADHD. Be gentle and polite and make everything go step-by-step. Activities such as getting up, eating meals, watching TV, and doing homework should all be done calmly and skillfully. Don't say, "Hurry up and get ready for school!" Instead, say, "Hi honey, time to get up and go to the kitchen to eat."

Chart a daily schedule for the affected child and help the family to follow that *dinācharya* (daily routine). Sweetly remind the child of things they forget, like a parrot. Get the child involved in sports and other activities that can keep them involved and relax their muscles at the same time.

Have a family rap session, where everyone meets and discusses their feelings. Then the affected child will start to discuss his or her feelings. The response to the child should be kind and appreciative.

Please don't be in a panic if your child is labeled 'hyperactive.' Ayurveda has some simple, direct, and practical remedies, and provides a great protocol for childcare through diet and herbs that will allow your precious flower to grow beautifully and bloom. Should the ADHD condition affect the education or family stability, medical intervention may be required.[74]

---

74. Helpful diagnostic information for ADHD is contained in the Diagnostic and Statistical Manual of Mental Disorders, Fifth Edition by American Psychiatric Publishing, 2013. You can find a good summary here: https://en.wikipedia.org/wiki/Attention_deficit_hyperactivity_disorder.

# Chapter 51

# Sleep and Dreams

Summer 2011, Volume 24, Number 1

ACCORDING TO SANKHYA'S PHILOSOPHY of the creation of man and the universe, the whole universe is a creation of Purusha and Prakruti. Purusha is choiceless, passive awareness, while Prakruti is creative potential and primordial matter. Purusha doesn't need any sleep, because it is the full awakening of awareness. In that pure awareness, we are not aware that we are aware. The moment you become aware that you are aware, that is the beginning of the dream.

I have decided to write an article, which is also a dream. This whole world is the dream of Purusha. Prakruti is the beautiful creative bed, and on that bed of Prakruti, Purusha is lying and dreaming. An ancient sūtra from *Vishnu Sahasranāma* states, *'Vasudeva shavasanat vasati akhilam vishvam'*: "It is the dream of Vasudeva (Purusha) that creates this whole world."

Within ahamkāra (self-identity), the three *mahā gunas* (qualities) are present in an unmanifested form. When sattva, rajas, and tamas are equal and balanced, it is pure mahat (intelligence). Then, for the purpose of experience, sattva creates the concept of an observer, rajas creates the concept of observation, and tamas creates the objective world. Our mind is the pure essence of sattva, split from ahamkāra. This mind has three states: *jagrat, svapna,* and *sushupti.* The wakeful state (jagrat) is associated with sattva, the dream state (svapna) is related to rajas, and deep sleep (sushupti) to tamas.

Jagrat, the wakeful state, functions with more of a sattva quality, which is clarity and purity. Sattva creates individual consciousness and the concept of an observer. The moment we become conscious of consciousness, it creates a center—this is the observer. This observer projects outside of itself because of the rajasic quality. The movement of observation is rajas, and it relates to the dream state. When awareness flows from one point to another, it becomes attention, and that flow of attention is perception. Perception is the process of rajas carrying awareness through the doors of perception (the senses) to meet with the objective world, which is tamas. The visible world is an expression of tamas, which is inertia, matter. Tamas relates to the state of deep sleep.

Sattva is the observer, rajas is observation, and tamas is the thing to be observed. The moment the observer (sattva) touches the thing to be observed (tamas) via observation (the medium of rajas), that gives us experience. In that experience, our awareness becomes materialized or crystallized. Experience is the precipitation or residue of awareness, so it is always of the past. Every experience nourishes ahamkāra. The bigger the experience, the bigger the experiencer; the smaller the experience, the smaller the experiencer. If ahamkāra does not identify with the experience, then awareness can remain in the present moment, becoming bliss.

## Table 12: The Three States of the Mind

| State (Sanskit) | Guna | Consciousness | Mind | Senses |
|---|---|---|---|---|
| Waking (Jagrat) | Sattva | Conscious | Active mind | Sensory impressions |
| Dream (Svapna) | Rajas | Subconscious | Active mind | Sensory impressions |
| Deep Sleep (Sushupti) | Tamas | Unconscious | Inactive mind | No sensory impressions |

You cannot experience the truth. You can only experience reality. Truth is universal, timeless, causeless, boundless, pure Purusha. Reality is sattva meeting tamas via rajas. The meeting point of these three gunas gives shape to the truth in the form of reality. Reality is a personal affair. It is a product of time and space, of cause and effect. Reality in Albuquerque is different from the reality in New York or New Zealand. Reality now is different from yesterday's reality.

*Yadā tu manasi klānte karmātmānah klamān vitāh*
*Vishayebhyo nirvartante tadā svapiti mānavah*

*Charaka Samhita, Sūtrasthana, ch. 21, vs. 25*

This beautiful sūtra states that our body, mind, and senses become tired of being consciously active because of our daily activities, thoughts, feelings, and emotions. Then the mind withdraws from the sensory world and enters the *sushumnā nādī,* which is the central canal of the spinal cord.

Passing through several lighter stages of sleep, we enter into a dark timeless zone called deep sleep, where the mind becomes relatively unconscious and inactive. We are cut off from the sensory world. In deep, dreamless sleep, there is no color, no light, and no form. Tarpaka kapha, prāna vāta, and sādhaka pitta are active, but the mind doesn't think about or feel anything. In deep sleep, the person is close to his own being–there is only being, no becoming. Deep sleep is not possible with dreams. Dreams are due to rajas, which is movement.

All sensory faculties are affected in deep sleep. For example, smell, taste, and sight are suppressed and the person cannot smell, taste, or see anything in the external world. However, touch and hearing are least affected, which is why touching a person or calling his or her name can easily arouse someone who is sleeping.

In between jagrat and shushupti, there is a transitional period, in which we are neither awake nor asleep. We enter into a subjective world. This junction between wakefulness and deep sleep is dreaming. Sleep is not a constant process, rather it fluctuates from wakeful to deep sleep to dreaming, to light sleep, back to dreaming and then to deep sleep, and so forth.

Sleep and wakefulness occur alternately within the daily sleep cycle during the whole life of the individual. During sleep, the brain is still active and the body still performs most of its functions. Externally sleep can appear to be a very passive state, but internally it is active. The heart rate, respiration, kidneys, gastrointestinal tract (GI), and other organs are still active in deep sleep. The kidneys are still performing filtration, and the GI tract may still be digesting the previous meal. Similarly, the brain is also active during sleep. The brain undergoes rejuvenation and reorganization rather than inhibition.

Sleep can be defined as a state of consciousness that moves from alert wakefulness to a loss of critical activity and response to the events in the environment, accompanied by profound alteration in the function of the brain. Sleep is not a continuous uniform phenomenon. There are ups and downs, fluctuations, and variations in the nature and depth of sleep. Even in the same person, the depth and nature of sleep will vary.

> **WHAT IS SLEEP?**
>
> At Stanford University, I visited William Dement, the retired dean of sleep studies, a co-discoverer of REM sleep, and co-founder of the Stanford Sleep Medicine Center. I asked him to tell me what he knew, after 50 years of research, about the reason we sleep.
>
> "As far as I know," he answered, "the only reason we need to sleep that is really, really solid is because we get sleepy."
>
> *Secrets of Sleep* by D. T. Max, National Geographic Magazine, May 2010

The nature of sleep varies according to a person's prakruti and vikruti doshas. For a vāta person, sleep is light and interrupted. Pitta people find it difficult to go to sleep, but once they fall sleep, they have relatively sound sleep. They are intermediate sleepers. Kapha people have deep prolonged sleep.

Vāta is mobile, light, and cold and if there is cold weather or a cold room, a vāta person cannot get to sleep. The same is true about noise coming into the bedroom. The light quality of vāta creates light sleep. The dryness of vāta leads to constipation and drowsiness with insufficient sleep. Pitta is hot, sharp, penetrating, and liquid. If the room is too hot or there is a light on, a pitta person will not sleep well. A pitta person needs a dark, quiet room and comfortable temperature, not too hot or cold. Kapha is heavy, dull, and slow or static. Kapha people can sleep comfortably in almost any room, cool or warm and with or without a bed. Sleep can vary in these ways.

## The Rhythm of Sleep

The rhythm of sleep varies according to an individual's age and his or her prakruti and vikruti. One's diet and habits, the environment, the season, work responsibilities, stress, and daytime sleep can also change it. Sleep requirements vary according to age as well.

In adults, the maximum depth of sleep comes at the end of the first hour or two. In children, there are two periods of deep sleep: one period is between the first and second hours, while the second period is between 8–9 hours after going to sleep. So children often go to sleep right away for one and two hours, then they start tossing and turning and have phases of rapid eye movement, and then they go into deep sleep for the remaining hours.

The Ayurvedic understanding of sleep is that older people usually need less sleep than younger adults. Elderly people sometimes feel they don't sleep enough, as they may only sleep for 4-5 hours per night. However, because of physical weakness or fatigue that may accompany aging, they often feel they need more sleep than this.

| Age and condition | Sleep Needs[a] |
|---|---|
| Newborn (0-3 months) | 14 to 17 hours |
| Infants (4-11 months) | 12-15 hours |
| Toddlers (1-2 years) | 11-14 hours |
| Preschoolers (3-4 years) | 10-13 hours |
| School-age children (5-12 years) | 9-11 hours |
| Teenagers (13-17 years) | 8-10 hours |
| Adults (18-64 years) | 7-9 hours |
| Older Adults (65+ years) | 7-8 hours |

a   https://en.wikipedia.org/wiki/Sleep#Recommendations

## Stages of Sleep

*Stage 1, light sleep.* It is the beginning of the sleep cycle, the junction between the jagrat and sushupti stages. This stage lasts for about 5-10 minutes. Theta waves (4-7 Hz) are present, producing a slow brain wave pattern. By comparison, when still awake, there is a predominance of alpha waves, which range from about 8-13 Hz. Stage 1 sleep is governed by prāna vāta and sees the calming down of prāna.

*Stage 2, the junction between light sleep and deep sleep.* There is a predominance of sigma waves, also known as sleep spindles (11-16 Hz). This second stage accounts for about 50% of the time a typical adult spends asleep. Body temperature drops, heart rate slows, and breathing deepens and becomes parasympathetic. Stage 2 sleep is governed by sādhaka pitta.

*Stage 3, deeper sleep.* There are an increased number of delta waves (0.5-4 Hz). There is still a deep, slow breathing pattern. This is the inhibition of sādhaka pitta and a predominance of tarpaka kapha. This third stage generally lasts for about 20-30 minutes per sleep cycle.

*Stage 4, deepest sleep, with more than 50% delta waves.* The whole brain becomes slow, as this stage is governed by tarpaka kapha. It typically lasts for about 20-30 minutes per cycle. During this stage, tarpaka kapha and prāna vāta can stimulate each other, which is why bedwetting or sleep walking can occur during this fourth stage.[75]

*Stage 5, rapid eye movement (REM) sleep phase, in which there is an increase in respiration and brain activity.* This is the svapna state of mind. While voluntary muscles are paralyzed, dreaming occurs at this stage. Vascular engorgement of the genitals in this stage can result in dreams of sex. REM sleep can comprise 20% to 25% of total sleep time.[76]

---

75. These first 4 stages are all non-REM sleep. Stages 3 and 4 have recently been combined into stage N3, under the 2007 American Academy of Sleep medicine (AASM) Guidelines, with the first two stages now referred to as stages N1 and N2.
76. There are two main types of sleep: non-rapid eye movement (NREM) sleep (also known as quiet sleep) and rapid eye movement (REM) sleep (also known as active sleep).

There is more deep sleep earlier in the night, whereas there is a greater amount of REM sleep later in the night. A sleeper constantly transitions between stages of sleep. Sleep begins in stage 1 and progresses into stages 2, 3 and 4. After stage 4 sleep (deep sleep), stage 3 and then stage 2 sleep are repeated before entering REM sleep, stage 5. Once REM sleep is over, the body usually returns to stage 2 sleep. Sleep cycles through these stages approximately 4 or 5 times throughout the night. Most dreaming occurs in REM sleep. Although dreams also occur in stages 3 and 4, most people do not recall those dreams.

## Table 13: Three Stages of Sleep

| 1 | 5-10 minutes | Theta waves. Gradual cessation of prāna vāta |
|---|---|---|
| 2 | 10-25 minutes | Sleep spindle brain activity. Rapid, rhythmic brain waves. Temperature drops, breathing, and heart rate slow down. Cessation of sādhaka pitta. |
| 3 | 20-30 minutes | Delta waves. Slow brain activity. Deep sleep induced by tarpaka kapha |
| 4 | 20-30 minutes | Delta waves. Governed by tarpaka kapha. However prāna may become active, causing bedwetting or sleepwalking. |
| 5 | Initial occurrence can be very short but each cycle becomes longer, lasting up to an hour as sleep progresses | Rapid eye movement (REM) stage of sleep, which indicates activation of prāna. It is the dream stage, respiration becomes faster, and repressed emotions activate, causing some to have dreams of sex in this stage. |

# The Physiology of Sleep

In normal sleep, the eyes are closed, the jaw is relaxed, and muscles are relaxed; there is a deep parasympathetic breathing. The person breathes into their belly. During the wakeful state, most people breathe into their chest, called sympathetic breathing. Ayurveda says that sleep is due to excess tarpaka kapha secretion in the majjā dhātu, and that slows down the activity of prāna vāta and sādhaka pitta. Logical intellectual activities slow down and physical motor activities slow down as well.

During sleep, the srotāmsi are still active, but some srotāmsi are much less active than when awake, while others remain in a similar state of activity. Many reflexes are elevated, whereas responsiveness is lessened. People cannot remember any physiological events during their sleep. For example, rasa and rakta vaha srotas are somewhat inactive, as pulse rate, cardiac output, blood pressure, and heart rate are all reduced. In prāna vaha srotas, there is slow breathing, which sometimes becomes shallow. This diminished rate of respiration indicates that prāna vaha srotas also slows down.

In deep sleep, the activity of agni is reduced by 10-15%. Thus, one's basal metabolic rate, which is governed by jathāra agni and dhātu agni, becomes slower.

Māmsa vaha srotas is completely relaxed, as all voluntary muscles are relaxed during sleep, and meda vaha srotas also slows down. Mūtra vaha srotas activity is reduced, so the volume of urine is less than during the day. The specific gravity and concentration of urine is raised because globular filtration diminishes. Bodhaka kapha and thus salivary secretions are diminished, as is lacrimation.

Majjā vaha srotas is intermittently relaxed and active. The eyeball, a part of majjā, is rolled up outwardly, eye lids are closed, and pupils are contracted when a person is in a deep sleep. However, there are periods of rapid eye movement when dreaming occurs.

### Historical Theories of Sleep

We discussed the Ayurvedic theory of sleep earlier in this article. Even today, we have not yet found the exact cause of sleep. Historically there have been many theories that try to explain sleep. From the late 1800s to the mid-1900s, one prevalent theory was that of cerebral ischemia or lack of blood supply to the cerebral cortex. In the 1950s, Mangold and Sokoloff did studies on cerebral metabolism that showed an increase of blood flow during sleep, putting to rest the cerebral ischemia theory. I. P. Pavlov believed that sleep is conditioned inhibition.

These were followed by biochemical theories such as the accumulation of acetylcholine creating sound sleep or the accumulation of lactic acid in the tissues causing fatigue. Other theories include studies of reserpine, serotonin, and the amino acid precursors of serotonin, 5-hydroxytryptophan (5-HTP) and L-tryptophan, and their role in sleep. Others focused on the reduction in muscle tone experienced during sleep, positing that the afferent impulse to the cerebral cortex creates sleep. This theory is interesting because oil massage does cause the muscles to relax and reduce their tone and transmission of the afferent impulse, which can lead to sleep. In Ayurvedic terms, this relaxes vyāna vāyu and prāna vāyu, creating sleep. Today, most sleep researchers agree that sleep has restorative, memory processing, and preservative functions.

## Dreams

Sleep is a biological need and a psychological requirement because of these rejuvenating, relaxing, and revitalizing functions. Sleep creates a total reorganization of the brain structure. Our brain cells' neurons undergo changes in deep sleep. Dream sleep has a different function.

What happens in our day-to-day activities? There are a lot of incomplete or unresolved thoughts, feelings, and emotions. These are all stuck in our brain tissue and, during second and fifth stages of sleep, the brain cells create a dream state so that these incomplete actions and unresolved emotions can be completed.

A dream is a discharge of an incomplete action. After a dream, the brain becomes orderly. Ayurveda says that the dream state (svapna) is rajasic. Wakefulness (jagrat) is sattvic, whereas dreamless deep sleep (shushupti) is tamasic. However, in a deep sleep, we are close to our being, close to our pure Purusha or soul.

Yogis practice *yoga nidrā,* which is psychic sleep, according to Vedic science. Because deep sleep is a way of being close to the inner source of being, when you sleep with awareness and maintain that awareness in the deep sleep state, you will become enlightened; that kind of sleep becomes a form of samādhi. Sleep is not samādhi, but samādhi is like sleep when it occurs with total awareness. In that awareness, there is no judgment, no criticism, no likes, or dislikes. In this awareness, there is a complete cessation of ego, because to some extent we forget our ego or identity in a deep sleep. Hence, the Ayurvedic approach to sleep is one of the gateways to becoming enlightened. In deep sleep, even a king and a beggar are the same. The moment they wake up, they become king and beggar again. This is due to identification.

There are different dream states. In these dreaming states, systemic vāta dosha may activate prāna vāyu, systemic pitta dosha may stimulate prāna vāyu, or systemic kapha dosha may disturb prāna vāyu, leading to three different categories of dreams.

## Vāta Dreams

Dreams of falling, being attacked, being pushed, or of always doing something in the dream as well as being frozen with fright, seeing the death of a loved one, or being locked up or flying are vāta dreams. Certain animals such as snakes, camels, and flying birds are related to vāta. Dreams about the autumn season are about vāta. In vāta dreams, the person is trying to fulfill a desire.

These dreams are about a person falling or being attacked. In some cases, kapha or pitta may attack vāta dosha and prāna vāta may receive the dream. It is a successful or unsuccessful effort of the dosha or higher consciousness to convey the message to the lower consciousness.

## Pitta Dreams

From the hot and sharp qualities, pitta people will teach or will be learning, even in the dream state. They will also release their anger through sex, killing someone, being inappropriately dressed, being nude in public, by arriving too late, or by eating in dreams. They will dream of summer, fires such as burning buildings, problem solving, or failing in some way because of their desires for success. They tend to see frogs and cats in their dream as well as wild animals like tigers.

## Kapha Dreams

Kapha dreams are very romantic. They dream about swimming, finding money, enjoying romantic sex, or being in the snow. They also dream about eating candy, doing the same thing repeatedly, or arriving too late, satisfying unconscious needs. They can also see themselves as dead. Kapha dreams will be about the spring or winter season, seeing the ocean or a lake, and animals like elephants, swans, or lions.

Ayurveda classifies dreams according to the doshas. Other dreams are spiritual dreams. An example may be a dream in which you see a teacher or deity whom you worship. Devotion can come in the form of a dream. In a dream, the mind goes beyond the past and present, seeing into the future. Suggestions about the future are given in some dreams. In this way, we can classify dreams.

One can meditate upon a dream; make your own dream diary. That way, by studying the patterns of your dreams, you can understand underlying etiological factors, such as your khavaigunya or weakness. I had a patient who told me, "Dr. Lad, for three days I have had a repeated dream about the back of my house, where there is a lake that is on fire." I could see that the lake represented the bladder, the fire is pitta, and the three days were her vāta pushing pitta in the bladder. Her bladder was giving her the message she has high pitta in the bladder and is likely to get cystitis or a bladder infection.

Other dreams can indicate death. To dream of teeth falling out means someone near you will die. Or seeing a cremation in your dream can mean that someone is going to die. There are also cultural dreams. In the Indian tradition, if someone dreams that people are rubbing sindhu on his forehead and flour over the body, it indicates that person will die. If a person dreams of a hole in the wall, that individual is likely to get tuberculosis in the lung cavity. If someone sees holes in a pole or pillar, it means that the person has osteoporosis or will likely get a medical fracture.

## Categories of Sleep Disorders

There are many environmental factors that induce insomnia. Insomnia may be due to noise (vāta), too much movement or travel (vāta), changing time zones or a change of altitude (vāta), cold weather or a cold room (vāta), too much heat in the room (pitta), or eating hot, spicy food (pitta).

There are different categories of sleeplessness. Dissomnias are sleep disturbances or excessive sleepiness and include types of insomnia, hypersomnia, narcolepsy, sleep apnea, brief limb jerks, and restless leg syndrome. Parasomnias include night terrors, nightmares, sleepwalking, and disorders related to mental illness. There is also sleep pattern disruption associated with medical illness such as endocrine disorders or pulmonary disease.[77]

There are various causes of insomnia and other sleeping disorders:

- Dietary factors – foods that the person finds hard to digest can cause indigestion and result in insomnia
- Lack of exercise
- Strenuous exercises before bed
- A bath immediately before bed
- Daytime sleep, such as an afternoon nap or siesta
- Sleep apnea
- Narcolepsy
- Restless leg syndrome
- Illnesses that cause pain, such as rheumatoid arthritis
- Mental illness
- Psychological factors such as anxiety, worry, and stress
- Drinking coffee, tea, and other caffeinated beverages

Drugs can cause drug-induced insomnia from consumption of alcohol, recreational drugs, or pharmaceuticals. For instance, if people drink whiskey, they will likely wake up at 2 o'clock in the morning as the liver tries to metabolize the alcohol. Certain medications can also cause insomnia.

---

77. *Taber's Cyclopedic Medical Dictionary*, 20th Ed., 2005, Venes, Donald, editor; page 2013.

## Doshic Types of Insomnia

Vāta insomnia is more likely with cold temperatures, excess travel, noise, excessive exercise, and consumption of vāta-aggravating foods such as raw foods, pinto, adzuki, or black beans. It is typically worse in the fall season. In vāta type of insomnia, the person often wakens every hour or two and usually has many dreams or nightmares. As a result, the person wakes up fatigued and feels drowsy during the day. This often results in constipation and difficulty in concentrating. Vāta tendencies towards constipation, bloating, arthritis, and rheumatism can create vāta insomnia. Excessive sexual activity can also cause insomnia.

Pitta insomnia is often caused by hyperacidity, staying up late at night, a bedroom that is too hot or exposed to light, or excessive consumption of foods such as citrus, sour fruits, chili pepper, coffee and other caffeinated beverages, red wine, or hard liquor. It is worse in summer season. In pitta type of insomnia, it is difficult for the person to get to sleep and they often waken during 'liver time,' which is around 2 AM. If the person doesn't get to bed by 10 PM or so, they get a burst of energy and tend to burn the midnight oil. They are often night owls who like to read, work, or watch TV at midnight. Pitta types like to read one or two chapters before bed. They generally need a completely dark and silent room to go to sleep.

Kapha insomnia is mild. The person goes to sleep right away but may wake up at dawn and have early morning insomnia. Kapha insomnia is usually related to overeating, which can cause breathlessness, snoring, sleep apnea, restless leg syndrome, seasonal affective disorder, mild depression, and/or kapha-type emotional dreams.

## Management of Sleep Disorders

To have naturally healthy sleep, we should receive periodic massage. Abhyanga is Ayurvedic oil massage and it will help to induce sound sleep. For better sleep, rub bhringarāja oil onto the scalp and soles of the feet before going to bed.

Milk is a good source of tryptophan, which can increase sound sleep. Drink a cup of warm milk about an hour before bedtime. Alternatively, vāta types can have garlic milk, pitta types can choose shatāvarī milk, and kapha people will benefit from turmeric milk. These medicated milks are made by boiling the herb in the milk for a few minutes and then allow the milk to cool a little.

The layout of your bedroom is another important factor. Don't sleep under ceiling beams or dividers. Your feet should not point towards a doorway. There should not be much of a gap between the headboard of the bed and the wall—a few inches distance is okay, but a larger gap can create insomnia.

Your sleeping position is also important to consider. Lying on your right side is calming, but lying on your back or left side can be okay. If you lie on your back or side, do So'hum meditation, inhaling with "so" and exhaling with "hum." With a peaceful mind watching the breath, you can go straight to sleep.

### Herbal Protocol for Sleep

"Herbal Formulas for Sleep" has some helpful herbal formulas for sound sleep, according to one's prakruti and vikruti.

Each of these remedies can be taken an hour before bedtime along with a cup of warm milk or the medicated milks listed above. These are simple but effective remedies to help induce sound sleep. Additionally, put an ounce of the Ayurvedic herb jatamamsi in a little silk bag and place it under your pillow to create sound sleep.

If you take melatonin, there should be complete darkness. If there is a little light, it will create more drowsiness. It is a 2 multi-functional hormone that has many usages, but side effects include headaches, an altered sleep pattern, mood swings, itching skin, tachycardia, and depression. One should be careful not to take more than a 10 mg dose of melatonin. Melatonin side effects are usually temporary, so if you stop the medicine, within a week these can clear up.

### Table 14: Herbal Formulas for Sleep

| Vāta | Pitta | Kapha |
|---|---|---|
| Dashamūla 5 parts<br>Ashvagandhā 4 parts<br>Tagara 3 parts<br>Jatamāmsi 3 parts<br>½ teaspoon of this mixture nightly | Shatāvarī 5 parts<br>Gudūchī 3 parts<br>Jatamāmsi 3 parts<br>Shankha Pushpī 2 parts<br>½ teaspoon of this mixture nightly | Punarnavā 5 parts<br>Sarasvatī 3 parts<br>Chitrak 2 parts<br>Tagara 2 parts<br>½ teaspoon of this mixture nightly |

# Chapter 52

# Sleep Disorders

Fall 2011, Volume 24, Number 2

IN THIS ARTICLE, we will examine the following conditions as they relate to sleep disorders:

- Chronic Fatigue Syndrome (CFS)
- Depression
- Migraine
- Sleep Apnea
- Snoring
- Bedwetting
- Restless Legs Syndrome
- Sleepwalking

Any dosha can disturb sleep if it becomes high in majjā dhātu and mano vaho srotas. Sādhaka pitta is present in the cerebral-cortical area, tarpaka kapha in the medulla area of the brain, and prāna vāta governs sensory stimuli and motor responses. If any of these are increased, the individual's sleep pattern can become disturbed.

## Chronic Fatigue Syndrome

Chronic fatigue syndrome (CFS) is an uncommonly common condition these days in clinical practice. In CFS, an infectious mononucleosis virus can disturb rasa dhātu and particularly the lymph nodes in the neck area, which can become inflamed and swollen. Sthāyi and asthāyi rasa are affected, which causes āma and in turn results in sroto rodha (clogging of the channels). There are inflamed and swollen lymph nodes with low-grade fever, sore throat, and aches and pains. The person feels as if he is "dead on his feet," with extreme fatigue, and is often confined to bed for long periods. Ojas can become severely depleted.

CFS and sleep disorders can go together, as poor sleep depletes ojas. Sound sleep is necessary to restore and even build ojas. Hence, those with constitutionally low ojas can become susceptible to diseases if they get insufficient sleep.

To heal, the person should follow the following guidelines:

- Don't over-exert oneself
- Have enough restful sleep
- Eat home-cooked meals
- Don't eat foods with additives or preservatives, or canned food
- Take multi-vitamins
- Take care of allergies: food intolerances and *prāna sroto dushti* are particularly common in CFS
- Take this herbal formula TID with warm water: dashamūla 500 mg, ashvagandhā 400 mg, vidārī 300 mg, and jatamāmsi 200 mg[78]
- If there is fever, sore throat, or upper respiratory congestion, take sitopalādi 500 mg and mahāsudarshan 300 mg
- Good Night Sleep Tea[79] contains chamomile, skullcap, and tagara. It is particularly beneficial for this condition.
- If there are more pitta symptoms, one can take the following formula TID: shatāvarī 500 mg, gudūchi 300 mg, sarasvatī 200 mg

## Depression

If a person doesn't get proper sleep, it can lead to depression. In this condition, the individual keeps anxious and sad feelings inside.

In our daily life, we can see two types of depression. 'Healthy depression' comes from realistic feelings of pain, sadness, disappointment, guilt, anger, anxiety, or physical or psychological trauma. Suppression of these feelings or keeping one's feelings inside will create depression. This can lead to sleeplessness and insomnia and, in turn, the sleeplessness and insomnia can lead to depression. Effect becomes cause and cause becomes effect.

All healthy people feel this type of depression in their life. It comes and goes. The person is capable of functioning normally in relationships and in life in general. However, prolonged 'healthy depression' can produce chemical changes in the brain, leading to chronic depression. Therefore, don't take any depression lightly.

'Unhealthy depression' comes about when the individual is unable to function in one or more areas of life—relationship, work or so forth. Prolonged, persistent bad feelings will produce chemical changes in the brain, leading to unhealthy depression. The person can suffer from insomnia, or can become more passive and less active, sleeping for greater amounts of time than normal. Sleeping during the day and insomnia at night is one common scenario.

78. This amount of herbs, combined together, is a single serving. Most often, herbs are taken for a period of time, such as a week or a month. Then your herbalist would formulate a larger amount using these proportions and give you enough of the mixture for the recommended time period and number of servings per day.
79. Vasant Lad's tea formula, sold at the Institute. The traditional formula is made with jatamāmsi, shankha pushpī, and tagara. Jatamāmsi and shankha pushpī are endangered and/or threatened species. See cites.com for more information. Our current formula is quite effective.

Lifestyle changes can help in cases of 'healthy depression' and short-term 'unhealthy depression:'

- Regularize the lifestyle by sticking to a daily routine
- Wake up early and watch the sunrise
- Go for a morning walk
- Increased periods of activity are better than prolonged periods of passivity
- Cultivate friendships and enjoy a social life
- Try not to take things personally
- Watch your life objectively and know yourself as you are
- Eat fresh food (steamed vegetables, basmati rice, mung dal, fruit, etc.)
- Don't eat leftovers, or canned and frozen food
- Do daily yoga, prānāyāma, and meditation or relaxation

One can easily handle short-term depression by adopting these lifestyle changes. The most important thing for someone suffering from depression is to love their life and not engage in comparison.

People who are depressed live in the past or future. They do not live in the eternal present. Meditation means to bring awareness to this moment, without comparison or judgement. It means to be here now. Now is peace and bliss. Meditation is not hollow; it is whole, complete. Therefore, meditation can be of great benefit for someone with depression.

## Treatments of Doshic Types of Depression

Vāta-type depression with fear, anxiety, and insomnia:

- Abhyanga (sesame oil massage of the whole body) followed by a hot shower
- Gentle yogāsana followed by calming prānāyāma
- Dashamūla 500 mg, ashvagandhā 400 mg, vidārī 300 mg, jatamāmsi 200 mg, TID
- Triphalā ½ teaspoon (tsp.) nightly
- Basti made from a tea containing 1 tablespoon (Tbs.) each of dashamūla, gudūchi, and brahmī
- Vacha oil nasya

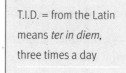

T.I.D. = from the Latin means *ter in diem*, three times a day

Pitta-type depression with competitiveness, failure, anger, hate, envy, or jealousy (someone with this condition can become suicidal and need medical help):

- Abhyanga (sunflower oil massage of the whole body) followed by hot shower
- Yogāsana followed by cooling prānāyāma
- Shatāvarī 500 mg, gulvel sattva 300 mg, kāma dudhā 200 mg, shankha pushpī 200 mg, TID
- Bhumi āmalakī ½ tsp. nightly
- Basti made from a tea containing 1 Tbs. each of gudūchi, shankha pushpī, and jatamāmsi
- Brahmī ghee nasya

Kapha-type depression with attachment, greed, possessiveness, hypersomnia, and emotional eating:

- Abhyanga (sesame oil massage of the whole body) followed by hot shower
- Vigorous yogāsana followed by heating prāṇāyāma
- Punarnavā 500 mg, chitrak 200 mg, kutki 200 mg, sarasvatī 200 mg, TID
- Bibhītakī ½ tsp. nightly
- Basti made from tea containing 1 Tbs. each of punarnavā and brahmī
- Anu tailam nasya or vacha powder nasya

Note that vāta and kapha types of depression are relatively easy to handle, but the pitta type of depression can become serious and may need medical help.

# Migraines

Migraine headaches are a vāta-pitta type of disorder. They are more common in women and in people with pitta constitutions, especially perfectionists, compulsive types, or type A personalities who are success-oriented and who live more in the head than the heart.

There are two main theories about the causes of migraine:

1. The blood vessels (rakta) expand due to the hot quality of pitta, exerting pressure on the nerve fibers (majjā), causing pain. This is the cause of pitta type of migraines.
2. The blood vessels (rakta) contract, due to the cold attribute of vāta, blocking flow to part of the brain (majjā). This causes pain and is the cause of vāta type of migraines.

One of the main causes of sleep disorders is aggravated vāta pushing pitta in rasa-rakta and majjā dhātus. People with disturbed sleep patterns are prone to migraine.

Migraines can cause visual impairment, because the eyeballs are an important part of majjā dhātu. The aura of the migraine begins in the eyes.

## Causative Factors of Migraines

- Disturbed sleep
- Emotional factors
- Food allergies and intolerances
- Coffee
- Chocolate
- Cola drinks
- Citrus fruits
- Sour foods

## Symptoms of Vāta-type Migraines

- Throbbing pulsating pain
- Cluster headaches
- Constipation
- Gas and bloating

## Symptoms of Pitta-type Migraines
- Sharp pain
- Excessive sweating
- Nausea
- Photosensitivity
- Flashes of light (ophthalmic migraine)

## Healthy Lifestyle Tips for Acute or Sub-Acute Migraines
- Sufficient sound sleep
- Avoid artificial sweeteners and MSG
- Avoid prolonged exposure to sunlight, or wear a hat and sunglasses
- No smoking or drinking alcohol
- Avoid excessive sexual activity
- Take time to relax
- Munch on magnesium, which means green leafy vegetables, pumpkin seeds, oats, barley, and soy beans
- Ensure you drink enough water
- Avoid foods to which you are allergic
- Cool the scalp by applying coconut oil medicated with brahmī oil
- Take a brisk walk or do other aerobic exercise in the early morning (kapha time)
- Rest, read, and relax during the middle of the day (pitta time)

## Management of Chronic Migraine Headaches
- The following herbal formula TID: dashamūla 500 mg, shatāvarī 300 mg, kāma dudhā 200 mg, tagara 200 mg, and jatamāmsi 200 mg
- One-half tsp. of bhumi āmalakī nightly with warm water
- Take Good Night Sleep Tea herbal mixture
- Do nasya daily: 1) vacha oil nasya for vāta types or 2) brahmī ghee nasya for pitta types
- Super Nasya Oil® is suitable for all constitutions
- Rub bhringarāja oil and brahmī oil on the scalp and soles of feet before bedtime

## Sleep Apnea

Sleep apnea is another important sleep disorder. It is characterized by abnormal pauses in breathing (apnea) or periods of unusually shallow breathing (hypopnea) during sleep.

One in ten Americans suffer from abnormal snoring. The person can stop breathing for between ten seconds to two minutes, typically for ten to fifteen times per hour. In my hospital clinical practice, I have observed patients stopping breathing for 30-40 seconds. The patient doesn't know that he is snoring or that he has stopping breathing.

Loud snoring, noisy breathing, gurgling, and harrumphing during sleep can all be associated with sleep apnea. Such snoring sounds can be terrifying to the person's partner. Those suffering from sleep apnea are usually obese. The patient may have nasal congestion, a snuffly nose, deviated nasal septum, or other such condition.

There are various factors that can cause these symptoms. For instance, noisy breathing can be due to food intolerances or food allergies. Sleep apnea can also be induced by cold medicines and other drugs.

### Lifestyle Recommendations
- Nasya with Super Nasya Oil® or vacha oil before going to bed
- Use nasal spray that relieves nasal congestion
- If overweight, reduce weight
- Don't drink alcohol (as it can increase sleep apnea)
- No smoking
- Avoid allergic foods
- Don't eat late in the evening and no late-night snacks
- Āsana and prāṇāyāma can be particularly beneficial, especially anuloma-viloma and kapāla bhāti prāṇāyāma
- Punarnavā 500 mg, sitopalādi 400 mg, tālīsādi 300 mg, abhrak bhasma 200 mg, trikatu 100 mg TID
- Before going to bed, inhale steam with 2 drops of eucalyptus oil

Sleep apnea is potentially a serious condition. It can induce a heart attack in some patients as well as cause other complications, so it needs to be properly managed. In particularly serious cases, this treatment may not be sufficient, so it will be necessary to see a medical doctor and have a sleep evaluation.

# Snoring

When a person sleeps on his or her back, gravity acts on the loose tissue in the upper respiratory passage and the tongue falls backwards into the throat. This can create snoring.

Snoring is particularly common in men, because they have a more oval vocal cord, due to the physiology of the Adam's apple, as opposed to women's more round vocal cords. It also frequently occurs in obese people and those with upper respiratory congestion.

### Causative Factors
- Sleeping on your back
- Obesity
- Upper respiratory congestion
- Heavy consumption of alcohol in the evening prior to sleep
- Sleeping pills and tranquilizers
- Insufficient sleep
- Stress
- A soft, saggy mattress
- A pillow that is too low or too high can exacerbate snoring

### Management
- Sleep on one side, especially the left side (as this promotes better digestion)
- Ensure sufficient sound sleep
- Sleep on a firm mattress

- Use an appropriate-sized pillow
- Elevate the head-end of the bed by placing a brick under it, raising it by about 2 or 3 inches
- Nasya with Super Nasya Oil® or other nasya appropriate for the constitution
- Inhale steam with eucalyptus oil
- No smoking
- Avoid drinking alcohol in the late evenings
- The following herbal formula is to be taken TID: sitopalādi 500 mg, tālīsādi 400 mg, mahāsudarshan 300 mg, and abhrak bhasma 200 mg
- One tsp. of bhumi āmalakī before bedtime will also help this condition.

# Bedwetting

This is a common condition for children. A family history of bedwetting is frequently present for those who wet their bed.

The main causes of bedwetting are:
- A small bladder
- Overactive prāna vāyu
- Respiratory allergies, which can cause insufficient sleep
- Psychological factors, such as stress, fear, or anxiety

Dealing with bedwetting is a delicate situation, as it can strongly affect the child's self-esteem. Do not humiliate or punish a child for wetting the bed, as this can increase his or her stress levels and thereby worsen the problem. It is important not to tell other people that your child wets the bed, as this can undermine self-esteem.

## Management
- No beverages just before bedtime
- No carbonated drinks
- Encourage the child to urinate before going to bed
- Before the child goes to bed, gently massage the lumbosacral area of the back, the hypogastric region on the front, and the scalp and soles of the feet. Use oil or cream, or just do dry massage if that is more practical
- Check out if there are allergies and get those managed
- Check if the child snores and, if so, treat the cause of the snoring
- Train the child to hold onto his or her urine as long as possible

Nowadays, there are wireless moisture sensors with an alarm attached, and the sensor can be placed in the child's underwear. This can be shocking, so I do not think this is suitable for children under age five. It may help older children who have this condition.

Externally, apply vacha paste to the belly button. Internally, give sesame-jaggery candy, made from one tsp. of ground sesame seeds and ½ tsp. of raw sugar or jaggery mixed together. This is called *tila-guda rasāyana*.

Also, boil one cup of milk and ½ cup water with 5 whole pippalī in it. Keep it cooking until the water evaporates and the mixture reduces to one cup in total. Then give this mixture to the child to drink an hour or so before bed. Alternatively, give the child a cup of warm licorice milk to drink a few hours before bedtime.

Gulpha marma is a set of marma points that can be gently massaged with vacha oil before bed. Connected to the kidneys, ureter, and bladder, gentle massage will calm down undue stimulation of apāna vāyu.

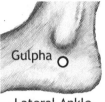

Gulpha ○

Lateral Ankle

Scary stories and horror movies can aggravate bedwetting by increasing vāta dosha, so these things should be strictly avoided. Scary dreams can cause the child to pass urine in his or her sleep. Giving 200 mg each of brahmī, jatamānsi, and shankha pushpī can have a helpful tranquilizing effect and thereby minimize bedwetting.

○ Gulpha

Medial Ankle

I have observed that children who have worms can suffer from bedwetting. Therefore, it can be beneficial to de-worm the child by giving 200 mg each of vidanga, palash, kamilla, and krumi kathar. Also clean the perineal area before bed with a cotton swab dabbed in neem oil.

## Restless Foot / Leg Syndrome

This chronic disorder may be due to the increased mobile (chala) and irregular (vishama) qualities of vāta dosha. The feet and legs are the lower extremities, so they come under the physiological functioning of apāna vāyu.

Chronic constipation, diverticulosis, irritable bowel syndrome (IBS), kidney stones or stones in the bladder or ureter, renal colic, pregnancy, iron-deficiency anemia, and intake of stimulants such as caffeine or tobacco are all etiological factors that may activate the mobile and irregular attributes of vāta in māmsa and majjā dhātus, thereby contributing to restless foot/leg syndrome.

Many times, restless foot/leg syndrome may be due to an internal itching sensation or intolerable creeping sensation in the lower extremity. This sensation can be so strong that there is an irresistible urge to move the leg. It can also be drug-induced.

This syndrome occurs mainly at vāta times (dawn and dusk) or at the end of the day when the patient goes to bed tired or fatigued. The condition is worse in cold climates. Modern medicine still does not know an exact etiology for this condition. One has to thoroughly investigate the patient's history and family health history, and rule out other conditions such as thyroid disorders, renal colic, anemia, and so forth.

One may be able to discern a relationship between restless foot/leg syndrome and coffee intake or other factors. Then one can treat the cause of the condition.

### Management
* Snehana – massage with sesame oil
* Svedana – soak feet for five to ten minutes in a bucket of warm water with a mustard seed tea bag. (2 Tbs. of slightly crushed mustard seeds in a piece of cheese cloth.)

- The following mixture TID before food: ashvagandhā 500 mg, vidarī 300 mg, jatamāmsi 200 mg, and yogarāja guggulu 200 mg
- One half tsp. of gandharva harītakī at bedtime, to maintain the normal movement of vāta dosha (anuloma)
- Rub a mixture of 50:50 mustard oil and vacha oil on the soles of the feet before going to bed
- For pregnant woman with this condition, give one cup of warm milk with a tsp. of ghee (clarified butter)
- If the condition is due to the side-effects of a psychotropic drug, use an antidote such as nutmeg. A good mixture is jatamānsi, nutmeg, and mustā.
- If due to anemia: 200 mg each of loha bhasma and abhrak bhasma, or 4 tsp. of loha āsava after food. Also, take natural sourced iron, such as Floradix®, currants, raisins, beets, or carrots.
- If due to caffeine, eliminate coffee or other caffeinated drinks and increase protein and grain drinks, such as kefir and soups made with barley, quinoa and so forth
- Tranquility Tea is a natural alternative to valium, a frequently prescribed drug that has many undesirable side effects
- Beneficial yogāsana include palm tree pose, standing on one leg, eagle pose, leg lifting, plough pose, and locust pose. These poses should be maintained for at least one minute each. Lotus pose (*padmāsana*), easy cross-legged pose (*swastikāsana*), and accomplished pose (*siddhāsana*) are also helpful for restless foot/leg syndrome.

# Sleepwalking

This condition is called somnambulism, which translates as sleeping ambulance. It is an autonomic action performed during sleep due to high vāta in majjā dhātu. The person has little or no recollection of any sleepwalking the following day.

Sleep is induced by tarpaka kapha, sādhaka pitta, and prāna vāta. When tarpaka suppresses prāna, prāna vāyu can get disturbed and stimulate the autonomic nervous system. The person appears to awaken partially, with open eyes but a blank facial expression. The patient is not fully aware. He or she may sit up, sit on the edge of the bed, walk in the bedroom, or even leave the room. Some can even get in their car and drive off! There is a real danger of physical trauma to the patient or to others.

Sleepwalking is surprisingly common in children, but rare in adults. It is more common in male children and female adults. The exact cause is not known. However, women can suffer from this condition during the menarche age, as hormonal changes may trigger the hypothalamus, which governs autonomic actions.

Psychic children who are also oversensitive can have an overactive autonomic nervous system. Thus, they can experience sleepwalking or other sleep disorders. Night terrors may accompany sleepwalking, so scary stories and horror movies should be avoided.

## Management

- The first thing is to prevent injury by removing sharp or dangerous objects from the bedroom
- Lock the door and windows in the room
- Place a safety gate at the top of any staircase
- Don't keep any fire or water hazards
- Hide the car keys
- Keep the patient under observation
- Avoid horror movies or scary stories before bedtime
- Where appropriate, another person should sleep on the side of the room closest to the door
- Rub bhringarāja oil on the scalp and soles of feet at bedtime
- The following herbal mixture can be given TID: ashvagandhā 500 mg, brahmī 400 mg, shankha pushpī 300 mg, and jatamāmsi 300 mg
- Nasya with brahmī ghee or vacha oil
- Place a silk bag (4 inches by 4 inches) of jatamāmsi root under the pillow
- Massage Mūrdhni, Sthapanī, Oshtha, Jatru, and Hasta/Pāda Kshipra marma points with nutmeg oil (see illustrations page 460)
- Mantra, *yantra,* homa, and havana therapy can be beneficial if done under expert guidance

# Chapter 53

# Dementia and Alzheimer's Disease

Summer 2012, Volume 25, Number 1

ACCORDING TO AYURVEDA, three important doshas govern every individual's unique psychophysiology. Vāta dosha is the principle of movement. Pitta is the energy of transformation that maintains metabolic activity. Kapha is the building block materials of the body. The functional aspects of the body are governed by these three doshas, whereas the structural aspects are the seven dhātus.

Rasa dhātu is plasma or serum, which does nutrition. Rakta dhātu is blood, including the red and white blood cells, and these govern oxygenation, the life function. Māmsa dhātu is the muscle tissue, which provides the body's power, locomotion, and plastering. Meda dhātu is adipose tissue (fat) and cholesterol, which have the important functions of lubrication and storage of energy for future usage. Asthi dhātu is the bone tissue, which offers protection, supporting the body and giving longevity. Even though a person may die, his bones remain. Majjā dhātu is the nerve tissue and bone marrow, and its prime function is communication. Shukra and ārtava dhātus are the reproductive tissues in men and women respectively. These seven dhātus govern all the body's structural aspects.

## The Functioning of Mano Vaha Srotas

The mind is a separate channel (srotas), but it is intimately connected to majjā dhātu, the nerve tissue. Dementia and Alzheimer's disease are disorders that mainly affect majjā dhātu and mano vaha srotas, the channel of the mind.

The illustration at right is a depiction of mano vaha srotas. When you look at a tree, you are touching the tree through awareness. Similarly, when looking at a star, you are actually touching the star with your attention. Unless you pay attention to an object, that object does not exist for you. The circuit of awareness has to be completed.

Your attention touches the object and brings back to you the details of that object. The moment that image is touched by prāna, prāna creates sensation. If you are paralyzed, you have no sensation, so sensation is very important. Awareness becomes sensation due to prāna, so awareness + prāna = sensation. Prāna carries that sensation to the manas, where the mind feels it. Feelings are awareness + prāna + mind. Those feelings about the object are carried by prāna to buddhi. The function of buddhi is reasoning and logical thinking. *Buddhi samam pashyati* means buddhi sees things exactly as they are. It churns the sensations and feelings, and concludes, "This is a tree; not a mountain or a house."

Buddhi extends that information to smruti, the memory, which records it. Smruti has previous experiences of objects and compares the current image with past images. "Yes, this looks like a tree." Reasoning becomes recognition and this is sent on to *chitta,* mindstuff or mental energy. Through chitta, we see the innermost image of the object. These images can be colorful, with different shapes and dialogue. Much as a video camera creates a video recording, these images are created within the machinery of chitta.

The image created on the retina is inverted like a pinhole camera. The image created by prāna is a sensory image. The image created by manas is full of feelings. The image created by buddhi is a reasoned image. The image created by smruti is recognition. Chitta creates the inner image, an image of intimacy, with the help of ahamkāra, the image-maker. Ahamkāra makes the image through the image-making machinery of chitta in the form of *vritti.*[80] The vritti is then projected to *atman,* the soul, which is the flame of awareness.

There is a meeting point of chitta's generated image with the soul. At that meeting, the soul becomes one with the image and we receive pure knowledge of the object. To know is to become one. This intimacy is why they state *chitta vritti druksukham, tadasmi'hum tadasmi'hum*—I am that, I am that. This all happens in a fraction of a second.

When the knowing is over, a division takes place between the knower (ahamkāra) and the known (the object). Ahamkāra creates the concept of knower and takes credit for knowing. Ahamkāra always separates the object from the soul and creates division and separation. That is why every experience nourishes the experiencer. To remain with the pure state of knowing is meditation.

In our day-to-day life, awareness becomes perception, and then perception becomes sensation due to prāna. Then sensation becomes feeling, feeling becomes recognition, recognition becomes recollection, recollection becomes the inner image, and finally there is knowledge of what is perceived. That is the complete functioning of mano vaha srotas.

## Two Disorders of Mano Vaha Srotas

In Ayurvedic medicine, dementia is called *buddhi bhramsha* and Alzheimer's disease is called *smruti bhramsha.* In cases of dementia, the functions of buddhi (intellect) are affected, whereas in Alzheimer's it is mainly smruti (memory) that is involved. These are both major organic psychiatric disorders.

Dementia and Alzheimer's have similar symptoms. Alzheimer's is a form of dementia and other types of dementia can lead to Alzheimer's disease. In other words, someone with dementia may get Alzheimer's, or they may not. To give an idea of the practical difference, a dementia patient will find his or her own way home, whereas an Alzheimer's patient will get lost.

---

80. Anything that moves or changes chitta.

## The Process of Knowing

- Prana – Sensation
- Manas – Feelings
- Buddhi – Reasoning
- Smruti – Recognition
- Chitta – Image of Intimacy
- Ahamkara – Image-maker
- Soul – Awareness becomes one with the object, in the process of knowing

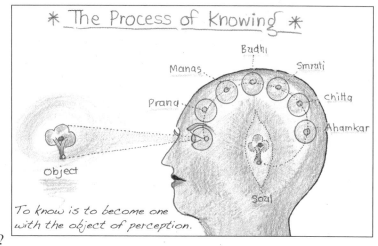

The Process of Knowing

To know is to become one with the object of perception.

## General Etiology

What is dementia or senility?

Every thought creates a neuroelectrical, neuromagnetic circuit. Hence, thinking creates a groove or pathway along the brain cells. Where there is a groove, there is a *samskāra*. Every thought or memory creates a scar on the mind and the total number of scars is samskāra. If there is undue emphasis on one fragment of life, this creates repetitive, mechanical thinking. The thoughts become repetitive and this mechanical thinking damages the brain cells, causing senility.

If we look at the etiological factors, vāta provocation is the main cause of dementia and Alzheimer's. These are both vāta disorders, possibly also involving blockage by kapha dosha or irritation from pitta dosha. Vāta prakruti, vāta vikruti, and a vāta-aggravating diet and lifestyle are common factors involved in the development of dementia.

If systemic vāta dosha undergoes accumulation and provocation, and then spreads, it is attracted towards a khavaigunya (defective space). This vāta dosha can deposit into majjā dhātu and mano vaha srotas, where it affects the functioning of chitta. Images become distorted. This can affect buddhi, resulting in impaired intellectual functioning, or smruti, causing defective memory. This is what happens in dementia and Alzheimer's disease respectively.

Changes happen in the brain. Sādhaka pitta is hot and sharp, tarpaka kapha is oily and heavy, and prāna vāyu is dry and mobile. Increased prāna vāta becomes more mobile and dry, which causes the oily quality of pitta and kapha to become sticky. This sticky (picchila) quality creates a buildup of senile plaque, which is a key reason for the development of these disorders.

### CATEGORIZATION OF PSYCHIATRIC DISORDERS

Psychiatric disorders are divided into one of three categories and several subcategories, as follows:

**Major Disorders**

a) Organic
- Acute, e.g., delirium
- Chronic, e.g., dementia, Alzheimer's disease

b) Functional, Acute
- Bipolar Disorder
- Severe Depression
- Psychosis
- Schizophrenia

**Minor (Functional, Chronic)**
- Mild depression
- Anxiety
- Hysteria
- Phobias
- Psychoneurosis
- Obsessive or compulsive behavior
- Sexual deviation
- Alcoholism and drug dependency
- Psychosomatic disorders

**Mental Disability**
- Intellectual disability (formerly called mental retardation)

These diseases are more common in women than men, with a ratio of about 2:1. They most commonly occur in people over the age of 60 (vāta age). Those cases were previously called senile dementia.

Hereditary factors (*bīja dosha*) are important. There is a specialized protein called apolipoprotein, which results in too much liquid accumulating in the blood vessels. The blood vessels lose their elasticity and flexibility, becoming hard and rigid like a lead pipe. High cholesterol and high triglycerides lead to a buildup of plaque, which further hardens the vessels. This is called cerebral atherosclerosis. The brain doesn't receive sufficient nutrition (rasa dhātu) and oxygenation (rakta dhātu), so it is like a slow heart attack to the brain. That patch of the brain suffers molecular death of the brain cells, resulting in memory loss. (see illustration page 429)

**STAGES OF DEMENTIA**

1. Unimpaired individual experience but minor cognitive impairment

2. Mild cognitive decline

3. Mild memory loss (friends and family notice the problem)

4. Moderate cognitive decline and memory loss

5. Moderately severe cognitive decline and memory loss

6. Severe cognitive decline and memory loss

7. Very severe cognitive decline and major memory loss; person loses the ability to respond to their environment

A previous trauma to the head, such as a head injury or cerebral concussion, compression, or contusion, can cause a khavaigunya in the brain and lead to dementia. A deficiency of neurotransmitters (such as acetylcholine, serotonin, or melatonin) may also play a part, as these are the precursors of sādhaka pitta and a chronic deficiency of one or more of these can result in dementia.

Environmental factors also play a significant role. Toxicity from cooking in aluminum pots, smoking, alcohol, and other sources have all been considered possible factors in the development of dementia and Alzheimer's disease. Certain types of drugs or medication, such as barbiturates, bromide, or alcohol toxicity, can create dementia or Alzheimer's.

Anything that creates inflammation can damage the brain cells and result in dementia. This includes encephalitis, meningitis, and other viral and bacterial infections. The importance of inflammation is now being more widely recognized by modern medicine, and there are some promising results from the trial of an anti-inflammatory drug in the treatment of Alzheimer's disease.

Note that all these etiological factors can create khavaigunya leading to dementia and possibly Alzheimer's disease, and can worsen the effects of any existing defective space.

## Dementia

Buddhi bhramsha (dementia) is a deterioration of intellectual functions. Dementia is not a disease per se, but a syndrome with a wide range of symptomatology. The word 'dementia' means to make insane, with impairment of intellectual functions and memory. It has a slow onset and the person develops poor memory, abstract thinking, bad judgment, clouding of the consciousness, disorientation, depression, agitation, insomnia, and paranoid ideas.

# Alzheimer's Disease

Smruti bhramsha (Alzheimer's disease) is a displacement or depletion of memory. Alzheimer's disease is a major, chronic, organic disorder that is the most severe form of dementia. It is a progressive, degenerative illness that causes an incurable loss of cognitive functioning. It accounts for approximately 60-70% of all cases of dementia.

Alzheimer's disease is a vāta disorder in which there is a steady degenerative process in majjā dhātu, the brain tissue. It results in progressive loss of memory, lack of recognition, personality changes, and diminished mental power. There is a loss of neurons and synapses in the brain tissue of the cerebral cortex that affects intellectual functioning. This atrophy gradually spreads all over the cortex. It is regarded as an incurable disorder.

## Types of Alzheimer's Disease

Late-onset Alzheimer's due to senility is the most common form. Old age is the age of vāta dosha. Because of increases in the dry, light, cold, and rough qualities, the brain doesn't function as well and memory is impaired.

Early-onset Alzheimer's is due to a genetic mutation that is inherited, and it can begin as young as 30 or so. This is a serious disorder that can cause a debilitating functional disability, but it comprises less than 5% of all Alzheimer's cases. Early-onset Alzheimer's is more common in pitta types.

## Specific Etiology of Alzheimer's Disease

All the etiological factors for dementia in general are relevant for Alzheimer's disease. However, some additional causes may also be relevant.

Modern medical science still does not know the actual causes of Alzheimer's. However, excessive plaque and tangles in the brain cells appear to be important factors. Plaque and tangles are found in most people as they age, but they are much more plentiful in people with Alzheimer's.

Plaque is a deposit of amyloid protein that builds up in the intercellular spaces of majjā dhātu. Tangles are tau protein deposits that build up inside the cells of majjā dhātu. These tangles act as if they entangle the memory. The memory remains like a tangled tape, while the recorder keeps going, on and on.

Genetic factors seem to be related to both forms of Alzheimer's disease. A genetic mutation on chromosomes 1, 14, or 21 that runs in families is known to produce early-onset Alzheimer's. Additionally, a number of studies have linked the apolipoprotein E

> **STAGES OF ALZHEIMER'S DISEASE**
>
> 1. Early Stage - Mild dementia: loss of short-term memory, diminished judgment, inability to perform arithmetic calculations, difficulty comprehending abstract ideas
>
> 2. Mid Stage - Mild to moderate dementia: difficulty with speech and changes in labile personality, changes in habits, hard to remember the purpose of objects, urinary incontinence, wandering, lose their way home, seizures, psychotic behavior, depression
>
> 3. Late Stage - Severe dementia: inability to perform daily activities (eating, dressing, toileting, etc.), cannot remember how to walk and swallow food, immobile, bedridden, no communication, get respiratory problems because of inability to swallow food, may die of pneumonia.

(APOE) gene to late-onset Alzheimer's. Chromosome 19 generates this protein, while chromosome 21 generates the precursors of amyloid protein, which may also be involved. All these genetic factors create a khavaigunya that can result in the development of Alzheimer's disease. People with Down syndrome are at high risk of developing Alzheimer's disease because they have an extra Chromosome 21. Individuals who have suffered a minor stroke or head trauma are also at higher risk of developing Alzheimer's.

Autoimmune disorders are immunological illnesses in which tejas burns ojas. People who are bright, brilliant, and intellectual with a type A personality can burn out their ojas in this way. This can be another cause of Alzheimer's disease.

The herpes simplex virus lodges into the neuromuscular cleft and creeps into the nervous system, where it remains dormant. There is a high correlation between people with herpes simplex virus (which is pitta) and the onset of Alzheimer's disease. This may be another significant etiological factor.

## Progression of Alzheimer's Disease

**KEY SIGNS AND SYMPTOMS OF ALZHEIMER'S DISEASE**

- Increased plaque in the cerebral cortex (majjā dhātu) and grey matter (sādhaka pitta)
- Loss of mental power
- Very poor memory
- Poor concentration
- Inability to communicate
- Repeatedly asks the same questions that have already been answered
- Personality changes
- Repetitive unnecessarily actions
- Loss of bladder and bowel control
- Respiratory disorders
- Death usually due to pneumonia or heart or kidney failure

The main symptom in the earlier stages of Alzheimer's is a loss of recent memory. The person may be cooking and watching TV at the same time, and suddenly they notice the food has burnt. That individual might still have good memory of past events. Mood swings are another early symptom, as is spending a lot of time in abstract thinking, and decreasing amounts of time in reality. The extent and severity of symptoms varies from person to person. They may occur occasionally, for days together at a time, or month after month.

My friend's wife had Alzheimer's and she would tell me all her childhood stories. She would be very specific, telling me the exact date she fell, which step caused the fall, and then show me how she fell. As she was telling me this, she was there in the past. These people get carried away by their thoughts, with abstract thinking rather than concrete thinking.

In the next stage, the symptoms get more serious. The person starts to forget people's names and cannot even recognize his or her relatives. Commonly, a person with Alzheimer's cannot recall events and people after around age 40. For example, a mother may remember her daughter as a child, from when she was 30 years of age, and not as an adult.

These people can get lost coming home from work or the grocery store. They may forget to turn off the oven or stove, and they often misplace articles. Additionally, people with Alzheimer's recheck things to see if they have correctly performed a task. For instance, they lock the door, walk to the car, and then go back and check if the door is locked.

Another symptom of Alzheimer's is to repeatedly ask the same question again and again, even though it has already been answered. There is virtually no short-term memory. This gap in memory means they are missing *dhārana,* steady attention or concentration. There can be an endless repetition of unnecessary actions, such as opening and closing a drawer over and over again. Fiddling with the hands is also common or repeatedly running their fingers through their hair. The person also has trouble working with figures and paying their bills. They generally can't do even simple arithmetic.

A common physiological consequence is loss of bladder or bowel control. That happens when Alzheimer's causes the cerebral reflexes to go out of control.

As the disease progresses, the sufferers become more confused, frustrated, irritable, and restless. They are always moving about. These people must be watched; otherwise, they will wander away and possibly get into a dangerous situation. Failure to recognize their work colleagues, friends, and family members destroys the person's normal work and social life.

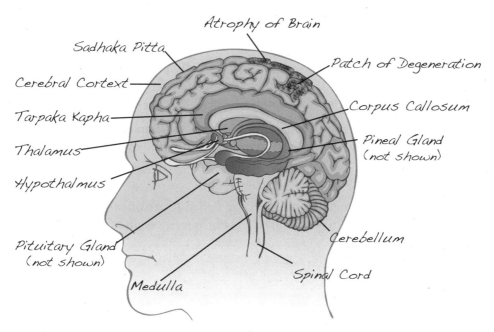

Dementia and Alzheimer's Disease
Buddhi Bhramsha & Smruti Bhramsha
Decreased Majja Dhatu

Atrophy of Brain

Sadhaka Pitta

Patch of Degeneration

Cerebral Cortex

Corpus Callosum

Tarpaka Kapha

Pineal Gland
(not shown)

Thalamus

Hypothalmus

Pituitary Gland
(not shown)

Cerebellum

Medulla

Spinal Cord

Dementia and Alzheimer's disease go together.

Aggression can be a particularly difficult symptom to deal with. Some people with Alzheimer's become violent because of irritability and agitation, which is due to increased pitta dosha.

In the final stages, patients forget whether they have eaten or not. Loss of motor control causes them to forget to swallow, choking on their food. Alzheimer's patients commonly die of pneumonia, heart attack, or kidney failure.

### Diagnosis of Dementia and Alzheimer's Disease

Diagnosis is done by taking a thorough medical history, personal history and family history, followed by an extensive neurological and psychological examination and a psychiatric examination.

Nowadays, computer topography is used. You can see a picture of the brain with any plaque showing as blue dots. A cerebrospinal fluid examination is used to see if there are protein markers or if there has been a stroke. Some people experience a stroke in their sleep and don't even know it has happened.

There is also a link between Alzheimer's and thyroid function. Generally, slow memory goes together with sluggish thyroid function. Not every hypothyroid person gets Alzheimer's, but most Alzheimer's patients have hypothyroidism.

Differential diagnosis is needed to distinguish the particular form of dementia that the person is suffering. And to discern between dementia and apathy, inattention, poor concentration, poor memory, shock, or the death of a loved one. For example, after the death of a spouse, the surviving partner can become very disoriented and shocked, and this may look like dementia.

## Treatment Protocol

Modern medical science does not yet know how to fully prevent and treat dementia and Alzheimer's. Ayurveda uses a variety of treatments to help reduce the symptoms. These include shirodhāra, nasya, netra basti, karna pūrana, abhyanga, and panchakarma.

Nasya (nasal administration) using vacha oil helps to stimulate prāna and calm down the doshas in majjā dhātu. Netra basti involves bathing the eyes with ghee (clarified butter). It nourishes the sclera and the sclera is connected to majjā dhātu. Abhyanga (oil massage) can be given regularly to pacify vāta dosha.

If the person has agitation, use tranquilizing herbs. A particularly good nervine tonic for a person with pitta prakruti (constitution), given ½ teaspoon three times daily, is:

Brahmī            500 mg
Jatamāmsi         300 mg
Shankha pushpī 300 mg
Sarasvatī         300 mg

For kapha prakruti:

Brahmī            500 mg
Jatamāmsi         300 mg

Shankha pushpī 300 mg
Jyotishmatī     200 mg
Vacha           200 mg

For vāta prakruti:

Dashamūla       500 mg
Ashvagandhā     400 mg
Shankha pushpī 300 mg
Brahmī          200 mg
Tagara          100 mg

Other herbal remedies that can be given are:

Sarasvatī arishta
Brahmī prash
Shankha pushpī syrup
Smruti sagar ras to improve memory

Standard recommended dosages can be given for each of these Ayurvedic remedies.

If there is a tendency toward constipation, give a teaspoon of triphala or bhumi āmalakī before bedtime.

An herbal remedy to aid the memory should be given. The formulas above for each constitution are beneficial, and 300 mg gotu kola and 200 mg ginkgo biloba can also be given in addition to the other herbs.

Many Alzheimer's patients do not get much sleep. They may stay awake for the whole day and night. We can give garlic milk, or nutmeg milk, or tagara, or Good Night Sleep tea®. Rubbing bhringarāja oil on the feet and scalp will also aid sound sleep.

In the earlier stages, certain yoga postures can help to improve circulation to the brain. These include camel, cobra, cow, boat, bow, bridge, and palm tree poses. (see page 450) Gentle yoga stretches aided by an assistant is the best approach. Gentle prānāyāma is also beneficial.

We also have to gradually upgrade the person's lifestyle. Use a large calendar so that the person can easily find out today's date. Make a schedule, so you can help them to brush the teeth, scrape the tongue, drink water or tea, and eat breakfast, lunch and dinner on time. While the person is eating, ensure they are swallowing.

Reminders about home safety are very important. Remove any sharp objects and fire hazards, cover electric outlets, and do not leave glass objects lying around.

Chanting a mantra with someone who can remember the chant is another helpful type of chikitsā for a dementia patient.

If the condition becomes more advanced, then the patient should be moved to a health-care facility with professional staff providing around-the-clock care.

An Alzheimer's patient in the earlier stages of the disease can be supported with appropriate diet, lifestyle, herbal remedies, prāṇāyāma, and meditation. In some cases, the person can show remarkable improvement.

However, once there are multiple lesions in the cortical area, there's nothing much that can be done to turn the illness around. In such cases, the brain looks like hard cheese. Hence, when the person moves into the final stage of the disease, it is beyond the help of Ayurveda.

At one time, a drug called tacrine[81] was used to improve brain function. However, it is toxic to the liver and has unpleasant side effects. If using drugs such as that one, get regular blood tests to monitor liver functions. Kutki will help to protect the liver, as do shankha pushpī and bhumi āmalakī. A good Ayurvedic formula to take care of the liver is 200 mg each of kutki, chitrak, neem, and turmeric. Give ½ teaspoon of this three times daily with a tablespoon of kumārī āsava or water.

## Prevention of Dementia

Alzheimer's disease is more common in the Western world, as opposed to Eastern countries such as India, where people eat a lot of turmeric in their diet. Turmeric helps to prevent atherosclerotic changes, so it is good to ward off Alzheimer's. It can be taken on a daily basis throughout one's life. People can just add turmeric powder into their food, or alternatively can swallow two or three capsules of turmeric a day. That will help to prevent atherosclerotic changes.

Eating some coconut on a daily basis has been found to nourish the grey matter in the cortical area of the brain, and helps to prevent further damage to the cerebral cortex. Hence, it is beneficial to Alzheimer's patients and to those wishing to prevent dementia. Other foods that nourish the brain include nuts such as soaked almonds, cashews, pistachio, charoli nuts (*Buchanania lanzan*), and walnuts. Drinking warm cow's milk with turmeric and ground charoli is regarded as very beneficial.

Overall, to help prevent dementia, one should follow an appropriate constitutional diet, lifestyle, and exercise program. Also, undergo periodic panchakarma (detoxification) and *rasāyana* (rejuvenation program). Take a daily nervine tonic for the mind (*see* above). Finally, ancient Ayurvedic texts say that it is good to drill and discipline your memory by learning a few lines of a poem or mantra each day. This can strengthen the memory and help to ward off dementia.

---

81. Trade name Cognex; withdrawn from US market in 2013. Retrieved October 13, 2018:https://www.livertox.nih.gov/Tacrine.htm.

# Chapter 54

# Depression

Spring 2013, Volume 25, Number 4

DEPRESSION IS A MOOD DISORDER marked by a loss of pleasure and interest in life. The word "depression" literally means "pressing down." The subject feels a sense of pressure, hollowness, or emptiness, and suffers from low self-esteem. The person's mandible feels heavy and the mouth droops down. There are decreased vital functions. For example, respiration becomes shallow and blood pressure drops.

Depression may include dyspnea (breathlessness) as well as major depressive disorders such as schizoaffective or bipolar disorder and sudden mood swings.

Prashna (questioning) plays an important part in the diagnosis of depression and psychiatric disorders. By questioning the person, we can find out his or her symptoms and see how recent the onset of the illness is.

Mano vaha srotas is the mental system, and it is governed by prāna vāyu, tarpaka kapha, and sādhaka pitta. Prāna vāyu directs respiration, produces vitality, and gives rise to interest and inspiration. These functions are diminished in depression. Tarpaka kapha gives groundedness, but tarpaka may be increased in depression and that can result in heaviness, indecisiveness, and a sense of being stuck. It can also cause low self-esteem. Sādhaka pitta promotes attention and discernment, but in certain types of depression, high sādhaka can result in wrong judgment, wrong conclusions, criticism, and self-hatred.

---

**CATEGORIZATION OF PSYCHIATRIC DISORDERS**

Psychiatric disorders are divided into one of three categories and several subcategories, as follows:

**Major Disorders**
 a) Organic
  • Acute, e.g., delirium
  • Chronic, e.g., dementia, Alzheimer's disease
 b) Functional, Acute
  • Bipolar Disorder
  • Severe Depression
  • Psychosis
  • Schizophrenia

**Minor (Functional, Chronic)**
  • Mild depression
  • Anxiety
  • Hysteria
  • Phobias
  • Psychoneurosis
  • Obsessive or compulsive behavior
  • Sexual deviation
  • Alcoholism and drug dependency
  • Psychosomatic disorders

**Mental Disability**
  • Intellectual disability (formerly called mental retardation)

# Different Doshic Categories of Depression

*Vāta type of depression is a transient depression that can include auditory hallucinations.*

## Main Signs and Symptoms of Vāta Type Depression

- Fluctuating, comes and goes like a breeze
- Symptoms worst in evening
- Fear and anxiety
- Restlessness, severe agitation
- Insomnia, waking often during the night
- Early waking
- Diurnal variation of mood – worse during dawn and dusk
- Indecisiveness
- Poor concentration
- Feeling of unworthiness
- Loss of appetite
- Weight loss
- Malnutrition
- Amenorrhea in women
- Occipital headache or cluster headache
- Backache
- Constipation
- Weeping silently in a private place
- Excessive talk
- Talking in a jerky manner (alternating fast and slow)
- Mood swings
- Furrowed brow
- Down turned corners of mouth
- Slumped posture
- Poor eye contact
- Loss of pleasure
- Diminished sexual desire
- Amenorrhea
- World looks dry and colorless

Vāta type is atypical depression and it can sometimes look like bipolar depression. It may be accompanied by auditory hallucinations, whereby the person hears voices. Someone with vāta depression will often talk in a jerky manner. The person can have loud laughter and also cry easily. Vāta people with depression tend to be hyperactive. Their denial of the depression can quickly turn the loud laughter into tears.

Vāta type of depression usually comes from some kind of trauma, shock, separation, or loss, such as losing a loved one. It may also be due to certain drugs, such as amphetamines, cocaine, LSD, and other psychedelic drugs. Disappointment and distressing circumstances are other causes of this kind of depression.

A person with severe vāta depression often gets only two or three hours of sleep each night, and daytime variations of mood. The person can have slowness of thought and indecisiveness. Feeling guilty or unworthy is due to increased vāta. Such a person may be found weeping silently in the closet. Women with this condition often also have amenorrhea.

*Pitta type of depression expresses as severe depression or depressive psychosis.*

## Main Signs and Symptoms of Pitta Type Depression
- Irritability
- Anger
- Sense of failure
- Feelings of worthlessness (uselessness, low self-esteem)
- Guilt and self-blame
- Self-denigrating ideas
- Self-critical
- Misdeeds or misconduct
- Recurrent thoughts of suicide or death
- Shift quickly from one idea to another
- Judgment
- Jokes a lot, has a fake smile, keeps sad feelings or feelings of failure inside
- Overconfident and overly optimistic
- Reacts with violence or aggression if questioned
- Photosensitivity
- Acid reflux
- Indigestion

This type of depression generally occurs in someone with a rigid personality and strict discipline. The person usually is over-confident and overly-optimistic, but prone to react with violence or aggression when crossed or questioned.

A person who is addicted to success and then has a business failure can become restless and frustrated. Pitta type of depression is often triggered by a failure in the person's career or relationship, such as losing a job, having a divorce, or experiencing a general sense of failure in life. Pitta depression may be part of a middle-age crisis, which hits during the pitta phase of life.

The use of pitta-provoking drugs (e.g., caffeine, aspirin, quinine, marijuana) is another reason for pitta type of depression, and it can also follow incidents of high fever (pitta-type of fever). It is related to diarrhea, rashes, urticaria, photosensitivity, and acid indigestion as well.

Most of the time, people with pitta depression will have a fake smile and keep their sadness or feelings of failure inside. They often tease and joke with others, making fun. However, their self-criticism and sense of worthlessness can lead to recurrent thoughts of death or committing suicide.

*Kapha type of depression is characterized by chronic depression with melancholia.*

### Main Signs and Symptoms of Kapha Type Depression

* Melancholia
* Feelings of heaviness
* Overeating
* Obesity
* Excessive sleep
* Dullness
* Slowness
* Sluggish actions
* Monotonous behavior
* Slow and sluggish talk
* Silence or monosyllabic speech
* Morbid moods
* Diminished interest in usual activities
* Social withdrawal
* Feelings of hopelessness
* World looks dull, gloomy, and grey

Kapha depression brings a sense of melancholia. It is usually chronic in nature and can be triggered by the use of anti-hypertensive drugs, corticosteroids, or contraceptives, as well as other kapha-increasing factors such as excessive sleep, fatty or fried food, dairy products, and so forth.

A depressed kapha person typically has an eating disorder, eats for emotional reasons and becomes heavy, dull, and depressed. They also sleep for emotional reasons. Because jathāra agni[82] is falsely stimulated by the depression and the person doesn't have true hunger, we have to regulate their diet. A kapha-reducing diet that avoids fatty food, dairy products, and other kapha-increasing foods is most important.

There are also some types of depression that are due to two doshas. In manic depressive psychosis, there is elation with hyperactivity, rapidly shifting from one idea to another. This is due to vāta pushing pitta. If there is vāta pushing kapha, there may also be periods of feeling up, but the person will generally feel dull and munch on candy, cookies, and chocolate.

## Modern Medical Treatments

Antidepressant medications are the most commonly used treatment for depression. The first category of these drugs is tricyclic antidepressants. The second category, which has become more widely used, is selective serotonin reuptake inhibitors (SSRIs). Serotonin stimulates synaptic receptors and has an anti-anxiety effect, which can help many cases of depression, but these medications also cause undesirable side effects such as insomnia, nausea, and headache.

---

82. The central digestive fire that includes agni in the stomach and small intestine.

Cognitive behavioral therapy is now a common medical treatment for depression. It is based on the idea that a person's thought patterns result in a particular mental state. The practitioner helps the depressed patient to change some of their thoughts, which can help to lift that person's mood and overcome the depression.

Some violent patients or those with severe depression may require electroconvulsive therapy. In such cases, the patient is informed that serious treatment is required.

## Ayurvedic Management Protocol

We have to understand the doshic cause of depression. There is more anxiety in vāta types and more anger in pitta types of depression. In vāta depression, there is an idea of guilt, unworthiness, and self-blame, whereas in pitta depression there is worthlessness, preoccupation (continually mentally doing something), irritability, and suicidal thoughts. In vāta depression there is insomnia, whereas in kapha depression there is excessive sleep. Many people with vāta depression suffer weight loss, while someone with kapha depression has a tendency to obesity.

Whenever we see a patient of depression, we can ask questions (prashna parīkshā) to assess the specific cause. For instance, you can ask whether the person has had the sense of depression for just the past couple of weeks, or whether it has lasted for months or years. Find out if there is a feeling of hopelessness, or if there is lack of pleasure in doing anything at all.

One should find out what is causing the person's depression. Help the individual to find the area of his or her life that causes the deepest sadness, hurt, guilt, or sense of failure.

Watch the person's activity level, to see whether the individual is hyperactive or hypoactive. Also, assess the social behavior. Look at the body frame and weight, to assess whether there is adequate or excessive nutrition.

Then give an appropriate dosha-pacifying diet, along with proper dinācharya (daily regimen) and rutucharyā (seasonal regime). It is best to prescribe a structured routine that includes non-competitive activities that enhance self-confidence and self-esteem. Daily exercise is important, including walking, hiking, running, swimming, and aerobic exercise.

> **7 PRACTICAL STEPS TO UNFOLD INNER HEALING**
> - Get up early and watch the morning sun
> - Cultivate good friendships
> - Talk about your emotions
> - Don't stay alone all the time
> - Love yourself
> - Regular yoga, pranayama, and meditation
> - Eat fresh foods and avoid negative behaviors that can promote depression

It is great to get outdoors for a walk and deeply breathe the fresh air. This kindles agni, improves circulation, and removes any cerebral hypoxia. Yogāsana, prāṇāyāma, and meditation can all be helpful in balancing the doshas and thereby managing depression.

The person's vital signs should be observed, by checking the pulse, blood pressure, heart, and clarity of perception. Support is offered by talking calmly and giving a gentle touch.

### Lifestyle Treatments

Psycho-education or psychotherapy is the main approach for lifestyle improvements. See the patient regularly, such as once or twice weekly. You may need to keep in touch with the patient by phone. If the patient is on antidepressant medications, don't stop these drugs. Let the psychiatrist decide about appropriate medication. The person may feel demoralized if they are told they have a mental disorder, so be supportive. Ask if there are any thoughts of suicide. If so, the patient may need monitored care and should be admitted for clinical care. Take all self-destructive thoughts seriously.

Depression is a self-limiting medical disorder with a good prognosis. Anti-depressant herbal protocols can be effective and these are not habit forming. There are also some practical hints to help a person with depression.

A depressed person should make the effort to get up early and watch the sunrise each morning. The early morning sun has a predominance of pink, orange, and golden-yellow colored rays. When these fall on the eyelids and forehead, these light rays stimulate bhrājaka, ālochaka, and sādhaka pitta and boost serotonin secretion. Therefore, a patient of depression can feel increased happiness, joy, and creativity from exposure to early morning sun. In the winter, they can feel worse depression, due to lack of light.

Depressed people should cultivate good friendships and enjoy a social life. There is nothing like a loving friend who has compassion. Whenever possible, a depressed person should go to a happy, cheerful ceremony or *yagña* (fire ceremony), or some kind of spiritual gathering. *Bhajans, kirtan,* or group chanting can all help a depressed person.

The patient should talk about their emotions with a trusted friend. They should not suppress or repress their emotions. Talking about their concerns can reduce the heavy burden on their shoulders.

The person should not remain alone or stay inside all the time. A room with no other people is the devil's workshop for someone with depression, leading to worse sadness and loneliness.

Love yourself. Some people project their depression onto the world and label themselves as depressed. Place the depression on the periphery of one's consciousness and go to the center of your heart. In other words, when you feel depression, turn and head for your center. There is a mirror inside you that will mirror both light and darkness. Unfortunately, a depressed person stands in front of their inner mirror and faces away from it. They see depression but don't see themselves. Turn 180 degrees and look at yourself in the mirror. When you watch yourself in the mirror, you can fall in love with yourself for the first time in your life. Love yourself by watching within, moment-to-moment. This is self-awareness.

Yoga, prāṇāyāma, and meditation are beneficial for someone with depression. The patient should do regular yogāsanas that are specific to the individual, including sūrya namaskāra (sun salutation). Lion pose (*simhāsana*) can help depression through its action on the mandibles.

The vital functions of prāna are supported by daily prāṇāyāma. The best prāṇāyāma for all types of depression are anuloma-viloma (alternate nostril breathing), ujjāyi (conch breath), and utgīt prāṇāyāma. If someone has bipolar disorder, anuloma-viloma prāṇāyāma can be especially helpful. One can do regular meditation on one's personal deity of choice (*ishtha-devatā*). So'ham meditation is good for all doshas.

Good foods for someone with depression to eat are fresh, whole-wheat chapattis (tridoshic), mung dal, urad dal, zucchini, squash, raisins, apricots, whole milk, and ghee. The person needs to avoid smoking, alcohol, drugs, staying up late at night, fasting, and frequent sexual activity, as well as the suppression of natural urges.

## Clinical Treatments

For major acute psychiatric disorders, e.g., bipolar disorder, severe depression, psychosis, schizophrenia, which are all classified in Ayurveda as *unmād;* Charaka has given a complete Ayurvedic protocol. Panchakarma, shodana, shamana, and rasāyana are needed. Additionally, they should be part of *agni hotra* fire ceremony using brahmī, jatamāmsi, vacha, and shankha pushpī. This herbal combination is offered to the fire. When the smoke is inhaled, the client absorbs the superfine elements through the cribriform plate and olfactory bulb. These act on the frontal and parietal lobes of the brain, balancing sādhaka pitta and tarpaka kapha. This is a form of subtle molecular therapy.

Ayurvedic herbal protocols and the use of panchakarma therapies can be most effective at managing depression.

Vyādhi pratyanika for depression (treatments specific to depression) are mainly shamana herbs:

| HERBAL PREPARATIONS |
|---|
| **Kalka** - crushed herbs made into a pulp or paste; a wet bolus |
| **Prash** - an herbal preparation cooked with ghee that results in a jam or jelly-like substance |
| **Arishta** - a fermented herbal concoction |
| **Tailam** - oil is boiled with a decoction and a fine paste of the herb(s) |
| **Bhasma** - medicinal ash |
| **Āsava** - a medicinal herbal wine |

- Sarpagandha is a general antidepressant and also reduces high blood pressure
- Dhattūra (belladonna) is a tranquilizer and analgesic
- Raupya (silver) bhasma protects the myelin sheath, rejuvenates the nervous system, and is anti-inflammatory
- Ashvagandhā helps with neuronal fatigue
- Brahmī improves oxygenation (and increases prāna)
- Yashthi madhu (licorice) acts on tarpaka kapha and helps to produce optimal acetylcholine
- Jatamāmsi is a nervine tonic and tranquilizer
- Vidārī improves the communication between post-synaptic and pre-synaptic neurons, thus reducing neuronal stress.
- Shankha pushpī helps to release serotonin

Administration of strong nasal medications (nasya) is used to awaken the sensory pathways and bring clarity of perception. Vacha powder, vacha oil, brahmī oil, fresh onion juice, and ginger-jaggery nasya are all commonly used to bring alertness. Similarly, strong añjanam[83] can be applied to the eyelids.

Once the patient's severe condition is under control, give shigru leaf juice vamana to a kapha patient, virechana with nishottara for a pitta type, or dashamūla tea basti to a vāta patient.

The best rasāyana (nervine brain tonics) are brahmī prash, brahmī arishta, shankha pushpī syrup, aravindāsava, and sarasvatī arishta.

Marma points for depression are mūrdhni, brahmarandhra, sthapanī (ājñā), oshtha, hanu, jatru, and hasta and pāda kshipra.[84] Use vacha or sandalwood essential oils on these points. See illustrations page 460.

The best mudrās for depression are jñāna mudrā, ankusha mudrā, agni mudrā, and surabhi mudrā. Further recommendations are shown beginning on page 442.

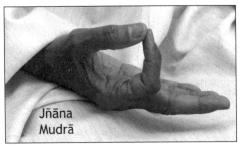
Jñāna Mudrā

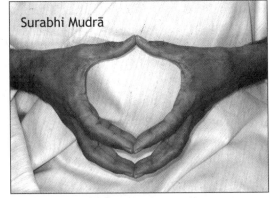
Surabhi Mudrā

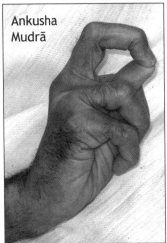
Ankusha Mudrā

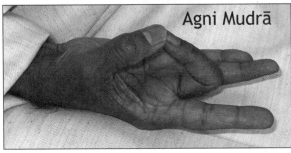
Agni Mudrā

## Complications

If there is insomnia, get the person to rub bhringarāja oil on the soles of the feet and scalp before bed, and also give the following herbal protocol before bedtime to induce natural sound sleep: 200 mg each of ashvagandhā, jatamāmsi, shankha pushpī, and tagara.

One has to manage any constipation that occurs. It may either be drug-induced or dosha-induced constipation. Half to one teaspoon of triphala is to be given nightly before

---

83. A specialized herbal eyeliner applied to the eyelid or eyelashes.
84. Hasta (Hand) Kshipra affects the occipital lobe of the brain and Pada (Foot) Kshipra the frontal lobe.

bedtime. Alternatively, someone with high vāta can use gandharva harītakī, while a pitta individual may use bhumi āmalakī.

## Depression in Children

Depression is common in infants when separated from their mother during the first two years of life. In fact, depression in children is widely seen when a child is separated from either parent, because children need both a mother and father. If a child is separated from either parent, or there is loss of love, lack of affection, or even lack of nutrition, that can definitely make the child depressed.

A depressed child will often cry a lot and have hyperactive motor activity, so he or she can get easily panicked. These children should be treated using Ayurvedic remedies such as brahmī prash or arvindāsava, oil massage, and by giving tender, loving care.

Depression in children can take a long time to heal, because childhood is the kapha age. Proper care and prompt action by parents and medical professionals are essential to ensure a successful outcome. Be patient with a depressed child, encourage them with their homework, and take care of their general health.

## Conclusion

One practice that can help is not to take things personally. Whatever you are facing in life, it is painted on the canvas of your consciousness. Look at life as a whole, objectively, and learn the art of self-knowing. Maintain moment-to-moment awareness and watchfulness of thoughts, feelings, and emotions.

An Ayurvedic health practitioner should express warmth, love, and compassion, and show interest in a patient with depression. Be totally optimistic, while guarding against excessive cheerfulness. This can help the person to see things as they are.

Most depressed people have lost interest in things, so speak encouragingly and admire their talents, to inspire them. This will also help the person to feel appreciated and a bit more enthusiastic.

Depressed people usually don't have much pleasure in life, so whenever you visit such a patient, Ayurveda says to give a little gift, such as a bunch of flowers. This will help to unfold pleasure in that person's life.

---

**VĀTA HERBAL MANAGEMENT**

| | |
|---|---|
| Dashamūla | 500 mg |
| Ashvagandhā | 400 mg |
| Tagara | 200 mg |
| Yogarāja guggulu | 200 mg |
| Sarasvatī | 200 mg |
| Sarpagandha | 200 mg |

Give this mixture three times daily with brahmī ghee.

Gandharva harītakī - one teaspoon each evening

Vacha oil nasya

Abhyanga (oil massage) with sesame oil or vāta-pacifying tailam*

Dashamūla tea basti every week

Repeat the mantra: "Aum Aim Namah"

Avoid cold foods, such as chilled salads, as well as raw vegetables and beans

* Boil 1 part of herbs (equal parts of dashamūla, balā, vidārī) and 16 parts of water and reduce water to 4 parts. Then add 4 parts of sesame oil to decoction and simmer until water is completely evaporated. Cool before applying to skin.

Every day is a new day in our life; it will never come again. Enjoy every day fully and completely as it comes to you.

Herbal management for each doshic type of depression is shown in the sidebars.

**PITTA HERBAL MANAGEMENT**

| | |
|---|---|
| Shatāvarī | 500 mg |
| Gulvel sattva | 400 mg |
| Brahmī | 300 mg |
| Kaishore guggulu | 200 mg |
| Moti bhasma | 200 mg |
| Sarasvatī | 200 mg |
| Shankha pushpī | 200 mg |

Give this mixture three times daily with brahmī syrup or brahmī prash.

Nishottara - one teaspoon at night, as virechana

Brahmī ghee nasya

Abhyanga with coconut or sunflower oil, or pitta-pacifying tailam*

The best rasāyana is one teaspoon of shatāvarī kalka twice daily with milk

Repeat the mantra: "Aum Hrīm Namah"

Avoid hot, spicy food

* Boil 1 part of herbs (equal parts of shatāvarī, gudūchī, brahmī, jatamāmsi, shankha pushpī) and 16 parts of water and reduce water to 4 parts. Then add 4 parts of sesame oil to decoction and simmer until water is completely evaporated. Cool before applying to skin.

**KAPHA HERBAL MANAGEMENT**

| | |
|---|---|
| Purnarnavā | 500 mg |
| Kutki (katukā) | 200 mg |
| Trikatu | 200 mg |
| Sarasvatī | 200 mg |
| Rāsna | 200 mg |
| Vacha | 200 mg |

Give this mixture three times daily.

Bibhītakī - one teaspoon nightly, as virechana

Vacha powder nasya

Abhyanga with mustard or sesame oil, or kapha-pacifying tailam*

Dashamūla and punarnavā basti

Repeat the mantra: "Aum Klīm Namah"

Avoid meat, dairy products and other heavy foods.

* Boil 1 part of herbs (equal parts of of punarnavā, kutki, chitrak, trikatu) and 16 parts of water and reduce water to 4 parts. Then add 4 parts of sesame oil to decoction and simmer until water is completely evaporated. Cool before applying to skin.

# Chapter 55

# The Role of Emotions in Disease Manifestation

Fall 2013, Volume 26, Number 2

SIT QUIETLY AND CLOSE YOUR EYES, not thinking or evaluating, just being aware. Then you will feel that your body is expanding, or else becoming smaller and smaller. Why do these experiences happen?

When your awareness becomes all-inclusive ("I am everything"), it expands. Then, when your awareness becomes all-exclusive ("I am not this, I am not that"), it becomes smaller and smaller, like an atom. You can go either way by either including everything in your awareness or excluding everything from the awareness.

The expansive state of awareness is freedom, and that freedom is love. When you sit quietly and focus on your breath, allowing the mind and thoughts to go on expanding, this all-inclusive awareness flows through the media of *ākāsha* (ether). When you close your eyes and become aware of your hands and feet, you can feel the whole body, and an inch beyond the physical body you will see a bluish-purple halo or aura. That is your etheric body. This etheric body is only visible in a meditative state. Through the etheric body, you are connected to the cosmos.

In the tiny space within a cell, and in the spaces between cells, there is a substance called ether. The same substance exists between two galaxies or two universes. The universal ether includes the earth, moon, sun, stars, and planets. Therefore, the space between two cells in a human body is the same space as exists between two galaxies.

When the etheric body passes from the outer space to the inner space, awareness flows through the doors of the senses and becomes perception. When *prāna* touches perception, it creates sensation, so that awareness becomes sensation. Then the mind comes and touches the sensation and creates feeling. Without the mind, you cannot feel. Then the intellect does reasoning and the memory does recognition. Memory reacts to the feeling in the form of thought, and thought plus feeling is emotion.

These emotions have a function. Any emotion that happens in the etheric field has to be digested and processed into pure intelligence, pure love. However, that usually doesn't happen, because our mind is attached to the emotion or the intellect tries to reason it out. Any unresolved emotions are stored in the subconscious mind, whereas resolved emotions just disappear.

This flow of awareness is a journey through prāna, the *jñānendriya* (the sensory faculties), manas (the mind), smruti (memory), buddhi (the intellect), chitta (the subconscious mind), and ahamkāra (the ego), right through to the true self, the being.

In this journey of awareness to the self, the movement of awareness becomes perception, then sensation, and then feeling. Then thought takes charge of the feeling and creates emotion. Ideally, the emotion should be processed by buddhi into pure intelligence. However, if it is not fully processed in buddhi, the unresolved emotion gets stored in the deeper layers of chitta, which is the storehouse of all emotions and the image-making machinery.

We all have our own self-image, the central image, which is known as the ego. The "I" or "me" is the center and around that "I" are several images: the image created by sound, the image created by touch, and the images made by sight, taste, and smell. The five *tanmātrās*—*shabda, sparsha, rūpa, rasa,* and *gandha* (sound, touch, sight, taste, and smell)—create these tanmātric or sensory images, which undergo crystallization if they are not fully processed.

## Table 15: Emotions and Tastes

| Taste | Positive Attributes | Negative Emotions |
| --- | --- | --- |
| Sweet | Love and compassion | Attachment |
| Sour | Discrimination | Judgment and criticism |
| Salty | Enthusiasm, romance | Undue craving and lust |
| Pungent | Stimulating | Anger, hate and jealousy |
| Bitter | Austerity, celibacy | Cynicism, brutality |
| Astringent | Simplicity, bringing together | Emotionally cold and stuck |

Emotions are subtle and all-pervading, spreading throughout the mind and body. However, as they become crystallized, specific emotions have an affinity to certain internal organs. For example, the emotions of grief and sorrow accumulate into the lungs, whereas anger has an affinity to the hepatic parenchyma in the liver. These unprocessed emotions accumulate into the respective organs, creating potential weaknesses in the organs, tissues, and related systems. These potential weaknesses in the tissues carry the dormant seeds of a future disease, called a khavaigunya (defective space).

Repressed emotions affect the dhātu agni. When dhātu agni is imbalanced, it affects tissue nutrition. Therefore, the repressed emotions first create functional changes, such as gas, bloating, blood sugar fluctuations, high or low blood pressure, changes in sleeping patterns, breathlessness, and tachycardia. Over time, these manifest as structural, pathophysiological changes. Examples of structural changes include diverticulosis, hemorrhoids, hernia, myocardial hypertrophy (dilatation of the heart), narrowing of the bronchial tree, and tumor formation. The illustration shows the affinity of certain emotions to the main bodily organs.

## Emotions and the Bodily Organs

An emotion is a psychological feeling, but it comes in order to help open the door to divinity. Let go of any emotions and become completely aware, right from the beginning until the ending of the emotion. In that journey of awareness, you'll learn a great deal about which emotion is related to which organ.

*The Brain.* The emotions of curiosity and confusion accumulate in the brain. Brahmī, jatamāmsi, and shankha pushpī can be given as a *rasāyana* for mano vaha srotas to kindle mental agni and process emotions.

*Thyroid.* Lack of communication, feelings of guilt, not telling the truth, betrayal, and unrequited love all accumulate in the throat area in the tissues of the thyroid gland. That can result in thyroid dysfunction and similar disorders. Unrequited love can cause communication problems, whereas received love brings clarity, compassion, and happiness. We can use kaishore guggulu, yashthi madhu, and goraksha chincha guggulu to help process feelings of guilt, and betrayal, and to support thyroid functions.

When the inner person doesn't meet with the outer person, it means one doesn't show one's true self. Therefore, the throat *chakra* is a place of isolation. Unrequited love means there is no appreciation, such as, your partner doesn't return "I love you." Whereas rejection means there is no acceptance.

*Lungs.* The lung parenchyma are the seat of sighing, grief, sorrow, passion, and self-abuse. Smoking will definitely affect the pulmonary parenchyma and create pulmonary disease. Similarly, these emotions can also result in pulmonary disorders. Sitopalādi (an expectorant), talisadi (a decongestant), pushkaramūla (an analgesic), and pippalī (a rasāyana or rejuvenative tonic for the lungs) will help to clear emotions stuck in the lung tissue, such as grief and sorrow.

*Heart.* The seat of worries, lack of love, abandonment, rejection, and dishonor. All these feelings accumulate within the connective tissue of the myocardium and can result in atrial fibrillation, flutter, extra systole, mitral valve prolapse, or even a heart attack. Ayurveda uses arjuna, punarnavā, ashvagandhā, and shringa bhasma to process worries, lack of love, rejection, and dishonor, and these herbs can also help to control tachycardia and other heart disorders, allowing the person to live a healthy and happy life.

*Stomach.* This organ is the seat of nervousness, depression, and annoyance. Shatāvarī, shankha bhasma, kāma dudhā, and pravāl panchāmrit will help to eliminate these emotions and maintain the optimal functioning of digestion, absorption, and assimilation.

*Liver.* The hexagonal tissues of the hepatic parenchyma are the seat of anger, frustration, jealousy (from being afraid of losing something), and envy (burning because of seeing someone else's success).

*Gallbladder.* This is the seat of hate.

These emotions cause the liver or gallbladder to weaken and the person can get hepatitis or a similar disorder. Specific herbs to cleanse and balance the liver and gallbladder include kutki, shankha pushpī, and shigru (drumstick). These herbs are all hepato-detoxifiers, so they will open the hepatic parenchyma and help to cleanse the liver and gallbladder of emotions.

*Spleen.* The seat of attachment, greed, pride, and hopelessness. Because of these emotions, splenic disorders can occur leading to autoimmune diseases, in which the immune system goes against its own bodily cells. We can use neem, turmeric, and mahasudarshan to detoxify the spleen tissues.

*Kidneys.* The seat of fear, anxiety, insecurity, and terror. Use punarnavā, gokshura, shilājit, and ushīra as rasāyana to treat the renal parenchyma and to process these emotions.

*Male Sexual Organs.* Related to sexual desire, lust, and embarrassment. Good herbs for rejuvenation of the male sex organs are ātmaguptā (kapikacchū), ashvagandhā, and the compound mākaradvāja.

*Female Sexual Organs.* Also related to sexual desire, lust, and embarrassment. Herbs that are beneficial for the female sex organs include kumārī (aloe vera juice), shatāvarī, and ashoka.

Sex plays an important role in life and relationships. It can unfold true love, happiness, and joy, and help to release emotions. However, sex often becomes a problem because people have sex at the wrong time, in the wrong place, or with the wrong person. That can result in lust, sexual perversion, or embarrassment, which can lead to low libido, premature ejaculation, or pain during coitus.

## Emotions and the Doshas

Generally, vāta emotions are quick to occur and are also quickly forgotten. Pitta emotions are intense, and they take time to resolve. Kapha emotions are slow and steady, and are generally longstanding, deeply buried in the subconscious mind.

Emotions have an intimate relationship with the doshas, and each emotion has a prakruti. The table lists common emotions that relate to each dosha.

Emotionally disturbed vāta can cause narrowing, spasms, and atrophy. Emotionally disturbed pitta can create irritation, inflammation, ulceration, perforation, and hemorrhage. Emotionally disturbed kapha may result in cold, catarrh, congestion, hypertrophy, and creation of neoplasm (tumor).

We need to create a treatment protocol according to the principles of *dosha pratyanika* (specific to the doshas), *vyādhi pratyanika* (specific to the disease), *dhātu pratyanika* (specific to the tissues affected), and *avayava pratyanika* (specific to any related organs). Any herbal remedy should include at least one herb to pacify for the aggravated dosha, one herb specific to the disease or disorder, one to support the dhātu or its related srotas, and one to support any affected organ.

# EMOTIONS AND THE ORGANS

**Brain**
Shock
Excessive
Curiosity
Confusion

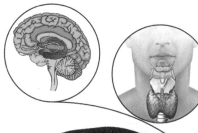

**Thyroid**
Lack of Communication
Guilt
Unrequited Love
Betrayal

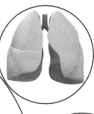

**Lungs**
Sighing
Grief
Sorrow
Passion
Smoking

**Heart**
Worries
Abandonment
Lack of love
Rejection
Dishonor

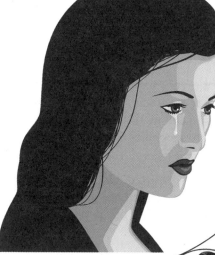

**Liver/Gallbladder**
Anger
Hatred
Frustration
Agony
Envy

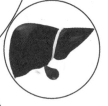

**Stomach**
Nervousness
Depression
Disgust
Annoyance

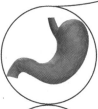

**Spleen**
Attachment
Greed
Hopelessness
Pride

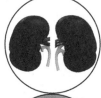

**Kidneys**
Fear, Terror
Anxiety
Insecurity

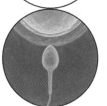

**Sex Organs**
Embarrassment
Lust
Sexual Perversion

447

## Summary

There is no person without emotion. Emotion is the reaction of past memory to the present challenge. Emotions always pull a person into the past or future. They also produce the idea of the future as modified past. The past has happened—it is dead.

Certain emotions are associated with the future, whereas others are more linked to the past. There may be a fear of the unknown future, yet that fear is based on the past.

## Emotions and the Doshas

| Vāta | Pitta | Kapha |
|---|---|---|
| Fear | Anger | Attachment |
| Anxiety | Hate | Greed |
| Insecurity | Envy | Possessiveness |
| Nervousness | Jealousy | Annoyance |
| Loneliness | Frustration | Depression |
| Grief and Sorrow | Irritability | Lust |
| Terror | Criticism | Dull |
| Sighing | Pride | Gloomy |
| Betrayal | Rejection | Melancholia |
| Curiosity | Disgust | Sluggishness |
| Confusion | Hopelessness | |
| Appalled | Embarrassment | |
| | Guilt | |
| | Craving for power, prestige, and position | |

If we stay solidly at one with "the now", there is no fear, anger, or other emotion. At that moment, there is no observer; only the intense energy of the emotion. A fraction of a second later, the observer comes along and tries to recognize the emotion. Then memory labels the emotion.

The moment we label the emotion, it is totally distorted. Once we label it "fear" or "anger", we pack it and suppress it. That which is suppressed has to come out in a modified form. These modified emotions are complex and affect our psycho-neuro-immunological responses, making the immune system overactive.

Pay complete attention to every emotion, and the moment the emotion arises in the consciousness, just observe it. Don't label it or judge it. To observe every emotion without labeling and judging is the greatest meditation.

Awareness is freedom and love. Everything flowers, so even the emotions flower. The flowering of emotion is the ending of emotion. Emotion ends by itself, and turns into love and clarity.

In this meditation, all unresolved emotions are completely resolved and dissolved. Dissolution is the solution for emotions. This moment-to-moment awareness of every thought, feeling, and emotion is observation of the whole movement of your consciousness. Individual consciousness empties itself of these thoughts, feelings, and emotions and becomes vast, dissolving into universal space, which is unconditional love.

Keep every emotion in motion; then it will open the door and light will come in. You are that light. Light is love, and you are that love. Every emotion has a function. The purpose of emotions is to bring awakening.

# Appendix

## Basti

A basti is a method to deliver medications given by enema primarily to treat vāta dosha, which is the main etiological factor in the manifestation of diseases. The Sanskrit word basti means bladder, referring to the bladder filled with medicated substances used for the enema. There are multiple types of enema substances including herbal teas, herbal teas that include healing oils, warm water and warm oil.

In general, when Dr. Lad refers to a basti, he is talking about a medicated enema.[85] However, there are other types of bastis. Uttara basti is a vaginal douche that delivers medicated substances to the vagina. (See chapter 47, "Female Health Issues" starting on page 371 for information on these treatments.) In addition, there are topical bastis that use a wheat-flour dough ring placed on specific areas of the body. Once this ring is in place and sealed, a warm medicated oil or other substance is poured into this ring to slowly penetrate the skin over a period of time, typically 30 to 40 minutes. These types of bastis include:

- Basti basti (bladder basti); first mention page 384
- Netra basti (eye basti); first mention page 12
- Kati basti (lower back basti); first mention page 11
- Nābhi basti (navel basti); first mention page 393
- Prushtha basti (thoracic spine basti); first mention page 267

Instructions for making the wheat-flour dough ring are on page 313 with further instructions on how to perform a netra basti.

### Herbalized Ghee

Instructions to make an herbalized ghee or oil are on page 312.[86] Herbalized ghee and oils are often used as medicated substances applied to the skin in bastis. The healing properties are absorbed directly through the skin.

### Herbal Tea Eyewashes

Herbal teas have healing properties that can be used with direct contact to the eyes. Instructions for them are found in chapter 41, "Glaucoma" on page 329.

---

85. There's more about basti on our website at https://www.ayurveda.com/resources/cleansing/basti.
86. Information about making ghee is on our website at https://www.ayurveda.com/recipes/ghee.

# Yoga Postures

Included here are examples of most postures mentioned in the text. The photos serve as reminders to the practitioner of the specific pose recommended. Dr. Lad has a great booklet about yoga and Ayurveda: *Ayuryoga: VPK Basics*. It contains information about the yoga postures he recommends as well as the full cycle of the Sun and Moon Salutations. [87]

| | |
|---|---|
| Accomplished Pose (Siddhāsana) | Legs Up The Wall (Viparīta Karanī) |
| Boat (Nāvāsana) | Lion Pose (Simhāsana) |
| Bow (Dhanurāsana) | Locust Pose (Shalabhāsana) |
| Bridge (Setu Bandha Sarvāngāsana) | Lotus Pose (Padmāsana) |
| Camel (Ustrāsana) | Palm Tree Pose (Tādāsana) |
| Chest-Knee Pose (Pāwanamuktāsana) | Peacock (Mayurāsana) (also called Cock or Rooster pose) |
| Child's Pose (Balāsana) | |
| Cobra (Bhujangāsana) | Plow Pose (Halāsana) |
| Corpse (Savāsana) | Shoulder Stand With Lotus Pose (Ūrdhva Padmāsana) |
| Cow (Gomukhāsana) | |
| Eagle Pose (Garudā) | Spinal Twist (Matsyendrāsana) |
| Easy Cross-Legged Pose (Sukhāsana) | Thunderbolt Pose (Vajrāsana) |
| Elevated Lotus Pose (Urdhva Padmāsana) | Tree Pose (Vriksāsana) |
| Frog Pose (Mandhukāsana) (*not shown*) | Triangle (Trikonāsana) |
| Leg Lifting (Uttāna Pādāsana) (*not shown*) | |

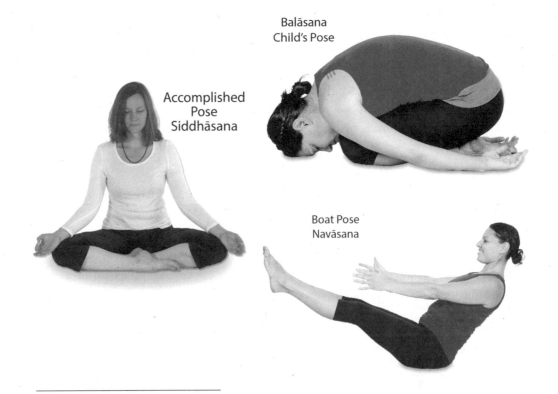

Balāsana
Child's Pose

Accomplished Pose
Siddhāsana

Boat Pose
Navāsana

87. Details are here: https://www.ayurveda.com/about/ayurvedic-press/ayuryoga-vpk-basics

# Yoga Postures

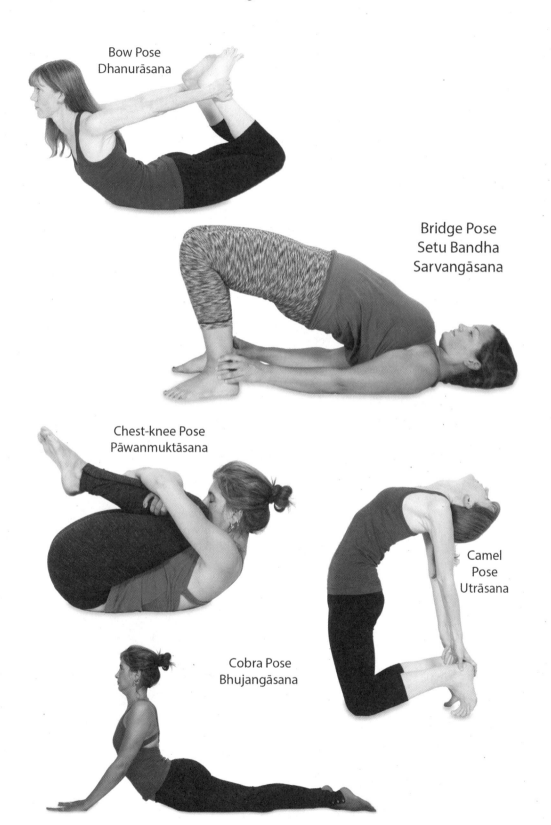

Bow Pose
Dhanurāsana

Bridge Pose
Setu Bandha
Sarvangāsana

Chest-knee Pose
Pāwanmuktāsana

Camel
Pose
Utrāsana

Cobra Pose
Bhujangāsana

# Appendix

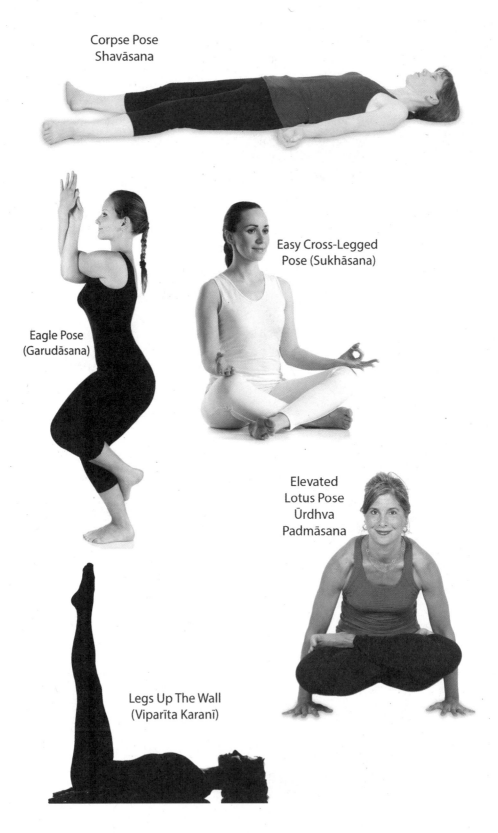

Corpse Pose
Shavāsana

Eagle Pose
(Garudāsana)

Easy Cross-Legged
Pose (Sukhāsana)

Elevated
Lotus Pose
Ūrdhva
Padmāsana

Legs Up The Wall
(Viparīta Karanī)

# Yoga Postures

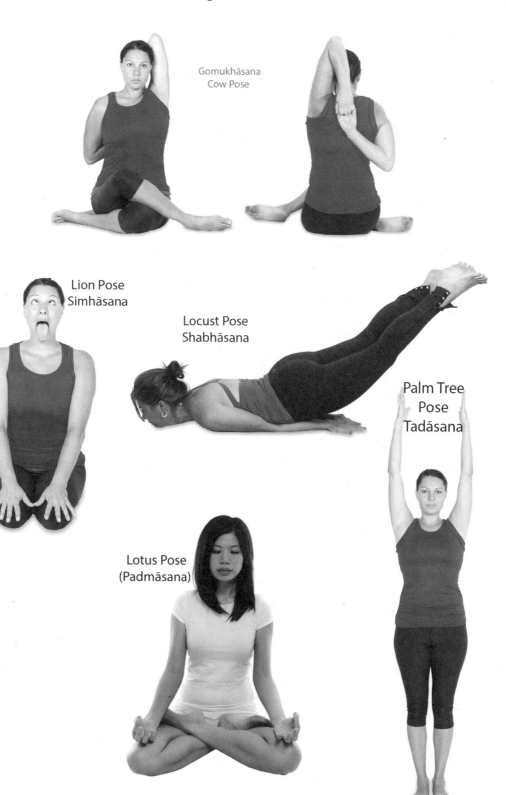

Gomukhāsana
Cow Pose

Lion Pose
Simhāsana

Locust Pose
Shabhāsana

Palm Tree
Pose
Tadāsana

Lotus Pose
(Padmāsana)

# Appendix

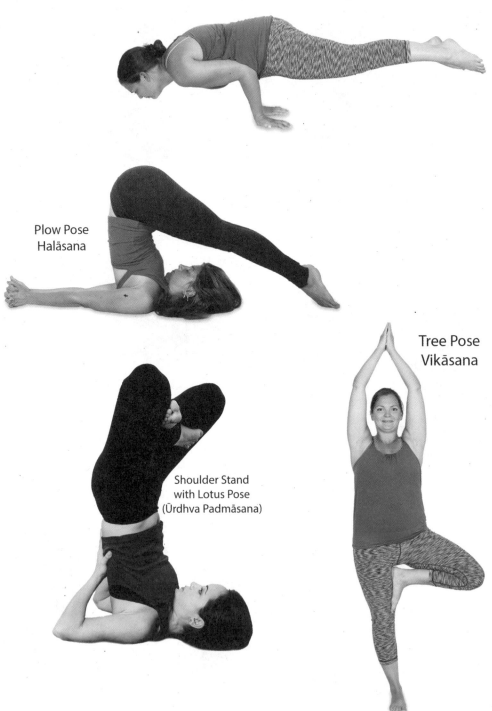

Peacock Pose
Mayurāsana

Plow Pose
Halāsana

Shoulder Stand
with Lotus Pose
(Ūrdhva Padmāsana)

Tree Pose
Vikāsana

# Marma Points

In ancient Vedic times, marma points were called bindu – a dot, secret dot or mystic point. Like a door or pathway, activating a marma point opens into the inner pharmacy of the body. Touching a marma point changes the body's biochemistry and can unfold radical, alchemical change in one's makeup. Stimulation of these inner pharmacy pathways signals the body to produce exactly what it needs, including hormones and neurochemicals that heal the body, mind and consciousness.

**From "Marma Chikitsā" on page 246, chapter 20, Backache and Sciatica**

Trik, Ūrū, Sakthi Ūrvī, Jānu, Gulpha, and Pārshni are marma points that are specific for treatment of this syndrome. Pārshni marma is a point at the central part of the heel that will relieve sciatica pain when it is pressed.

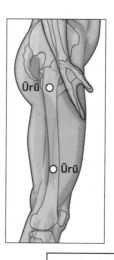

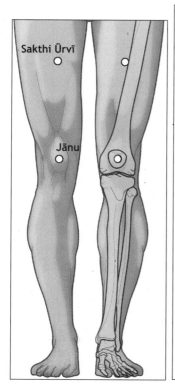

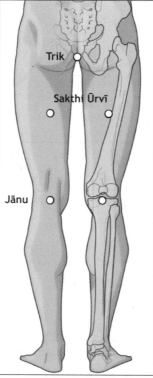

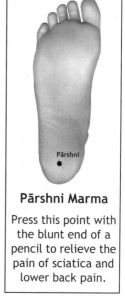

**Pārshni Marma**

Press this point with the blunt end of a pencil to relieve the pain of sciatica and lower back pain.

**From "Marma" on page 272 in chapter 32, Headache.**

Here are the locations of the points recommended in the text. Apply the appropriate doshic oil to the marma points shown in the illustrations below. Other points for headache include Ūrdhva Skandha (mid-point along top of shoulders, between neck and arm) and Hasta (Hand) Kshipra and Pāda (Foot) Kshipra.

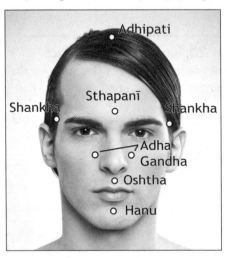

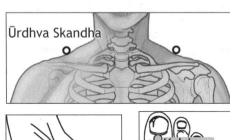

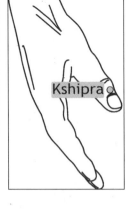

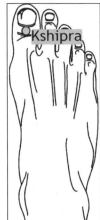

**From page 291, chapter 35, Epilepsy**

Mūrdhni, Sthapanī, Brahmarandhra, Oshtha, Hanu, Jatru, Agra Patra, and Pāda Kshipra marma points are treated, often using nutmeg essential oil.

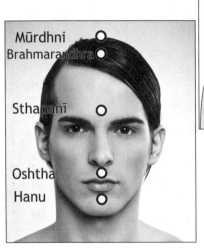

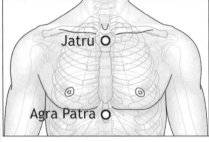

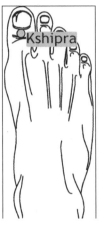

## From page 313, chapter 38, Maintaining a Healthy Brain.

Try this gentle marma facial treatment for brain balance

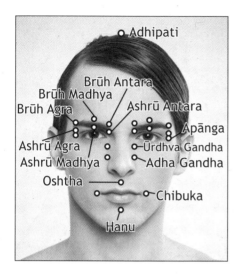

### GENTLE MARMA FACIAL TREATMENT

Have your client lie down face up and sit at the head of the client. Begin with gentle pressure on Adhipati marma using both thumbs. Then move from Adhipati to Bhrūh Antara above the eyebrows, then outward to Bhrūh Madhya, all the way across to Bhrūh Agra. Repeat this gentle, relaxing motion three times, pressing gently on each point as you pass. Repeat for the Ashrū points below the eyebrows.

Sweep the fingers across the eyebrows until the thumbs land in a natural depression at Apānga marma. Pressure should be held longer here, with a gentle counterclockwise rotation.

Next, pinch the eyebrows lightly at the inner point and release, repeating this technique towards the outer end of the eyebrows to stimulate all Bhrūh and Ashrū marmāni simultaneously. This technique can be repeated several times. Use caution not to pull the eyelid or place pressure on the eyeball.

Follow with pressure on the Ganda marmāni, moving the thumbs from Ganda marmāni downwards, until they fall in the natural groove at Chibuka. Hold for a moment. Stimulate Oshtha with the thumb and then circle the fingers around the mouth, giving emphasis to Chibuka again.

Move to Hanu marma at the chin and apply somewhat firm pressure with both thumbs. Grasp the chin between the thumbs and the index fingers and move from Hanu along the length of the mandible toward the ears. Repeat this motion three times. Move to Apānga, then return to Adhipati and hold the pressure for one minute.

## From "Trigeminal Neuralgia" on page 318, chapter 39, Neuralgia.

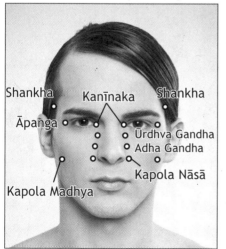

## From page 326, chapter 40, Multiple Sclerosis.

Patients with MS should receive gentle, cooling, calming, soothing treatments, including marma chikitsā therapy that incorporates these points.

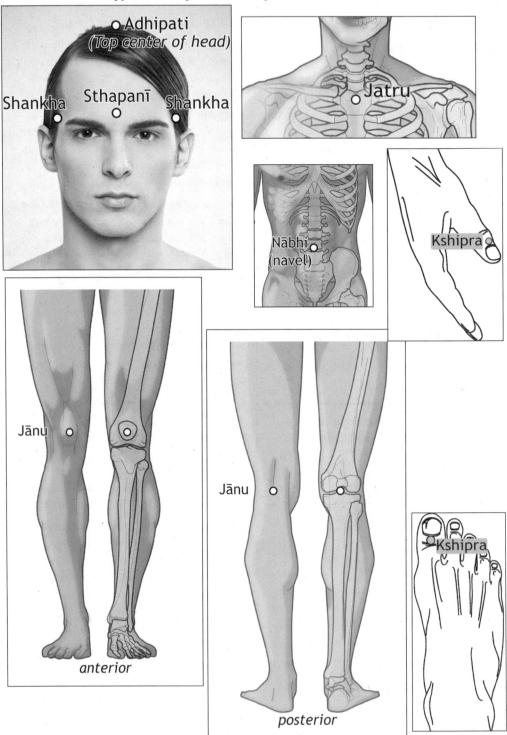

**From "Management (Chikitsā)" on page 370, chapter 47, Female Health Issues**

Marma chikitsā is also helpful and the best marmas for PMS are Nābhi, Bhaga, Sakthi Ūrvī, Jānu, Gulpha, and Trik. Nutmeg essential oil can be applied to these energy points.

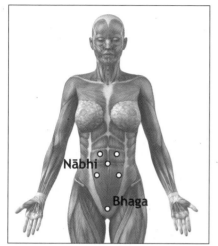

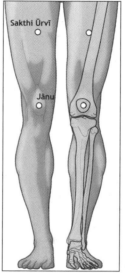

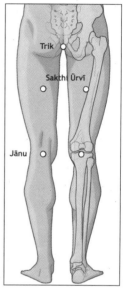

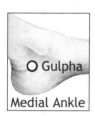

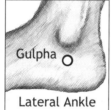

**From page 384, chapter 48, Endometriosis.**

Use nutmeg essential oil diluted in sesame oil and apply to each of these marma points. This marma chikitsā will help to minimize pain, normalize any retrograde apāna, and minimize displacement of the endometrium.

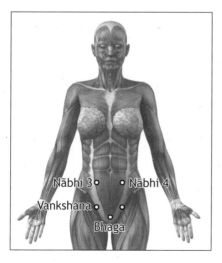

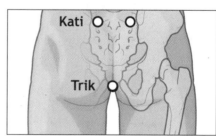

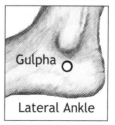

## From "Management" on page 422, chapter 52, Sleep Disorders

Massage Mūrdhni, Sthapanī, Oshtha, Jatru, and Hasta/Pāda Kshipra marma points with nutmeg oil.

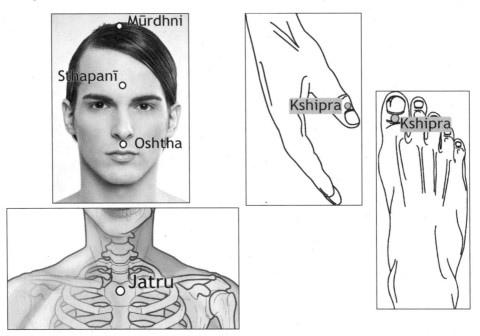

## From page 440, chapter 54, Depression.

Use vacha or sandalwood essential oils on these points for depression.

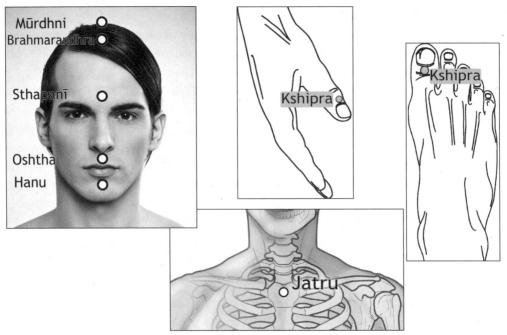

## About the Herbs and Other Substances Mentioned in This Book

### Table 16: Types of Preparations for Herbs and other Substances

| Type | Method |
| --- | --- |
| Āsava | a medicinal herbal wine[a] |
| Arishta | a fermented herbal concoction |
| Arka | a distillation of herbs suspended in water |
| Avaleha or leha | a semi-solid preparation made with jaggery, herbs and ghee or oil and honey |
| Vati | medicinal pills or tablets, also called gutikā |
| Bhasma | medicinal ash |
| Churna | a fine powder of herbs |
| Ghrita | preparations of ghee infused with a decoction and a fine paste of the herb |
| Guggulus | preparations having the exudate as the main effective ingredient |
| Kalka | crushed herbs made into a pulp or paste; a wet bolus |
| Kshira pāka | herbal preparations that are boiled in milk |
| Kvātha | a combination of coarsely powdered herbs; a decoction |
| Lepa | medicinal paste |
| Mandūra | preparations containing purified mandūra (Ferroso-ferric oxide) along with other herbs |
| Parpati | a rasa preparation using purified mercury and sulphur |
| Prash | an herbal preparation cooked with ghee that results in a jam or jelly-like substance |
| Rasa | preparations containing minerals as the main ingredients |
| Taila | oil is boiled with a decoction and a fine paste of the herb(s) |

a. Herbal preparations, as used in this table, can include other substances such as minerals, foods, etc.

## Herbs and Herbal Compounds

The herbs and compounds that are given here for Vasant Lad's formulas and recommendations are traditional combinations used in Ayurveda and the ancient texts. Some of these are unavailable or very difficult to obtain for a variety of reasons. Some have problems with contamination of heavy metals, others are endangered species, some are prevented from export by the government of India, others are not approved by the FDA for consumption, and some are simply not available in the USA. Many of these ingredients are not for sale by The Ayurvedic Institute.

Following is a list of the herbs and compounds, in alphabetical order, from the articles in this book.

# Appendix

Abhrak bhasma (compound)

Abhrak (*Talcum purification*[88])

Agaru (*Aquilaria agallocha*)

Agni mantha (*Clerodendrum phlomidis*)

Agni tundi rasa (compound)

Ahiphenam (resin) *Papaver somniferum*

Ajagandha (*Cleome viscosa*)

Ajvain (*Carum roxburghianum, Trachyspermum ammi, Carum copticum*)

Akarakarabha (*Anacyclus pyrethrum*)

Aloe Vera (see kumārī)

Alum (*Alumen*)

Āma pachak vati (compound)

Āmalaki (*Embelica officinalis*)

Amber (oil from multiple tree resins, primarily *Liquidamber orientalis*)

Amrita (see guduchi)

Amrita guggulu (compound)

Anantā mūlā *Hemidesmus indicus*

Anu thailam (compound)

Apamarga (*Achyranthes aspera*)

Aravindāsava (compound)

Arjuna (*Terminalia arjuna*)

Arka (*Calotropis procera*)

Arka patra, Arka pushpa (see arka)

Ārogya vardini (compound)

Asafoetida (*Ferula foetida*)

Ashoka (*Saraca indica*)

Ashvagandhā (*Withania somnifera*)

Ashvagandhā arishta (compound)

Asthi poshaka vati (compound)

Ātmaguptā (kapikkacchū) (*Mucuna pruriens*)

Avipattikar (compound)

Bacha nāga (*Aconitum napellus*)

Bachan (*Aconitum ferox*)

Bākuchī (*Psoralea corylifolia*)

Balā (*Sida cordifolia*)

Basil (see tulsi)

Bhallataka (*Semecarpus anacardium*)

Bhangā (see vijayā)

Bhringarāja (*Eclipta alba*)

Bhumi āmalakī (*Phyllanthus amarus*[89])

Bibhītakī (*Terminalia belerica*)

Bilva (*Aegle marmelos*)

Bitter Gourd (see karela)

Black Pepper (*Piper nigrum*)

Borax (see tankana)

Brahmī (*Centella Asiatica* is most common sometimes *Bacopa monnieri*)

Brahmī ghee (compound)

Brahmī prash (compound)

Calamus (see vacha)

Camphor (*Cinnamomum camphora*)

Cardamom (*Elettaria cardamomum*)

Cascara sagrada (*Rhamnus purshiana*)

Castor plant (*Ricinus communis*)

Catechu (see khadira)

Chamomile (*Matricaria recutita,* used internally in teas, etc.)

Chandana (*Santalum album*)

Chandrakalaras (compound)

Chandraprabhā (compound)

Chandraprabha vati (compound)

Chandrodaya vati (compound)

Chayavanaprash (compound)

Chitrak (*Plumbago zeylanica*)

Chitrakadi tailam compound (see chitrak)

Cilantro (see dhānyaka)

Cinnamon (*Cinnamomum cassia*)

Coriander (*Coriandrum sativum*) (see dhānyaka)

Cumin (*Cuminum cyminum*)

Dāruharidrā (*Berberis aristata*)

Dashāmūla [ten roots] (compound)

---

88. Black form is used in medicine.

89. Often erroneously known as Phyllanthus niruri, according to *Ayurvedic Medicine,* Sebastian Pole

Dashamūla arishta (fermented herbal concoction)

Dashānga paste (compound)

Deer Horn Ash (compound) (see shringa bhasma)

Deer Musk (*Moschus chrysogaster*)

Deodara (see devadāru)

Devadāru (*Cedrus deodara*)

Dhānyaka (*Coriandrum sativum*)

Dhattūra (*Datura metel f. fastuosa*)

Draksha āsava (*Vitis vinifera*) [herbal wine]

Dūrvā (*Cynodon dactylon*)

Echinacea (*Echinacea angustifolia*)

Eucalyptus (*Eucalyptus globulus*)

Evening Primrose (*Oenothera biennis*)

Eye of bamboo (*Bambusa vulgaris*)

Fennel (*Foeniculum vulgare*)

Flax seed (*Linum usitatissimum*)

Gandhak druti (compound)

Gandhaka rasayana (compound)

Gandharva harītakī (compound)

Garlic (*Allium sativum*)

Ghrita (ghee)

Ghrita madhu (compound)

Ginger Root (*Zingiber officinale*)

Ginkgo biloba (*Ginkgo biloba*)

Ginseng (*Panax ginseng*), Asian

Gokshura (*Tribulus terrestris*)

Gokshurādi guggulu (compound)

Goldenseal (*Hydrastis canadensis*)

Gomutra harītakī (compound)

Goraksha chincha guggulu (compound)

Gotu kola (*Centella asiatica*)

Gudūchī (*Tinospora cordifolia*)

Guggulu (*Commiphora mukul, Balsamodendron mukul*)

Gulvel sattva (Special preparation of gudūchī [*Tinospora cordifolia*])

Guñjā (*Abrus precatorius*)

Gurmar (*Gymnema sylvestre*)

Haridrā (*Curcuma longa*) [turmeric]

Harītakī (*Terminalia chebula*)

Hawthorn Berry (*Crateagus oxycanthus, Crataegus laevigata*)

Hema garbha (compound)

Hibiscus (*Hibiscus rosa-sinensis*)

Hing (*Ferula foetida/narthex*)

Hingvastak chūrna (compound)

Indra (*Citrullus colocynthis*)

Indrayava (*Holarrhena antidysenterica seed*)

Jaipāla, Jamalgota (*Croton tiglium*)

Jambul (*Syzygium cumini*)

Jatamāmsi (*Nastordachys jatamamsi*)

Jātīphalā (*Myristica fragrans*)

Jyotishmatī (*Cardiospermum halicacabum, Celastrus paniculatus*)

Kadhira (*Acacia catechu*)

Kaishore guggulu (compound)

Kākolī (*Lilium polyphyllum*)

Kāma dudhā (compound)

Kanchanar (kāñcanāra) (*Bauhinia variegata*)

Kānchanār guggulu (compound)

Kanthakārī (*Solanum xanthocarpum*)

Kapikacchū (*Mucuna pruriens*)

Kapittha (*Feronia elephantum*)

Karanja (*Millettia pinnata* or *Pangamia glabra*)

Karaskara (*Strychnos nux-vomica*)

Karela (*Momordica charantia*)

Kasturi (deer musk) (*Moschus moschiferus*)

Katukā (see kutki)

Khadira (*Acacia catechu*)

Khadiradi vati (compound)

Khurasani ova (*Hyoscyamus niger*)

Khus (*Andropogon muricatus*)

Kukkutanakhi (compound)

Kumārī (*Aloe barbadensis*) [aloe vera]

# Appendix

Kumārī āsava [fermented herbal wine (compound)]

Kushtha (*Saussurea lappa*)

Kutaja (*Holarrhena antidysenterica*)

Kutki [katukā] (*Picrorhiza kurroa*)

Laghu mālinī vasant (compound)

Laksha (*Cateria lacca*)

Lakshmī vilas (compound)

Lasunadi vati

Latākaranja (*Ceasalpinia bonducella*)

Lauha bhasma (compound)

Lavanga (*Syzygium aromaticum*)

Lavanga vati achusanam (compound)

Licorice Root (*Glycyrrhiza glabra*)

Lodhra (*Symplocos racemosa*)

Loha (*Ferrum*)

Loha āsava (herbalized wine)

Loha bhasma [iron ash (compound)]

Lotus (see padma)

Madana phala (*Randia dumetorum*)

Madhu (*Mel*)

Maha panchagavya ghrita (compound)

Maha rasnadi kvath (compound)

Maha tikta ghrita [bitter ghee] (compound)

Maha vāta vidhvamsa (compound)

Mahānārāyana oil (compound)

Maharasnadi kvātha (compound)

Mahasudarshan (compound)

Mahāyogarāja guggulu (compound)

Mākaradvāja (compound)

Manahshilā (*Arsenii disulphidum*)

Mandhūra bhasma (compound)

Manjishthā (*Rubia cordifolia*)

Mocharas/Mocha rasa (compound)

Moti bhasma [pearl ash] (*Mytilus margaritiferus*)

Multani mitti or mati (*Silicate of alumina, magnesia, and oxide of iron*)

Mustā (*Cyperus rotundus*)

Mūtrala (compound)

Nāgakeshara (*Mesua ferrea*)

Navjivan rasa (compound)

Neem (*Azadirachta indica*)

Nimbu (*Citrus bergamia*)

Nirgundī (*Vitex negundo*)

Nishottara (*Ipomoea turpethum*)

Nutmeg (see jātīphalā)

Nutmeg [essential oil] (*Myristica fragrans*)

Osha (*Ligusticum porteri*)

Pachak vati (compound)

Padma (*Nelumbo nucifera*)

Palash (*Butea monosperma*)

Panchamrit parpati (compound)

Panchamula (compound)

Parijatak, Parijata (*Nyctanthes arbortristis*)

Parpati (compound)

Pāshana bheda (compound)

Passionflower (*Passiflora incarnate*)

Patola Patra (*Trichosanthes dioica*)

Pātthā (*Cissampelos pareira*)

Pippalī [long pepper] (*Piper longum*)

Pradarāntak vati (compound)

Praval pañchāmrit (compound)

Punarnavā (*Boerhaavia diffusa*)

Punarnavādi guggulu (compound)

Pushkaramūla (*Inula racemosa*)

Raktachandana (*Pterocarpus santalinus*)

Rasa (*Hydrargyrum*)

Rasa parpati (compound)

Rasagandha (compound)

Rāsna (*Vanda roxburghii, Inula helenium*)

Rasnadi guggulu (compound)

Raupya bhasma (compound)

Red sandalwood (*Santalum album*)

Rose (*Rosa damascene*)

Saffron (*Crocus sativus*)

Saffron (*Mesua ferrea*), Indian

Sandalwood (*Santalum album*)

# Herbs and Herbal Compounds

Sandalwood (see raktachandana or chandana)

Sanjīvanī (compound)

Saptaparna (*Alstonia scholaris*)

Sarasvatī (compound)

Sarasvatī arishta [herbal wine (compound)]

Sarpagandha (*Rawolfia serpentine*)

Sat isabgol (*Plantago ovata*)

Senna (*Senna alexandrina*)

Shanka bhasma (compound)

Shanka pushpī (*Convolvulus pluricaulis choisy* or *Evolvulus alsinoides*)

Shanka vati (compound)

Shankha bhasma (compound)

Shankha pushpī *Evolvulus alsinoides*

Shankha (*Turbinella rapa, xanchus pyrum, or gastropoda*)

Shankha vati (compound)

Shardunikā (*Gymnema sylvestre*)

Shatāvarī (*Asparagus racemosus*)

Shigru [drum stick] (*Moringa pterygosperma*)

Shilājit (*Asphaltum*)

Shilājit guggulu (compound)

Shringa bhasma (deer horn ash) (compound)

Shuddha shilājit (compound)

Shuddha guggulu (compound)

Shulah vati (compound)

Shulahara vati (compound)

Shunthi (see ginger)

Simhanad guggulu (compound)

Sitaphal (*Annona squamosa*)

Sitopalādi (compound)

Smriti sagar ras (compound)

Sudarshan (*Crinum asiaticum*)

Sudarshan gana vati (compound)

Sūkshma triphalā (compound)

Sutshekhar (compound)

Suvarna (*Aurum*)

Suvarna mālinī vasant (compound)

Suvarna sutshekhar mātrā (compound)

Swayambhu guggulu (compound)

Tagara (*Valeriana wallichii*)

Tālīsādi (compound)

Tambra bhasma (copper ash)

Tankana (*Sodii biboras*)

Tapyadi loha (compound)

Tentu (*Oroxylum indicum*)

Tikta churna (compound)

Tikta ghrita [bitter ghee] (compound)

Tobacco (*Nicotiana tabacum*)

Tribhuvan kirti (ras/rasa) (compound)

Trikatu (compound of ginger, black pepper, pippali)

Triphalā (compound)

Triphala guggulu (compound)

Tulsi (*Ocimum sanctum*)

Tumbī *Lagenaria siceraria*

Turmeric (*Curcuma longa*) (see haridrā)

Ushīra (*Vetiveria zizanioides*) (see khus)

Vacha (*Acorus calamus*)

Vanga bhasma (compound)

Vangeshvara (compound)

Varuna (*Crateva religiosa*)

Vāsaka (*Adhatoda vasica*)

Vasant kusumakar ras (compound)

Vetiver (see ushīra)

Vidanga (*Embelia ribes*)

Vidārī (*Ipomoea digitata* or *Pueraria tuberosa*)

Vijayā (*Cannabis sativa*)

Visha garbha tailam (compound)

Wild Caraway (*Carum copticum*) (see ajvain, yavānī)

Yashthi madhu [licorice root] (*Glycyrrhiza glabra*)

Yavānī (*Trachyspermum ammi, Carum roxburghianum, Carum copticum*)

Yogarāja guggulu (compound)

# About the Author

AYURVEDA FINDS ITS HOME IN THE HEARTS of special beings whose dharma it is to preserve and maintain traditions of wisdom for the purpose of healing themselves and the world. Bridging the gap between the changing philosophies, sciences, and religions of the ages, it is passed down in the various cultures through these dedicated individuals. Vasant Lad's heart is one of the homes for that living flame, and his life and teachings are an expression of Ayurveda's true purpose in the world.

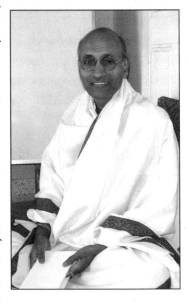

**Vasant Lad, BAM&S, MASc,** brings a wealth of classroom and practical experience to the United States. He received the degree of Bachelor of Ayurvedic Medicine and Surgery (BAM&S) in 1968 from the University of Pune, in Pune, India and a Master of Ayurvedic Science (MASc) in 1980 from Tilak Ayurved Mahavidyalaya in Pune. For 3 years, he served as Medical Director of the Ayurveda Hospital in Pune, India. He also held the position of Professor of Clinical Medicine for seven years at the Pune University College of Ayurvedic Medicine, where he was an instructor for many years. Vasant Lad's academic and practical training includes the study of allopathic medicine (Western Medicine) and surgery as well as traditional Ayurveda. In 1979, he began traveling throughout the United States sharing his knowledge of Ayurveda and, in 1981, he returned to New Mexico to teach Ayurveda. In 1984, he founded and began as Director of The Ayurvedic Institute.

Vasant Lad is the author of 11 books on Ayurveda as well as hundreds of articles and other writings. With over 500,000 copies of his books in print in the US, his work has been translated into more than 20 languages. His books include

*Ayurveda, The Science of Self-Healing* and *Secrets of the Pulse* and he is co-author of *The Yoga of Herbs* and *Ayurvedic Cooking for Self-Healing*. His work from Harmony Books, *The Complete Book of Ayurvedic Home Remedies,* is a compendium of classic Ayurvedic treatments for common and chronic ailments. The series of textbooks on Ayurveda. *The Textbook of Ayurveda: Fundamental Principles, Volume 1, The Textbook of Ayurveda: Clinical Assessment, Volume 2,* and *The Textbook of Ayurveda: General Principles of Management and Treatment, Volume 3* cover the topics he teaches in his residential Ayurvedic Studies Programs. He is co-author of a book on marma therapy, *Marma Points of Ayurveda*, and the author of *Applied Marma Therapy Cards,* a flash card study set for marma therapy. Additionally, he teaches the practice of pranayama, breathing exercises, on the DVD *Pranayama for Self-Healing.*

Vasant Lad presently is the Director of The Ayurvedic Institute in Albuquerque, New Mexico and teaches the Ayurvedic Studies Programs, Level 1 and 2 as well as advanced training programs in India each year. Vasant Lad also travels throughout the world, consulting privately and giving seminars on Ayurveda, its history, theory, principles and practical applications.

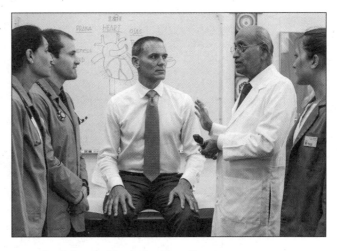

For more information about Ayurveda, Dr. Lad's books and his school, check our website Ayurveda.com or contact The Ayurvedic Institute, 11311 Menaul Blvd NE, Albuquerque, NM 87112-0008, (505) 291-9698.

# The Ayurvedic Press

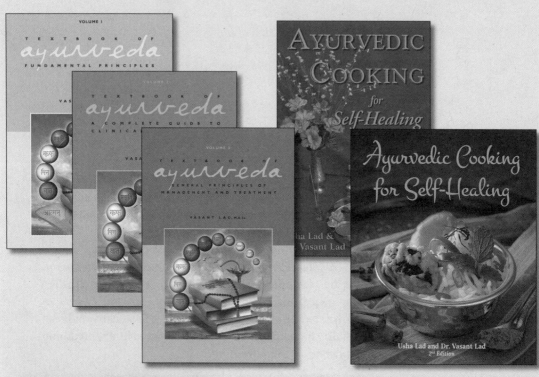

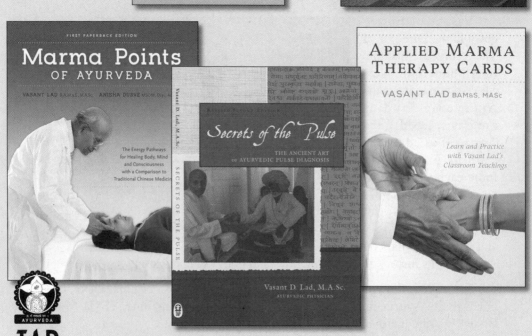

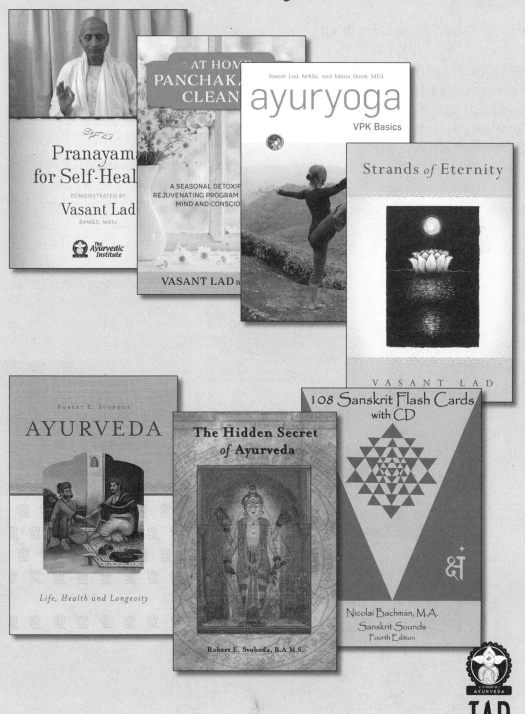

At **The Ayurvedic Institute,** we teach traditional Ayurvedic Medicine and provide ancient Indian therapies to help heal and maintain the quality and longevity of life.

Our **Ayurvedic Studies Program** is more than 30 years old and is a beautiful, academically rigorous, personally transformative journey! First-year students earn an **Ayurvedic Health Counselor (AHC)** certificate and 2nd-year students earn an **Ayurvedic Practitioner (AP)** certificate. They study Sanskrit, philosophy, pulse diagnosis, how to use nutrition as a kitchen pharmacy, herbology, marma therapy, body therapies, Ayurvedic Jyotish, pathophysiology, and more.

**Continuing Education,** professional and personal development options include weekend seminars, webinars and week-long intensives that people come back to year after year.

The **Herb Department** has Ayurvedic and Western herbs, audio and video tapes from our programs, books, incense, and a variety of Ayurvedic and other products.

The **Panchakarma Department** provides traditional Ayurvedic procedures for purification and rejuvenation that include oil massage, herbal steam treatment, shirodhara, cleansing diet, herbal therapy, and other treatments.

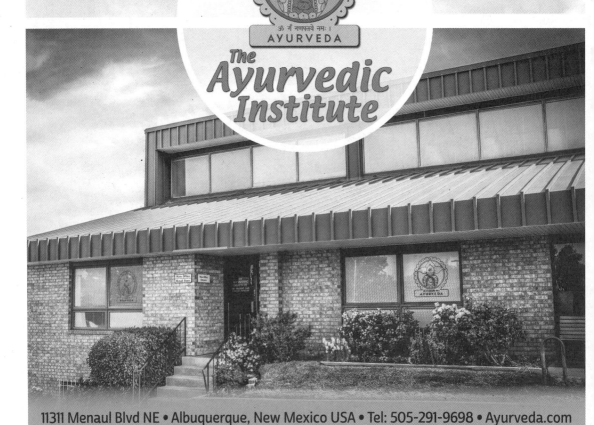

The Ayurvedic Institute

11311 Menaul Blvd NE • Albuquerque, New Mexico USA • Tel: 505-291-9698 • Ayurveda.com